Atlas of
clinical
ophthalmoscopy

G. SCUDERI   G. MORONE   R. BRANCATO

Co-ordinator
P. PIVETTI PEZZI

Atlas of clinical ophthalmoscopy

with 616 color and 90 black/white illustrations

Translated from Italian by
Frederick C. Blodi, M.D.
Medical Director, King Khaled Eye Specialist Hospital
Professor of Ophthalmology, University of Iowa

MASSON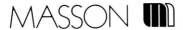

Milano • Parigi • Barcellona • Messico • San Paolo

Year Book Medical Publishers, Inc.

Chicago • London • Boca Raton

1987

Masson S.p.A.   Via Statuto 2/4, 20121 Milano
Masson S.A.   120, Bd Saint-Germain, 75280 Paris Cedex 06
Masson S.A.   Balmes 151, Barcelona 08008
Masson do Brasil Ltda.   Rua Borges Lagoa, 1044 - CEP 04038 - São Paulo
Masson Editores de Mexico   Dakota 383, Colonia Napoles, Mexico 18 DF

Original Italian title

Atlante di oftalmoscopia clinica

© Masson Italia Editori S.p.A. - Milano - 1986

Library of Congress Cataloging-in-Publication Data

Scuderi, Giuseppe, Prof.
  Atlas of clinical ophthalmoscopy.

  Translation of: Atlante di oftalmoscopia clinica.
  Includes bibliographies and index.
  1. Ophthalmoscope and ophthalmoscopy—Atlases.
I. Morone, Giulio. II. Brancato, Rosario. III. Title.
[DNLM: 1. Eye Diseases—diagnosis—atlases.
2. Fundus Oculi—atlases. 3. Ophthalmoscopy—atlases.
WW 17 S436a]
RE78.S3713 1987   617.7'4   87-14750
ISBN 0-8151-7737-2

©Masson S.p.A. - Milano

1987 English Edition by special arrangement with Year Book Medical Publishers

Printed in Italy

Authors

Emilio Balestrazzi *Associate Professor in Paediatric Ophthalmology*
Università "La Sapienza", Roma

Francesco Bandello *Assistant Ophthalmologist, Department of Ophthalmology*
Ospedale San Raffaele, Milano

Rosario Brancato *Full Professor in Clinical Ophthalmology Università di Milano*
Head, Department of Ophthalmology - Ospedale San Raffaele, Milano

Giuseppe Carella *Head, Department of Ophthalmology*
Ospedale Civile Generale, Piacenza

Adolfo Ghisolfi *Associate Professor in Paediatric Ophthalmology*
Università di Pavia

Ugo Menchini *Associate Professor in Clinical Ophthalmology - Università di Milano*
Head Assistant, Department of Ophthalmology - Ospedale San Raffaele, Milano

Giulio Morone *Full Professor in Clinical Ophthalmology - Università di Pavia*
Head, Department of Ophthalmology - Ospedale San Matteo, Pavia

Alfredo Pece *Assistant Ophthalmologist, Department of Ophthalmology*
Ospedale S. Raffaele, Milano

Paola Pivetti Pezzi *Associate Professor in Neuro-Ophthalmology*
Università "La Sapienza", Roma

Guglielmo Ranieri *Head Assistant, Department of Ophthalmology*
Ospedale Policlinico, Bari

Giuseppe Scuderi *Full Professor of Clinical Ophthalmology - Università "La Sapienza", Roma*
Head, Department of Ophthalmology - Ospedale Policlinico, Roma

Antonio Tazzi *Full Professor in Human Anatomy*
Università di Pavia

Foreword

It was indeed an honour to be asked to translate this beautiful atlas by my good friends from Rome, Pavia and Milan.

This book constitutes a proud continuation of the superb Italian contributions to ophthalmoscopy and to fundus photography. This tradition started already in 1858 with the atlas by Antonio Quaglino and the book by Gritti.

This volume is distinguished by its beautiful color photos and by excellent fluorescein angiograms which often explain in a more dynamic way the underlying situation or the basic pathologic process. Whenever necessary, photomicrographs which complement the clinical pictures and help us to understand the entire disease process are reproduced. The total pictorial presentation combines with the text to an excellent didactic package which should be of benefit not only to young ophthalmologists and residents, but also to internists, neurologists, pediatricians and family practitioners. May this book reach the wide audience it deserves.

I would like to acknowledge with gratitude the help of Dr. Carlo Traverso of Genova, staff ophthalmologist at the King Khaled Eye Specialist Hospital in Riyadh, Saudi Arabia, for helping me in some fine points of the Italian language. Thanks are also due to Ms. Nancy Chojnowski for her expert secretarial assistance.

FREDERICK C. BLODI, M.D.

Riyadh,
October 1987

Introduction

The invention of the ophthalmoscope at the middle of the last century and its introduction into the clinic have enormously contributed to the progress of ophthalmology; this event certainly represents a milestone in the evolution of medicine.

Helmholtz, the inventor of the instrument, had probably a genial intuition when he said that «The morphologic changes of retinal and vitreous pathology which so far had only been evident on the autopsy table can now be observed in the living eye».

The following decades with the improved technical aspects of the instrument not only confirmed its value and importance for ophthalmology, but also showed the indisputable usefulness of this method in other branches of medical science for the diagnosis and follow-up of many systemic diseases (vascular, metabolic, blood dyscrasias, endocrine, renal, neurologic, and other affections).

The use of this examination method became step by step so widespread and so important that it justified the statement (paraphrasing Leonardo da Vinci) «The eye is the window of human pathology».

And even today, in spite of the introduction of new and always more sophisticated examination methods into ophthalmology, ophthalmoscopy preserves intact the importance of its role. It is not only important in the realm of our specialty, but is indispensable for every physician, at least as far as recognizing the elementary lesions and fundamental clinical pictures of the fundus are concerned. On the other hand, the technical development has during the last centuries produced in addition to the traditional ophthalmoscopy new examination methods, occasionally more reliable, e.g., the biomicroscopy of the posterior segment of the eye, indirect binocular ophthalmoscopy, fundus photography, fluorescein angiography, fluorometry, etc.

The ophthalmic literature has been — and continues to be — rich in contributions which many authors have made to the multiple aspects of fundus pathology which, undoubtedly, vary and evolve, in time, with changing interpretations of human pathology.

The scientific achievements of Italian authors have been vast and substantial. They have contributed original ideas to the fundamental interpretation of the pathology and etiology of fundus conditions with monographs and publications of noteworthy relevance.

However, there is in Italy a dearth of complete fundus atlases which would keep the practicing ophthalmologist abreast of the developments in this most important aspect of our specialty.

There is only one truly monumental Italian work which is outstanding by the beauty of its pictures, the completeness and variety of pathologic conditions which have made it famous outside the confines of our country. I am referring here to the splendid book Fundus Oculi *by Quirino Di Marzio, published by Salomone in 1937. This book has been the reference source for generations of oculists; but, nevertheless, with the advent of fundus photography and the advances in pathology the book now has undoubtedly a more historical value. I have for many years thought to fill this gap in the Italian ophthalmic literature and finally the realization of this plan has come about with the publication of the present volume, the result of a collaboration between three different schools. I have pursued this goal because I was convinced that a collaboration and coordination of various clinical experiences and of different research interests will result in a more complete coverage of the discussions and illustrations, a more accurate critical and better approach to the didactic mission of the book.*

Two prominent ophthalmologic clinics have honored me by their support and collaboration:

— Giulio Morone, Chairman of the Department of Ophthalmology in Pavia, who has so much contributed to our specialty and whose investigations, mainly concerned with the microcirculation of the choroid and retina, have earned him international fame;
— Rosario Brancato, Director of the Department of Ophthalmology at the University of Milan (Hospital S. Raffaele), indefatigable brilliant teacher and investigator, who has channeled the scientific interests of his department into many directions but who is above all known in Italy and abroad for his important and significant contributions to the study of fluorescein angiography.

This atlas presents more than 600 color pictures, all of them originals, which were selected from several thousands of fundus photographs coming from our three institutions in Milan, Pavia and Rome. A considerable part of the photographic material comes from the Department of Ophthalmology of the University of Bari where during the many years of my directorship I founded and organized a modern and efficient laboratory of fundus photopraphy. I am delighted to thank the present Director, Professor Luigi Cardia, my valuable and dear collaborator, for having generously consented to put this photographic material of the institute at my disposal. I am also indebted to Dr. Guglielmo Ranieri, his assistant and my previous collaborator, for the patience of selecting and reproducing these ophthalmoscopic pictures.

The authors have always intended while writing this book to present illustrations not only acceptable from a technical point of view but also (and above all) to show typical aspects of the disease eliminating those features which are neither characteristic nor pathognomonic. If it is true that the ocular fundus provides often highly valuable clinical information, it is also true that the young specialist should have in front of him a reference picture in which, if possible, all the essential characteristics of the disease are illustrated. Whit this goal in mind and aiming at a better understanding the authors have integrated whenever necessary the fundus photo with fluorescein angiography and, occasionally, with histopathologic pictures for a better pathogenetic understanding.

I would like to express my thanks to all those who have directly and indirectly contributed by their valuable collaboration to the realization of this volume.

In the name of all the authors I would like to express our special gratitude to Professor Paola Pivetti Pezzi who has so brilliantly and with great intelligence and perseverance solved the arduous task of coordination.

Special thanks is also due to the publishing Company Masson which has given us complete assistance and has applied noteworthy technical expertise so that the book presents a publishing feat worthy of the best European traditions, also compared to the new publications in French and Spanish.
This book is written — and we hope that it elicits the appropriate interest — not only for the ophthalmologist, but also for neurologists, internists and family practitioners as a reference source which they can rapidly consult during their daily practice.
In summary then, this book is dedicated to the young ophthalmologists in whose hands lie the progress and future of our beloved specialty.

G. SCUDERI

From the Institute of Ophthalmology of the University "La Sapienza" of Rome
November 1985

Contents

Foreword VII
Introduction IX

Chapter 1 THE NORMAL OCULAR FUNDUS

G. MORONE, G. CARELLA, A. GHISOLFI, A. TAZZI

Schematic topography 1
Homogeneity, granularity and color 5
The retinal reflexes 9
The optic nervehead 10
The macula 15
The retinal vessels 16
The retinal periphery 30

Chapter 2 BASIC CHANGES

G. MORONE, G. CARELLA, A. GHISOLFI, A. TAZZI

Vascular changes 37
  Arteries 37
  Arterio-venous crossings 41
  Veins 45
  Neovascularization 50
  Microaneurysms 57
Retinal and choroidal hemorrhages 64
  Preretinal hemorrhages 66
  Intraretinal hemorrhages 67
  Subretinal hemorrhages 69
  Choroidal hemorrhages 70
Edema and exudates 71
Drusen 76
Changes in pigmentation 77

Chapter 3 CONGENITAL ANOMALIES AND MALFORMATIONS

R. BRANCATO, U. MENCHINI, A. PECE, F. BANDELLO

Albinism 81
Choroidal coloboma 82
Myelinated nerve fibres 82
Hypoplasia of the optic nerve 84
Coloboma of the optic nervehead 84
Pit of the optic nervehead 86
Drusen of the optic nervehead 86
Persistence of the primary vitreous and epipapillary membrane 90
Falciform retinal fold 91

Chapter 4 THE OCULAR FUNDUS IN AMETROPIA

G. MORONE, G. CARELLA, A. GHISOLFI, A. TAZZI

Hypermetropia 93
Astigmatism 94
Myopia 94

Chapter 5 DISEASES OF THE OPTIC NERVE

G. MORONE, G. CARELLA, A. GHISOLFI, A. TAZZI

Disc edema 103
Optic atrophy 112

Chapter 6 RETINAL DISEASES

G. SCUDERI, P. PIVETTI PEZZI, E. BALESTRAZZI, G. RANIERI

Occlusion of the central retinal artery and its branches 121
Occlusion of the central retinal vein and its branches 123
Retinopathies in systemic diseases 126
  Diabetic retinopathy 126
  Hypertensive retinopathy 136
  Arteriosclerotic retinopathy 138
  Retinal changes in arterial hypotension 141
  Retinal changes with blood dyscrasias 142
  Retinal changes in collagen diseases 146
  Retinal changes in inborn metabolic errors 147

R. BRANCATO, U. MENCHINI, A. PECE, F. BANDELLO

Retinopathy of prematurity 148
Congenital retinopathies 149
  Tuberous sclerosis (Bourneville's syndrome) 149
  Systemic neurofibromatosis (Von Recklinghausen) 149
  Retinal angiomatosis 150
Degenerative maculopathies 163

G. SCUDERI, E. BALESTRAZZI, P. PIVETTI PEZZI, G. RANIERI

Tapetoretinal degenerations 173
Peripheral retinal degenerations which may or may not cause a retinal break 177

Retinal holes and tears 185
Retinoschisis 192
Retinal detachment 194
Retinal folds 199
Retinal vasculitis 201
Eales disease 204
Acute posterior multifocal placoid pigment epithelio-
pathy (benign diffuse external exudative retinitis) ... 208

R. BRANCATO, U. MENCHINI, A. PECE, F. BANDELLO

Central serous retinopathy 211
Diffuse retinal epitheliopathy 211

Chapter 7 INFLAMMATIONS OF THE CHOROID AND RETINA

G. SCUDERI, P. PIVETTI PEZZI, E. BALESTRAZZI, G. RANIERI

Retinitis, retinochoroiditis, choroiditis, and choriore-
tinitis 219
Retinitis and retinochoroiditis 219
Choroiditis and chorioretinitis 220
Tuberculosis 224
Syphilis 226
Toxoplasmic retinochoroiditis .... 229 ·
Ocular infestation with Toxocara 232
Ocular cysticercosis .... 234 ·
Presumed ocular histoplasmosis .... 235 ·
Mycotic retinitis 236
Viral retinitis 238
Sarcoidosis 240
Behçet disease 240
Sympathetic ophthalmia 245
Vogt-Koyanagi-Harada disease 247
Serpiginous or geographic choroiditis 249
"Birdshot" chorioretinopathy 252

Chapter 8 DISEASES OF THE CHOROID

R. BRANCATO, U. MENCHINI, A. PECE, F. BANDELLO

Choroidal degeneration 253
Angioid streaks 253
Choroidal sclerosis 254
Choroideremia 254
Gyrate choroidal atrophy 254
Pseudo-inflammatory dystrophy of Sorsby 254
Choroidal detachment 258
Occlusion of the posterior ciliary arteries: the trian-
gular syndrome 259

Chapter 9 DISEASES OF THE VITREOUS

R. BRANCATO, U. MENCHINI, A. PECE, F. BANDELLO

Asteroid hyalosis 263
Synchisis scintillans 263

Chapter 10 TUMORS

G. SCUDERI, E. BALESTRAZZI, P. PIVETTI PEZZI, G. RANIERI

Retinal tumors 265
Choroidal tumors 270
Tumors of the optic nerve 279

Chapter 11 OCULAR TRAUMA

G. SCUDERI, P. PIVETTI PEZZI, E. BALESTRAZZI, G. RANIERI

Retinal contusions 285
Purtscher's retinopathy 290
Solar retinopathy 291
Retinal breaks 292
Choroidal ruptures 293
Intraocular foreign bodies 294
Trauma to the optic nerve 296

REFERENCES 297

INDEX 301

Chapter 1

The normal ocular fundus

SCHEMATIC TOPOGRAPHY

A critical review of the publications which necessarily should concern anybody who intends to write a modern and new atlas shows once again the difference in opinions, not only in terminology, but also in concepts concerning the topography of the ocular fundus.

The fovea, for example, is for some authors synonymous with macula and for others it is only the central zone of that area; other authors confuse it with the foveola.

Paramacular, peripapillary and juxtafoveolar are often only topographic assumptions in order to localize a pathologic change or a lesione.

The concept of fundus periphery is even more vague, more individualized and not quantitated with well established anatomical borders.

Out of these considerations and convinced that the increasing more sophisticated demands of fluorescein angiography and photocoagulation will not tolerate topographic vagueness and approximations, we have thought it advisable to precede the chapters on clinical ophthalmoscopy with a scheme which divides the fundus into sections that can be quantitated and related to definite and precise anatomical features (Figs. 1 and 2).

The classical monographs have led us into the habit of considering the fundus as a two-dimensional entity, a kind of concave panorama seen from above, the extent of which is quite limited because of the poor maneuverability and the inclination of the incident light from the ophthalmoscope. Today the biomicroscopic examination has given the fundus picture a three-dimensional character thereby allowing us to outline the anterior and posterior retinal profile, to individualize, and identify the contents, their essential character and frequently their nature; to quantitate the thickness of the tissue and the relative distance between the various layers; to follow in an anterior/posterior direction the prominent formations; to determine the depth of a lesion and to push the limits of our examinations to extremes previously beyond our reach.

From Helmholtz we have progressed to Goldmann; from the small to the big scope of exploration; from the illumination of the surface to the optical section; from surface view to biomicroscopy.

The modern methodological approach to conceptualize the ocular fundus must be radically changed. We have to think in three dimensions considering the choroid and retina with their pathologic changes as a spatial phenomenon which extends in three directions.

Consequently a topographical concept which is more detailed, more precise and more definitive is necessary, especially for the laser treatment which at the moment presents the most promising hope for the treatment of the most recalcitrant and controversial pathologic processes.

Fig. 1.

A   = Posterior pole: delineated by two ellipsoidal lines which encompass the optic nervehead and extend along the temporal vascular ▶
        arcades meeting temporally at a point which lies at the same distance from the fovea as the nasal disc margin. The smaller axis
        of the ellipse measures around 3.5 mm.

B   = Intermediate retinal zone. It lies between the border of the posterior ellipsoid and a line which theoretically connects the am-
        pullae of the vortex veins. The width of this zone is on an average 12.5 mm.

C   = The equatorial (posterior) part of the retinal periphery. It is the most peripheral retina still observable with the ophthalmoscope.
        Its extension is approximately 4.7 mm.

D   = The oral (extreme or anterior) retinal periphery. It can be seen with indentation. Its extension is about 5.8 mm and its most
        anterior margin corresponds to the anterior border of the vitreous base.

VV = ampullae of the vortex veins;

 *   = anterior border of the vitreous base;

 1   = tooth of the ora serrata;

 2   = bay of the ora serrata; 2b = sequestrated bay;

 3   = microcystoid degeneration;

 4   = oral pearl;

 5   = meridoneal crest;

 6   = oral pit (excavation);

 7   = oral excrescence.

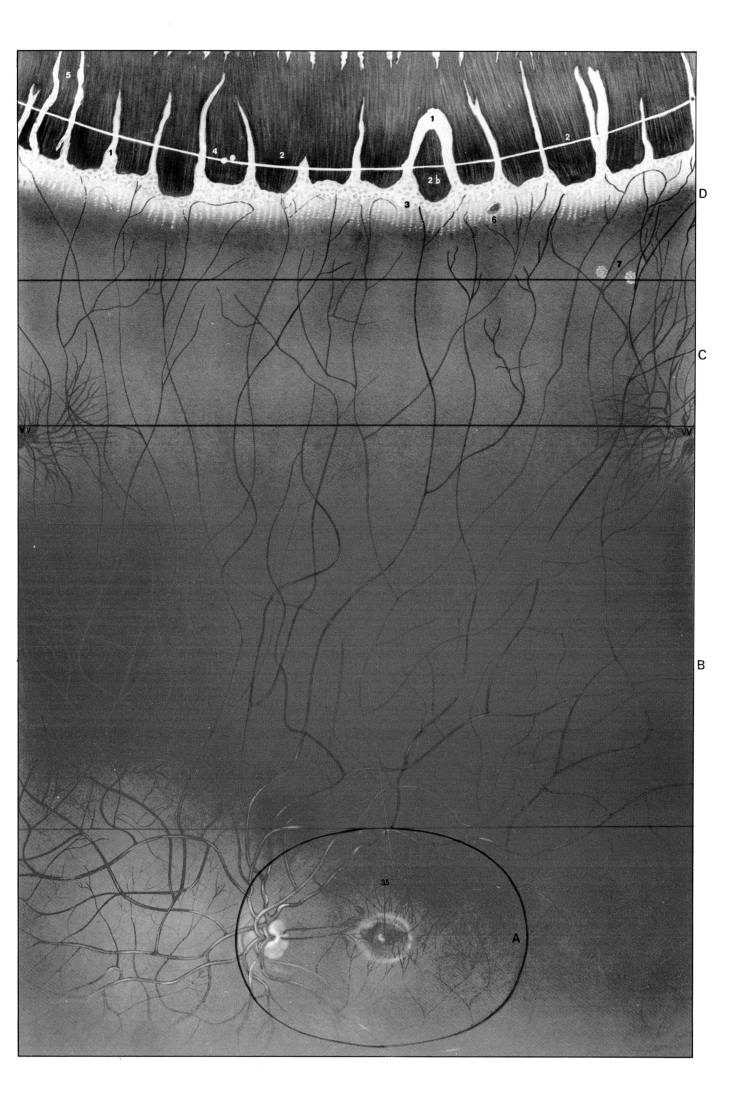

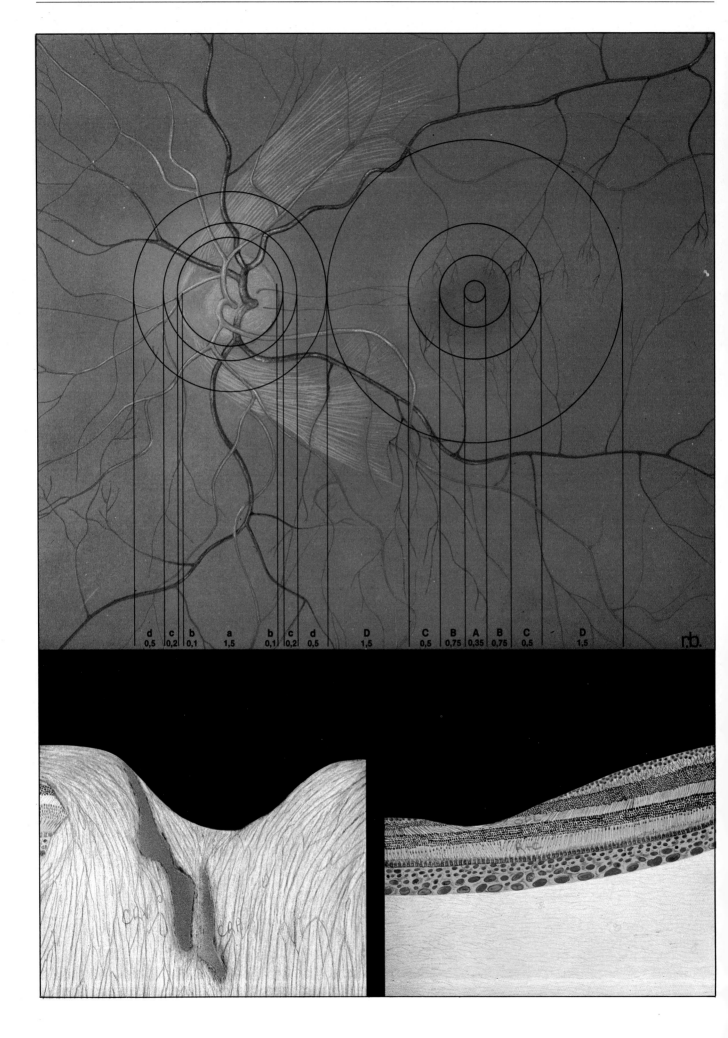

d	c	b	a	b	c	d	D	C	B	A	B	C	D
0,5	0,2	0,1	1,5	0,1	0,2	0,5	1,5	0,5	0,75	0,35	0,75	0,5	1,5

◄ **Fig. 2.**

Area of the optic nervehead	**Macular area**
a = area of the optic disc;	A = foveola;
b = juxtapapillary area;	B = fovea;
c = parapapillary area;	C = parafovea;
d = peripapillary area.	D = perifovea.

HOMOGENEITY, GRANULARITY AND COLOR

Peculiar characteristics of the normal ocular fundus are its relative homogeneity and definite granules visible with the ophthalmoscope.

The first is due to the fact that with a transparent retina the pigment of the epithelium and the dense network of the choriocapillaries hide the large choroidal vessels and obscure their pattern.

The second fact is probably due to the irregular and non-uniform distribution of the pigment within the pigment epithelial cells.

The granularity is more detailed at the posterior pole and more rarified and coarser in the periphery. Therefore the homogeneity is more uniform in the center of the fundus where the pigment is denser, while it becomes less pronounced in the periphery where the pigment is more dispersed so that the choroidal pattern may become visible (Fig. 3).

Varying the direction of the incident light of the ophthalmoscope it is easy to reveal a radiated striation converging towards the optic nerve head, and occupying an area about 7 mm around the disc.

This pattern is caused by the distribution of the optic nerve fibers which in the papillo-macular area assume a typical biconvex course (Fig. 4).

The color of the fundus varies in a normal Caucasian when observed with a polychromatic light of the usual electric ophthalmoscope from light orange to vivid red. This color is the result of two chromatic elements which influence each other to a varying degree: The first one is the oxyhemoglobin of the circulating blood in the choroid; the second one is the pigment in the choroid itself and in the overlying pigment epithelium. Therefore, the oxyhemoglobin and the pigment constitute the numerator and the denominator of a relationship which results in a variety of colors corresponding to the prevalence of one over the other (Fig. 5).

In a pigmented individual, and especially in the black races, the color of the fundus appears red-brown, whereas in a blonde individual, and especially in an albino, it appears light red. In the latter instance the macular area is usually occupied by a reddish spot with blurred outlines in which the underlying choroidal vessels cannot be identified, though they are perfectly visible in all other areas of the funds.

During life there is considerable change in the ophthalmoscopic picture. The water content of the cells decreases progressively so that the "soft" appearance of the ocular fundus in an infant changes into the more "dry" aspect in an adult and finally into the "arid" one in senescence. There is also over the course of the years a depigmentation of retinal pigment epithelium combined with a correspondig increase in choroidal pigment (Fig. 6). During infancy there is an intense pigmentation of the epithelium and a sparse pigment content in the choroid (producing the uniform red vivid color of the funds). With advancing age the pigment in the retinal pigment epithelium decreases making this structure more transparent so that the underlying choroid becomes visible. In the choroid the major part of the pigmentation is found among the vessels forming the characteristic mosaic of a reddish network contrasting with the grey-black background.

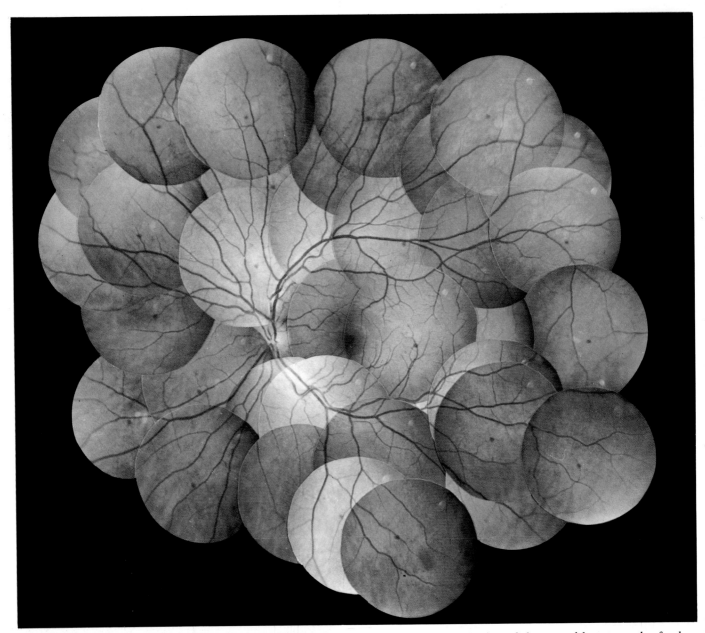

Fig. 3. Panoramic view of the normal human ocular fundus.

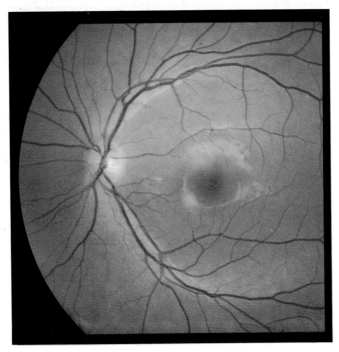

Fig. 4. Ophthalmoscopic picture of the course of the optic nerve fibers.

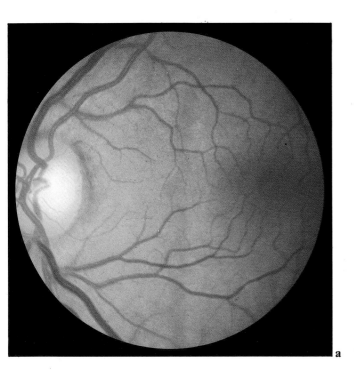 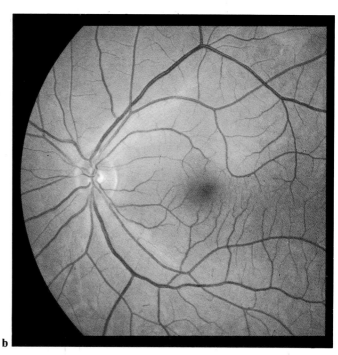

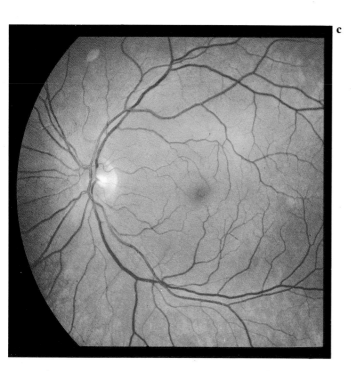 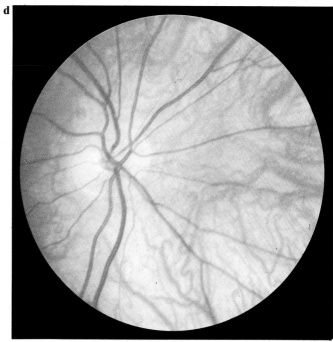

Fig. 5. a-d) Physiologic colors of the ocular fundus.
a) Black.
b) Dark brown.
c) Light brown.
d) Blonde.

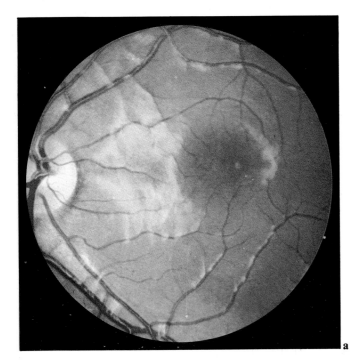
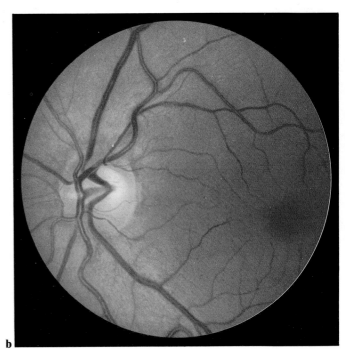
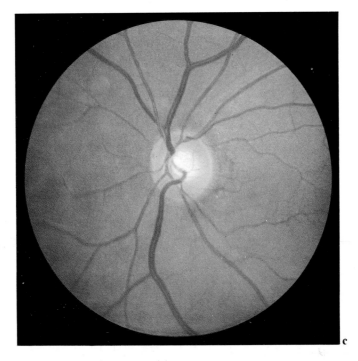

Fig. 6.   a–c) Physiologic variations of the characteristics of the ocular fundus (homogeneity, granular appearance, color and reflexes) in relation to age.
a) In children.
b) In adults.
c) In advanced age.

THE RETINAL REFLEXES

When the light of the ophthalmoscope strikes the fundus, which is a concave surface, a number of reflexes will be produced, the form and behavior of which may help us in identifying the fine structures.

These reflexes are produced by the incident light striking the internal limiting membrane which behaves here like an optical surface. The reflexes are fundamentally of two aspects: irregular and diffuse or regular and mirror-like. These two kinds of reflexes often combine in a varying and transient fashion. The specular reflexes in general outline the borders of a zone and define details of a surface. For example, the reflex from the fovea is characteristic because it delineates sharply with a more or less fine luminous ellipsoid line the margins of this area in the center of which the foveola is identified by its characteristic reflex (foveolar reflex).

From the foveola a conoidal reflex is created (similar to a head-light) extending to the borders of the fovea where it terminates (Fig. 7).

The reflex of Weiss is annular or arcuate and runs parallel to the disc margin, usually on the nasal side; it is due to the elevation of the internal limiting membrane in the area where the nerve fiber layer is thickest.

The reflex of Gunn consists of small ovoid spots usually located above and below the disc along the main nerve fiber bundles. All these reflexes are seen in the normal fundus, but it is certainly rare to see them all together in the same eye.

It is necessary to recognize them because their modifications could signify or exclude a pathologic condition. For example, the widening of the reflex of Weiss could precede the development of a disc edema.

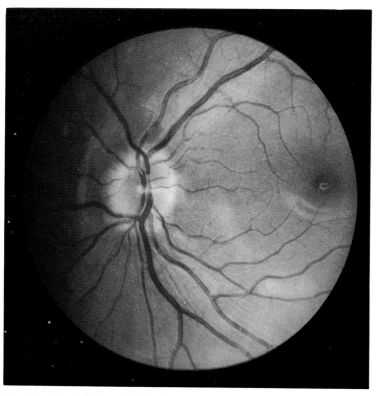

Fig. 7. Physiologic retinal reflexes.
Peripapillary nasal semilunar reflex of Weiss. Oval reflexes of Gunn along the nerve fiber bundles.
Partial foveolar reflex (below) delineating the fovea, in the center of which is the foveolar reflex identifying the foveola.

THE OPTIC NERVEHEAD

By optic disc we mean that part of the optic nervehead directly visible with the ophthalmoscope. It is therefore a two-dimensional concept. With papilla, on the other hand, we mean a histologic tridimensional structure, the optic nervehead crossing through the sclerochoroidal canal delineated posteriorly by the cribriform plate (Figs. 8 and 9).

In reality the ophthalmoscopic area of the disc is smaller than that of the papilla of which we actually only see the surface. The disc has a diameter of 1.5 mm (Fig. 10) and is usually round or slightly oval with the long axis vertically. It has a pink color with a slightly yellowish margin. The disc represents the most important landmark for ophthalmoscopic examination and is for the observer the principal point of orientation.

The color of the disc shows numerous physiologic variations. It is the result of light reflected from the retrolaminar myelin sheaths which is mixed with the red color from the capillaries in the optic nervehad. (Fig. 11). The optic nervehead is in a variable relationship to the structures through which it passes (from back to front: sclera, choroid and retina). A pale ring, rarely complete and more frequently seen on a temporal side, lies immediately around the disc and represents the scleral canal through which the nerve passes (Fig. 12). If the choroid and the retinal pigment epithelium do not reach the nervehead, but end at a certain distance from it, we may find in addition to the scleral ring a crescent shaped area in which the choroidal vessels and pigment are seen; this arcuate thin line consists of an accumulation of pigment derived from the pigment epithelium.

The optic nervehead shows in 85% of normal eyes in its center a funnel-shaped depression from which the central vessels emerge (Fig. 13). The shape and dimension of this depression vary considerably; it is frequently eccentric and lies nasally where it also has a steeper slope; it has a flatter slope temporally. It is an old dogma that the physiologic depression does, in contrast to the pathologic excavation, never reach the disc margin. The size of the depression increases somewhat with age and is more or less symmetrical in both eyes.

A considerable difference in the diameter of the two discs should raise the suspicion of a pathologic change. In the depth of the excavation the septated cribriform plate may be visible (laminar dot sign).

The ophthalmoscopic appearance and especially the color of the disc undergo considerable changes during life (Fig. 14). In early infancy (Fig. 14 a) the optic disc has a more greyish color compared to the pink appearance of the adult (Fig. 14 b). This has usually been explained by the yet incomplete myelinization of the optic nerve fibers and therefore less white light will be reflected than when the nerve is completely medullated.

In advanced age (Fig. 14 c) the disc appears paler than in a young adult; it is frequently accompanied by a temporal cone of chorioretinal atrophy.

It is quite likely that the choroidal vessels supplying the optic nervehead (Fig. 14 d), and presenting the main blood supply for the prelaminar area, become atrophic during this degenerative process which involves the peripapillary connective tissue and vessels. This leads to a decreased blood flow to the capillaries of the nervehead with subsequent partial atrophy of the axons closely dependent on the circulatory and metabolic properties of these vessels.

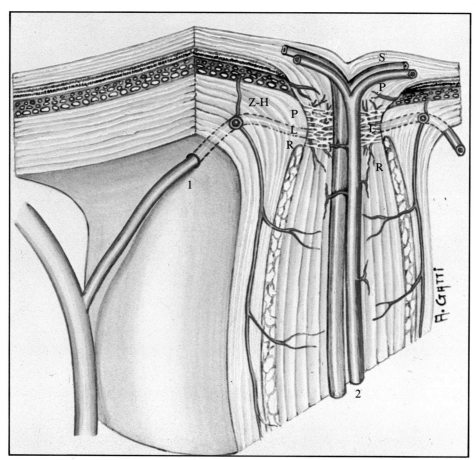

Fig. 8. Schematic drawing of the head and collar of the optic nerve.
There are two vascular systems: ciliary (1) and retinal (2). The vascular circle of Zinn-Haller (Z-H) around the optic nerve appears to indent the sclera.
Taking the cribriform plate as a reference plane we distinguish classically (Hayreh) four layers: retrolaminar (R), laminar (L), prelaminar (P) and superficial (S).

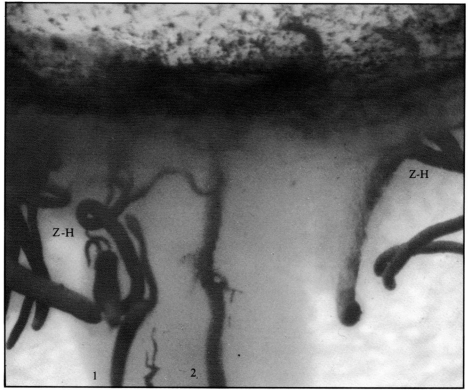

Fig. 9. Microscopic specimen of the head and collar of the optic nerve in transillumination after injecting a chromopolymer of neoprene latex. The two vascular systems-ciliary (1) and retinal (2) - are visible as well as the circle of Zinn-Haller (Z-H).

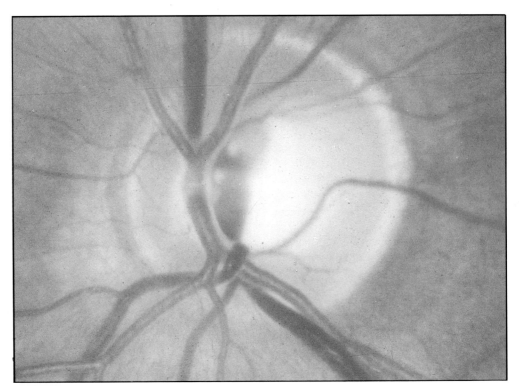

Fig. 10.   Ophthalmoscopic picture of a normal optic disc.

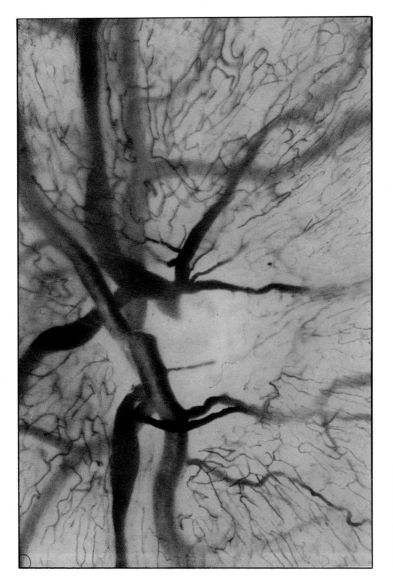

Fig. 11.   A microscopic specimen injected and seen in transillumination in order to demonstrate the various zones of arterial capillaries and veins for the optic disc.

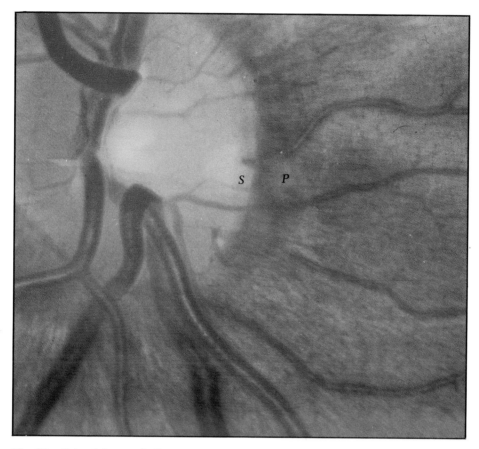

Fig. 12. Scleral (internal) (S) and pigment (P) ring on the temporal side where the optic nervehead goes over into the adjacent retina.

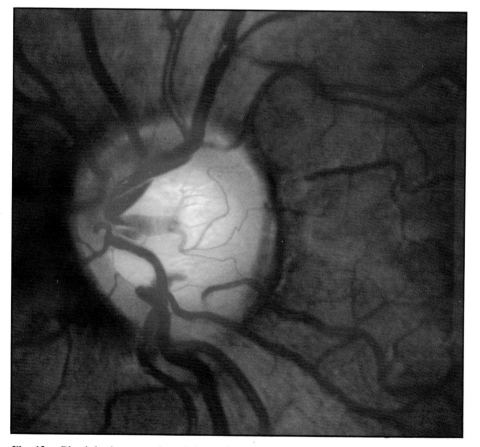

Fig. 13. Physiologic excavation of the optic nervehead in the depth of which the cribriform plate is visible (laminar dot sign).

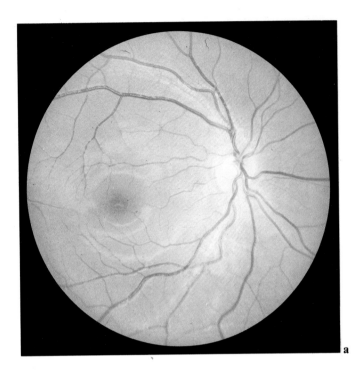
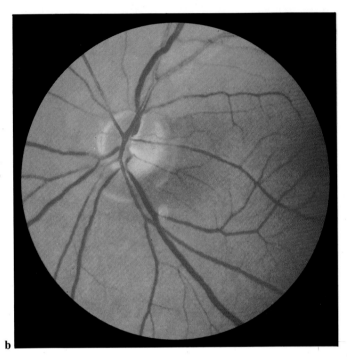

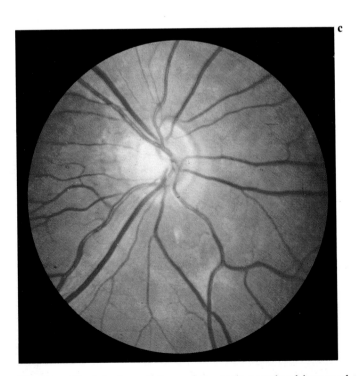

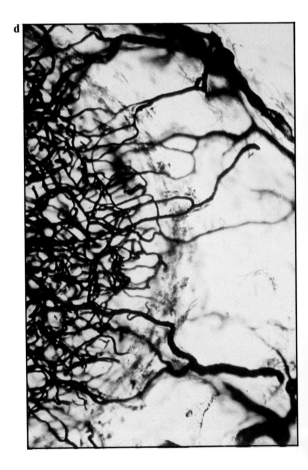

Fig. 14.   Physiologic variations of the optic nervehead in regard to age.
a) In children. **b)** In adults. **c)** In persons of advanced age. In the latter case
the characteristic peripapillary retinochoridal crescent is visible. It is probably
due to the degenerative involution of the anastomizing vessels between the
choroid and the optic nervehead, made evident in the microscopic specimen
of Fig. **d.**

THE MACULA

The macula is an eliptical area with the horizontal axis longer than the vertical one; it is darker in color than the surrounding retina and often delineated by an arcuate reflex. In the center is the foveola which is of a more vivid red color due to the thinning of the retina (Fig. 15 b). In a young person the fovea lies 4 mm from the disc margin if the eye is emmetropic (the distance is greater in the hypermetrope and smaller in the myope). It lies slightly below the horizontal meridian. The fovea also undergoes characteristic age changes: in the child (Fig. 15 a) the general soft appearance is even more clearly evident at the border of the fovea showing one or two concentric circular reflexes. This area also may produce reflexes.

In an older individual the dry tissue does not produce these reflexes any more; the fovea is in this age group not identifiable except by its variation in color (Fig. 15 c).

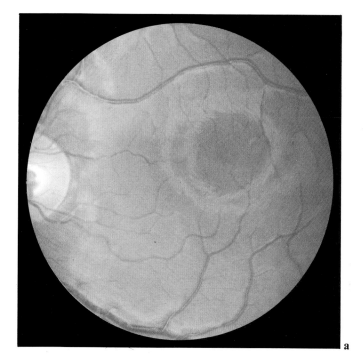 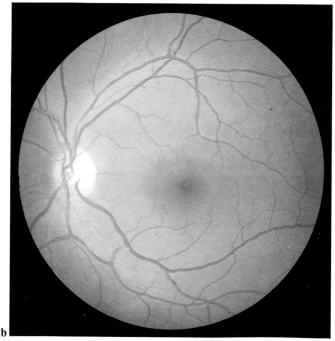

a b

c

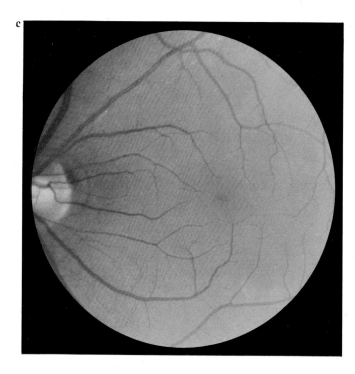

Fig. 15. a-c) Physiologic variations of the macula in regards to age.
a) In children.
b) In adults.
c) In advanced age.

THE RETINAL VESSELS

The variations in the distributions of the retinal vascular network are so great that there are actually no two fundi which look alike (Fig. 16).

The principal vessels course superficially in the nerve fiber layer dividing dichotomously into smaller and smaller branches and precapillaries, but always remaining in the same histologic layer. Two capillary networks stem from the precapillaries: One is superficial and remains in the nerve fiber layer, the other one is deep, denser and more complex. It lies in the area where the inner nuclear layer borders the outer plexiform layer. Anastomoses exist between the two networks, which are especially well visible on tri-dimensional models. The central retinal artery emerges from the depth of the physiologic optic cup (Fig. 17) and usually divides into two main branches, a superior and an inferior one. These two branches give origin to the temporal and nasal arcade so that each retinal quadrant is supplied by one main branch of the central artery (Figs. 18 a, b).

In general the veins follow quite closely the appropriate arteries. The veins are usually larger, darker and more tortuous than the arteries. The axial vascular reflex which is produced by the center of each vessel is more extensive on the arteries than on the veins; the venous reflexes are, however, more luminous (Figs. 19 a, b).

These reflexes are either produced by the outer layers of the vessel wall, by the convexity of the blood column within the vessel or by the mirror effect of the internal limiting membrane.

The branches of the retinal vascular tree frequently cross each other (Figs. 20 a, b). The artery always lies in a definite anatomical plane and the vein is forced to bend downward under the artery (it is rare that the vein lies above the artery). This relationship varies with the various zones of the fundus or with the age of the person. These relationships become closer in the adult and especially in old age when there is a denser intervascular adventitia. In general there are no crossings between artery and artery or vein and vein. The above described features representing the normal morphology of the retinal vascular tree show wide physiologic variations.

Figs. 21 a, b show an anomalous dichotomous branching of the inferior temporal artery which surrounds the fovea. A cilioretinal artery is present in about 20% of the eyes

(Figs. 22 a-c). It originates from the underlying choroid, exits at the temporal disc margin and extends in the retina. In view of the importance of the macular function a particular vascular pattern is present in that area. Fine vessels extend from the upper and lower vascular arcade and from the temporal border of the nervehead toward the fovea (Figs. 23 a, b). These extend up to the border of the foveolar depression, anastomose with each other and constitute a delicate perifoveal arcade delineating a central area of 300-400 μ in which there are no blood vessels at all (Figs. 24 a, b). Outside of the macular region where the capillaries are arranged in different depths of the retina the capillary network abruptly lies in only one plane and becomes progressively sparser from the posterior pole toward periphery (Figs. 25 a, b).

The capillaries of the retina and of the brain (but nowhere else in the body) show a characteristic arrangement next to the main vascular trunks (Fig. 26 a). Around the arterial trunks (never or rarely around venous vessels) (Fig. 26 b) there is a capillary-free zone which increases toward the retinal periphery and with advancing age.

It is the function of the retinal vessels coming from the central retinal artery to supply the inner retinal layers, whereas the outer layers (photoreceptors) are supplied from the choroidal vasculature. The latter can be evaluated ophthalmoscopically only under unusual circumstances of hypopigmentation of the retinal pigment epithelium (Fig. 27). The capillaries forming the choriocapillaries are perhaps the largest in the body (40-60 μ). They have the highest circulation rate of any organ (nine times more than that of the kidneys). In contrast to the retinal arterioles and perhaps as an explanation for their metabolic function the choroidal capillaries are fenestrated and constitute networks which are densest and most active in the foveal region (Fig. 28 a). This network is less dense in the perimacular area (Fig. 28 b), around the posterior pole (Fig. 28 c) and in intermediate areas (Fig. 28 d).

The peripapillary choriocapillaries (Figs. 29 a, b) contributes the vascular supply to the prelaminar part of the optic nervehead. This represents an area which is of particular physiologic and pathologic importance. These capillaries determine the irrigation of the neural components of the optic nervehead.

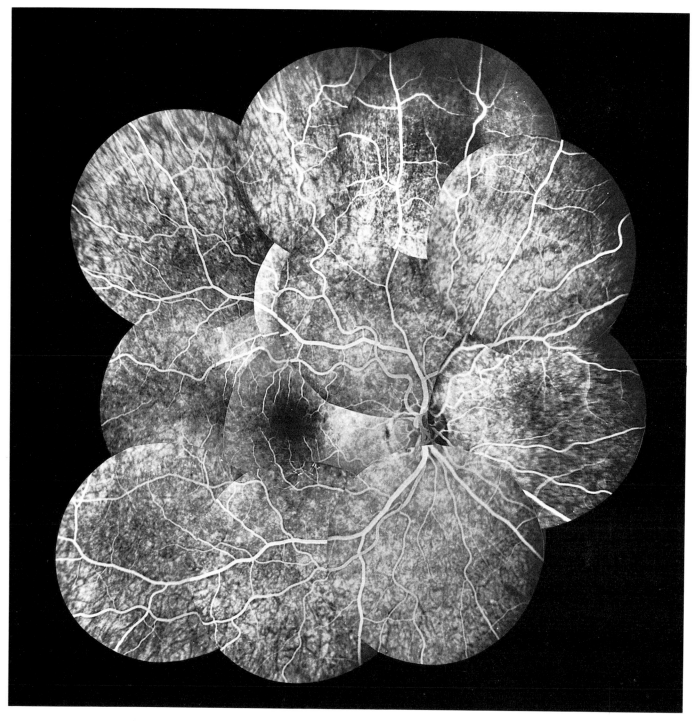

Fig. 16. Panoramic view of the retinal vascular pattern as seen on fluorescein angiography.

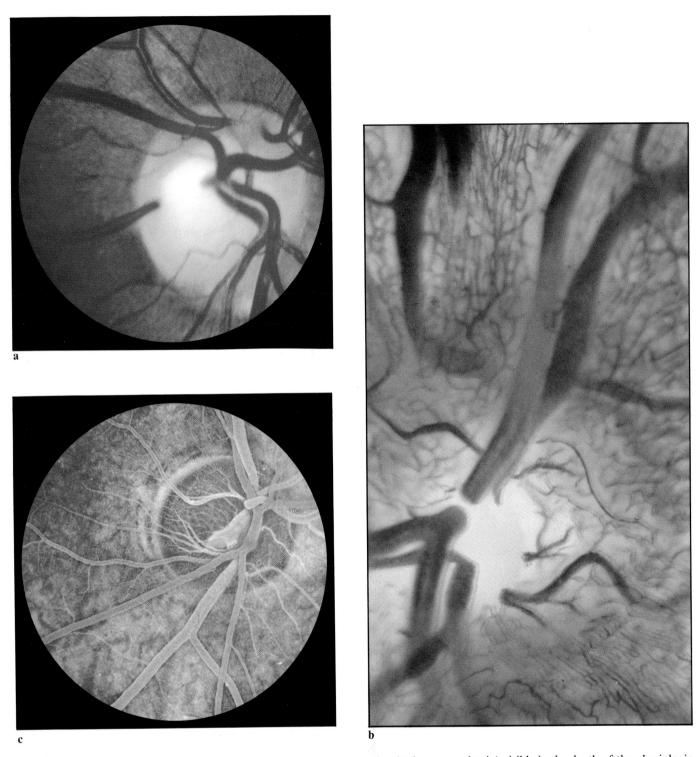

Fig. 17.   The central retinal vessel bundle (first branching of the central retinal artery and vein) visible in the depth of the physiologic excavation as seen with the ophthalmoscope (**a**), in a microscopic specimen (**b**) and on fluorescein angiography (**c**).
In **a** we see a cilioretinal artery which originates at the temporal margin of the disc.

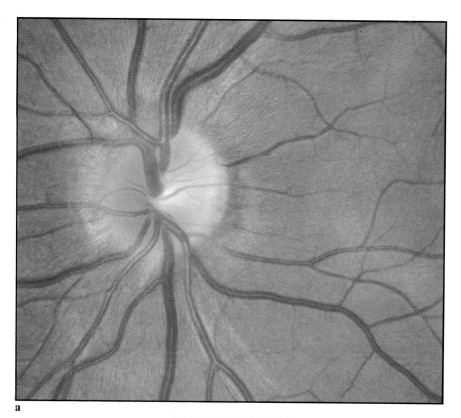

a

Fig. 18. First dichotomous division of the superior and inferior branches of the artery and vein, seen with the ophthalmoscope (**a**) and after injection of a polymer in a microscopic specimen (**b**). The quadrantic distribution of the four main branches becomes evident.

b

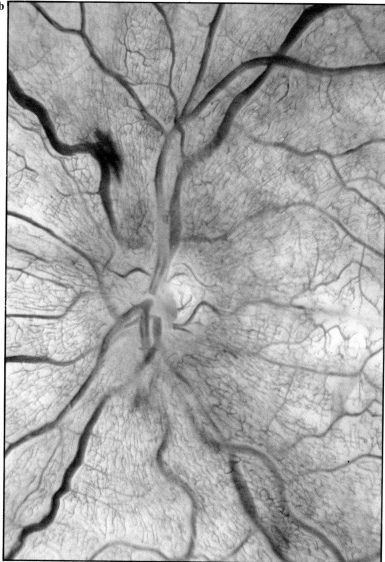

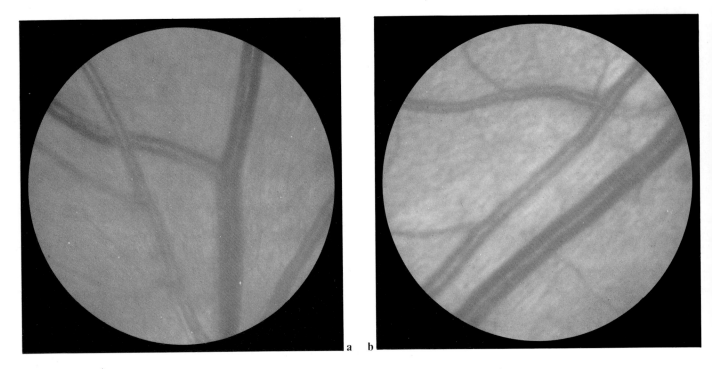

Fig. 19.   a) and **b)** Arterial and venous branches of the second order with the typical axial reflexes.

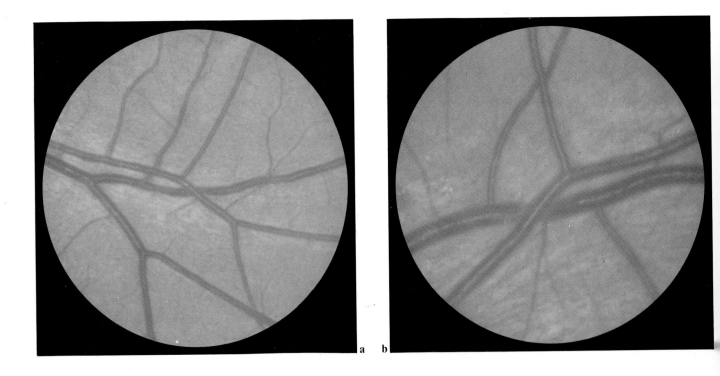

Fig. 20.   Typical arterio-venous crossing: the artery crosses over the vein (**a**). In **b** we see an indication of an adventitial intervascular tissue which is common to the two vessels.

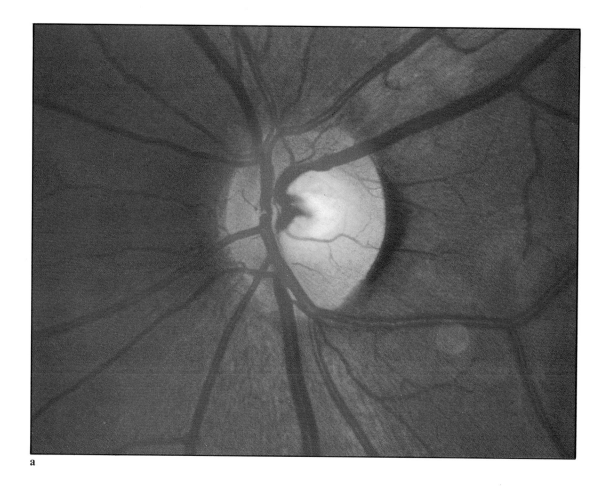

a

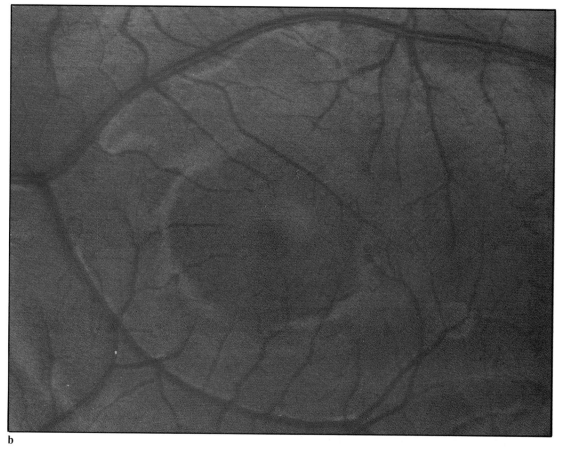

b

Fig. 21. **a)** and **b)** Anomalous branching of the infero-temporal artery which surrounds the fovea.

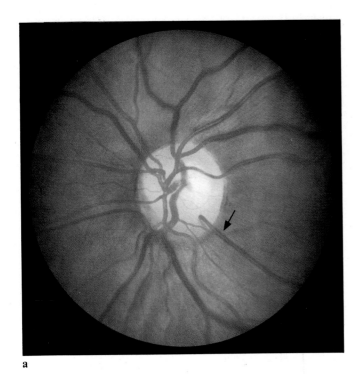

a

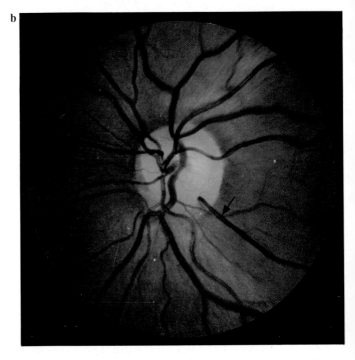

b

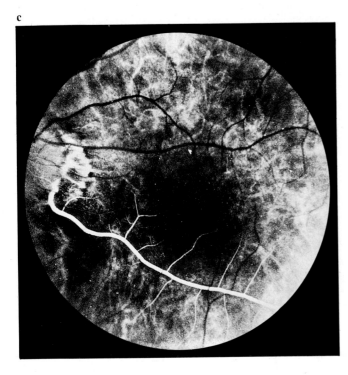

c

Fig. 22.   Cilio-retinal artery (arrow) seen with polychromatic light (**a**) and with red-free light (**b**); **c** fluorescein angiographic appearance of a cilio-retinal artery.

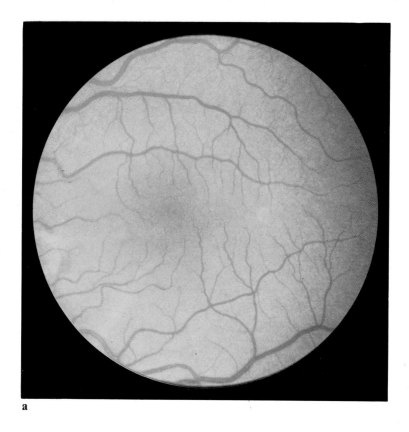

a

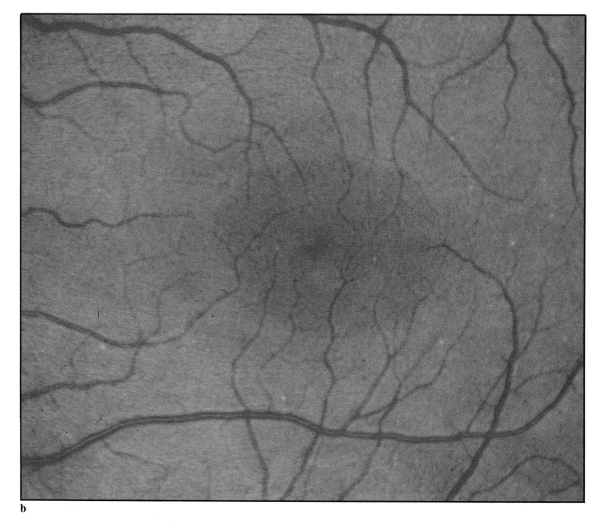

b

Fig. 23. **a)** and **b)** The vessels of the macular area (retinal photographs of different magnification).

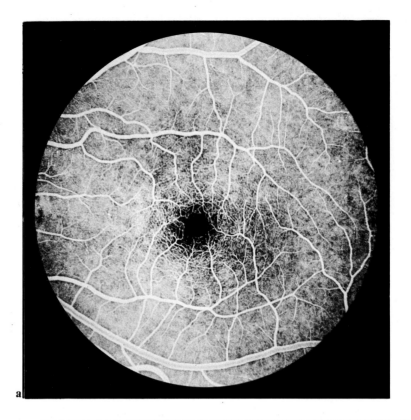

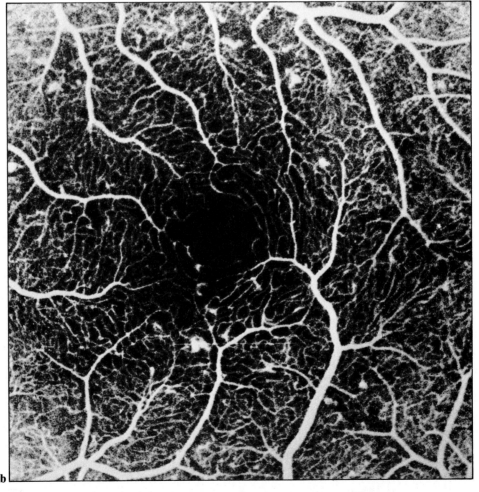

Fig. 24. **a)** Normal subject; **b)** Diabetic patient.
Fluorescein angiographic picture of the macular area. The vessels of the macula come from
the upper and lower vascular arcade, course toward the posterior pole to an arc which delineates
the central avascular zone.

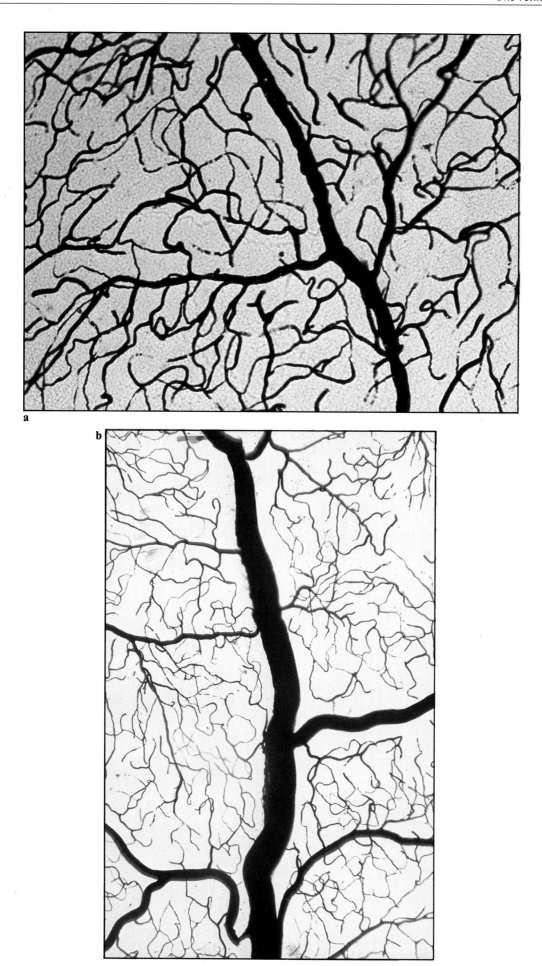

Fig. 25. Two-dimensional representation of the vascular network in the zone surrounding the foveola (**a**) and in the intermediate layer (**b**) (neoprene injection specimen).

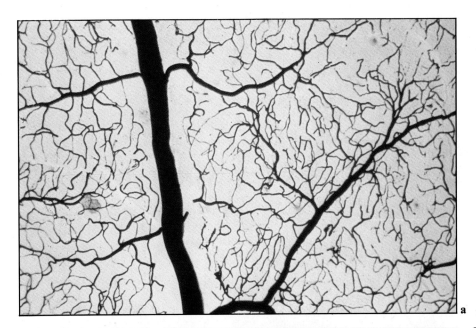

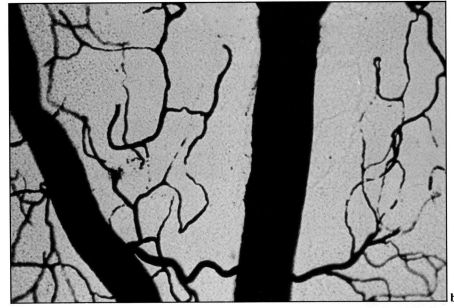

Fig. 26.   a) and **b)** Capillary-free zone around retinal arterioles (Indian ink injection).

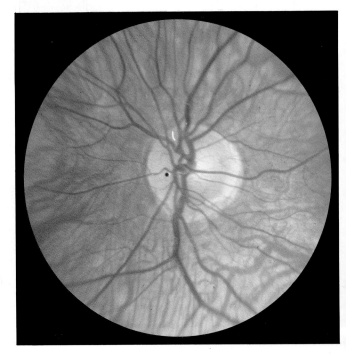

Fig. 27.   The network of choroidal vessels is well visible due to hypopigmentation of the pigment epithelium.

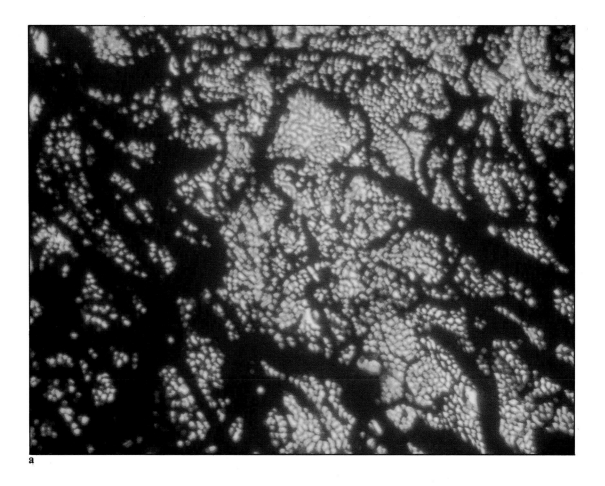

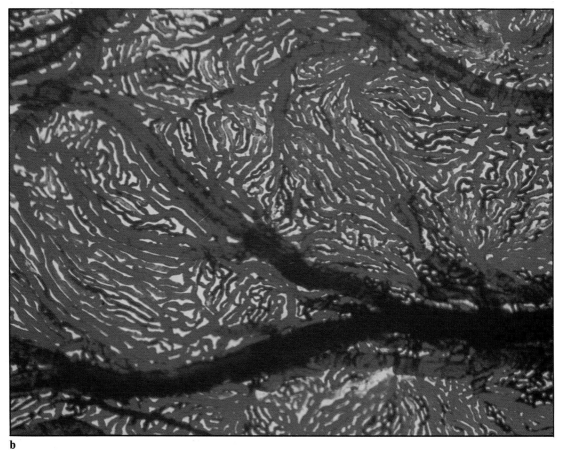

Fig. 28. **a)** and **b)** The choriocapillaries in the foveal zone (**a**), and in the perimacular area (**b**) (chromopolymer injection specimen).

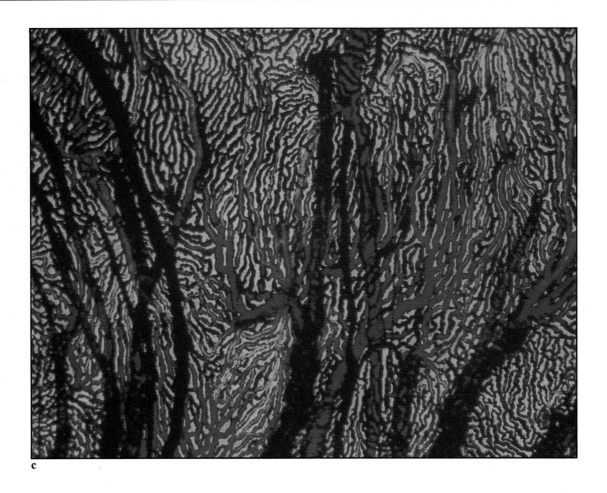

c

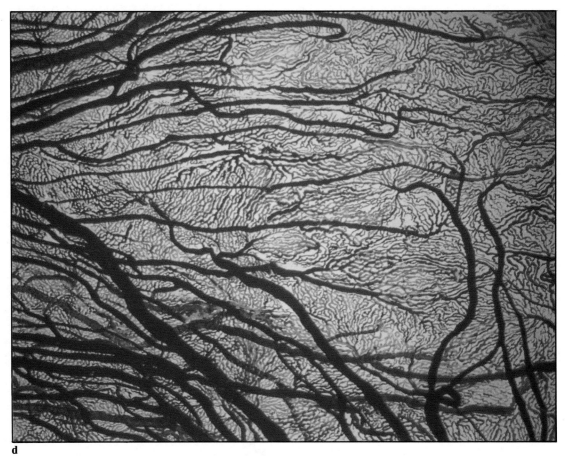

d

Fig. 28.   c) and **d)** The choriocapillaries around the posterior pole **(c)** and in the intermediate zone of the fundus **(d)** (chromopolymer injection specimen).

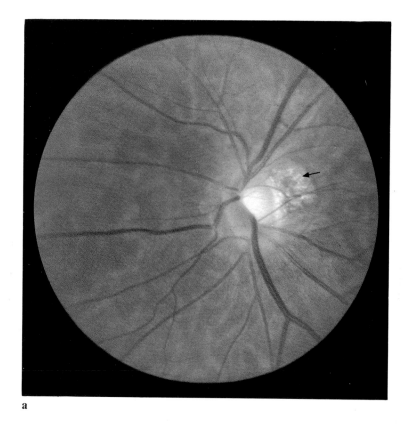

a

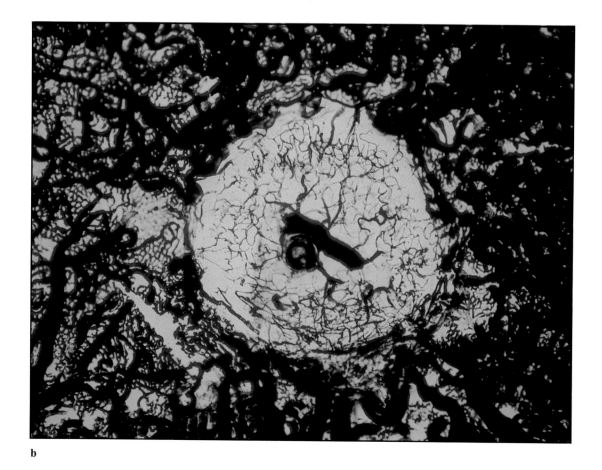

b

Fig. 29. The peripapillary choroid visible with the ophthalmoscope (**a**) (arrow); microscopic specimen demonstrating the anastomoses at the prelaminar part of the optic nervehead (**b**).

THE RETINAL PERIPHERY

By the term periphery we understand here the most anterior part of the fundus, the posterior limit of which is a line which ideally should connect the entrance points of the vorticose veins; its anterior border is the anterior margin of the vitreous base which presents a white line seen with indentation lying at about the middle of the pars plana (Fig. 1). The posterior (equatorial) part of the retinal periphery (Figs. 1, 30 a, b) is ophthalmoscopically characterized by the presence of pigmentary changes due to the thinning of the retina and to a decrease of pigment in the retinal pigment epithelium.

In this area the vessels divide rarely, are stretched, thinned and rectilinear.

The extreme retinal periphery (oral area) (Figs. 1; 31 a, b) has on indentation a characteristic white-greyish color, is opaque and slightly elevated.

The retinal vessels never extend beyond the ora serrata. On indentation the ora appears as a zig-zag line (from which it derivers its name) consisting of teeth surrounding bays the convexity of which is directed posteriorly. There are a number of physiologic variations seen in this area (Fig. 1); these are to be considered as normal and should be differentiated from pathologic alterations which are often seen in this zone and may lead to dangerous sequelae. It is for instance not unusual to see here small translucent cavities. These are innocuous and can be regarded as variance of the normal. Nevertheless, they are called ''cystoid degenerations''.

The teeth of the ora surround the bays and may be more or less pointed or prominent. The bays constitute a slightly arcuate indentation and may also present themselves as a more pronounced and deep excavation. When two adjoining teeth merge they may completely surround a bay which now appears like an island. This may clinically be mistaken for a retinal hole but its base is the ciliary body which has a darker color than the typical pink of the retina.

These areas (sequestrated bays) probably represent a danger point for a rhegmatogenous detachment and should be treated prophylactically. Spherules, the size of a pinhead, may be seen at the level of the teeth and bays. These increase in number with age. They are smooth, shining, refractile and are called pearls. Histologically they constitute the drusen of this zone.

Another morphologic variant is the meridional crest. These are transparent and irregular linear ridges which are irregular and run radially from the level of a tooth or a bay. They are in all likelihood caused by an excessive growth of embryologic retina, which accumulates to such a meridional fold.

We finally have to mention the excavations or pits of the peripheral retina. These are oval and constitute incomplete breaks of the retina. They are due to the disappearance of the external retinal layers and the presence of peripheral retinal excrescences; the latter constitute opaque, grey-white granules more or less elevated over the surface of the equatorial retina and the vitreous space.

The sparsity of pigment in the peripheral retinal pigment epithelium allows a good visualization of the vascular pattern of the underlying choroid (Fig. 33 a).

In contrast to the behavior of the retinal vessels the choroidal vessels increase in caliber from the posterior pole toward the periphery where the intervascular spaces also appear considerably wider. The choriocapillaries terminates abruptly at the ora serrata (Figs. 33 b, c) separating two vascular systems of different character.

The vortex veins constitute the main drainage vessels of the entire uvea (Fig. 33 d). A vortex vein represents the center of a fan consisting of the afferent vessels which give it the characteristic appearance.

The pink color of the vortex is more or less complete when all the afferent veins merge into the common collector channel, before or after the trunk has entered sclera.

We usually list four vortex veins, one per quadrant. In general these veins are more numerous (6-7 on an average). They represent primary drainage areas with strictly separated territories.

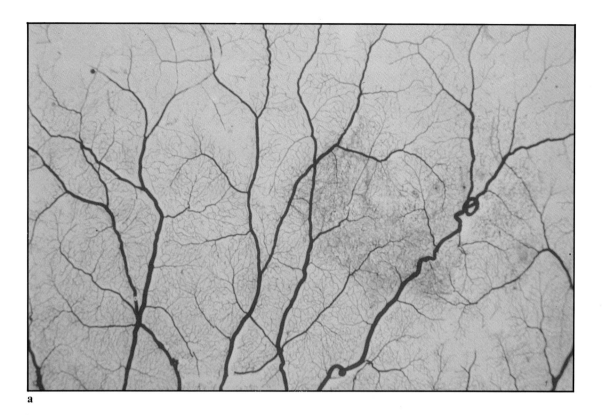

a

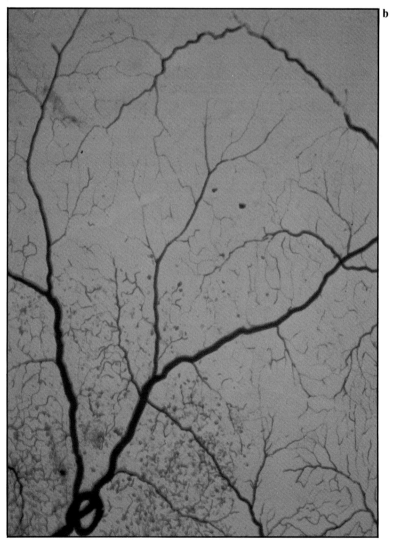

b

Fig. 30. The posterior (equatorial) part of the retinal periphery. Pigmented granules in the retina (**a**). Anastomosing loop at the most peripheral branching (**b**).

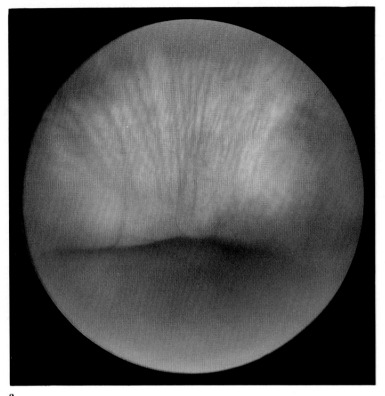

a

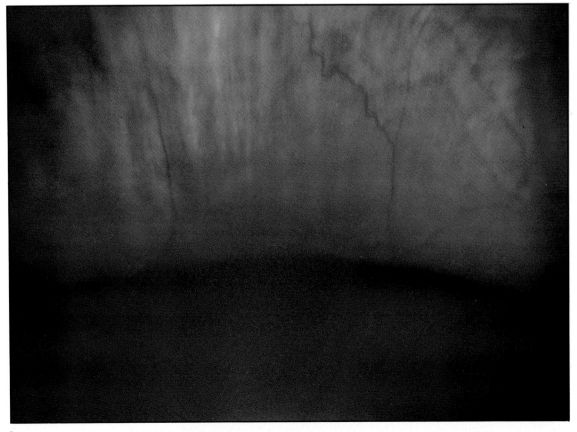

b

Fig. 31. a) and **b)** Anterior (oral) retinal periphery. The patient had been operated on for a retinal detachment: the indentation by the buckle makes the characteristic opalescence of that area ophthalmoscopically visible; it shows only a few blood vessels.

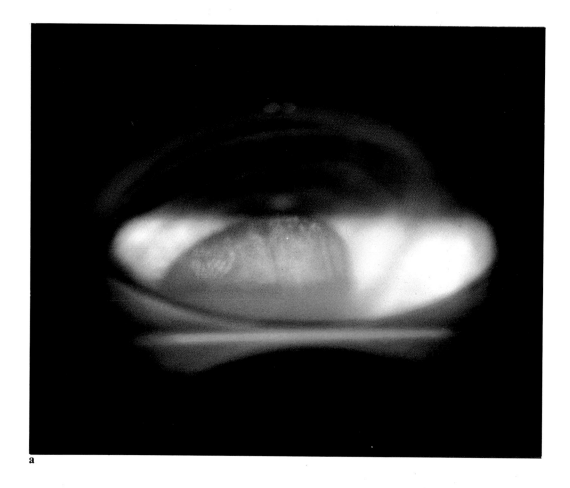

a

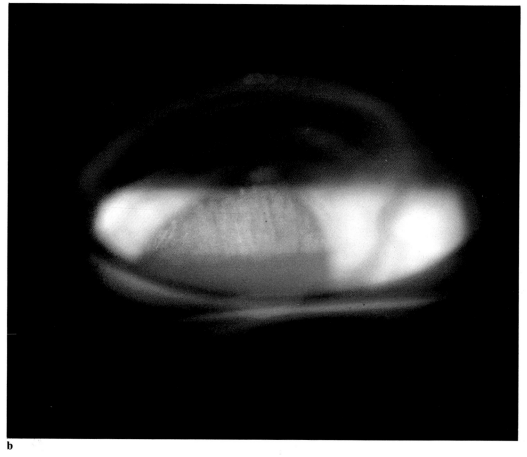

b

Fig. 32. **a)** and **b)** Biomicroscopic appearance of the ora serrata with the typical teeth surrounding the bays.

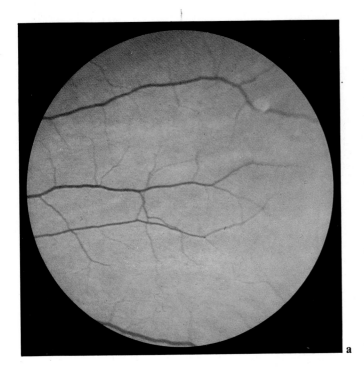
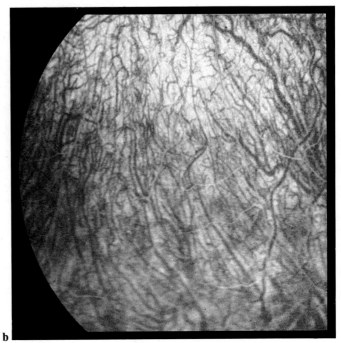

a   b

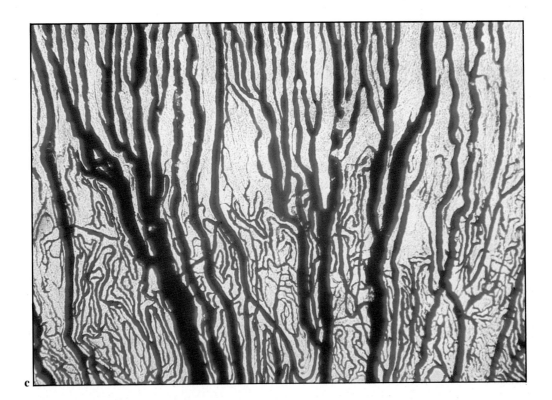

c

Fig. 33.   The retinal periphery. The framework of choroidal vessels is usually well visible in the peripheral areas because of the rarefaction of the pigment epithelial layer.
a) Ophthalmoscopic appearance.
b) Fluorescein angiogram.
c) and **d)** The microscopic specimens show clearly the sudden qualitative and quantitative changes in the capillary network at the ora serrata. The ora is not an abstract topographic line, but a real anatomical demarcation.
e) Microangiographic specimen showing two whorls of venous drainage converging to the vorticose veins of the appropriate area and separated by an area dividing the two irrigation zones.

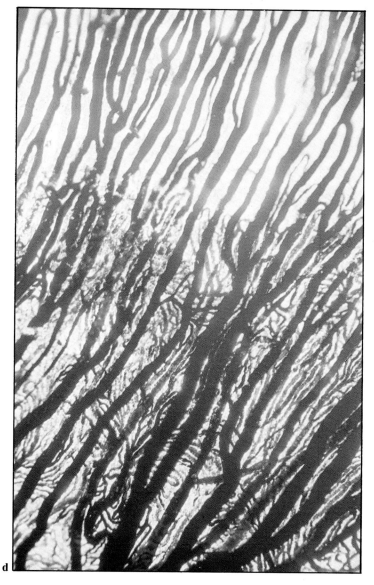

d

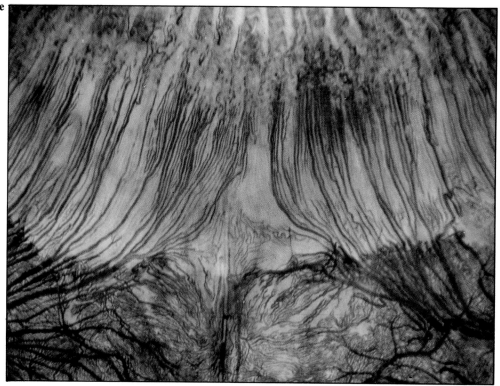

e

Chapter 2

Basic changes

VASCULAR CHANGES

ARTERIES

Dilatation and Tortuousity

The dilatation of an arterial vessel is usually accompanied by tortuousity. The vascular reflexes become more accentuated and acquire a metallic color (Fig. 34 a). The copper wire reflex can be seen in a tortuous vessel which still has normal caliber and a normal color of the blood column (Figs. 34 b, c). The silver wire reflex on the other hand is typical for a vessel with diminished caliber and with a blood column that appears pale because of the thickened vessel wall (Figs. 34 d and 35).

Attenuation

The diminution of the vascular caliber may be diffuse over the entire arterial tree (Fig. 35) or may be segmental (Figs. 34 e, f), i.e., affecting only specific zones of the retina or involving the same vessel which then acquires a fusiform appearance in which ectatic or ampulliform segments alternate with attenuations (similar to a rosary). The attenuation of the arterial caliber may be sustained by a spasm and could therefore be transient and temporary; or it may be the expression of a permanent fibrous change of the vessel wall

with a diminution of flow, generally a consequence of atheromatosis of the central retinal artery within the optic nerve.

Opacification

The loss of transparency of the arterial vessel wall is a frequent expression of retinal vascular pathology. We distinguish three degrees:

— light: the blood column appears intact though its color is duller than normal; the axial reflex is present and normal (Fig. 36 a);
— moderate: two pale lines appear which constrain the blood column (parallel opacification); the vascular reflex is altered (Fig. 36 b);
— severe: the blood column, if it is still present, is completely obscured (pipe stem opacification).

The thickening of the vessel wall alone is usually not sufficient to produce the third degree. Here we also find hyalinosis whit lipid deposits (Fig. 37).
Calcium salts and cholesterol crystals may also produce opacities in the arterial vessels (Fig. 38 a, b). An opacification parallel to the vessel is only found in larger arterioles and is generally an expression of fatty degeneration within the framework of an atheromatous plaque.
A final cause of arterial opacification is the presence of cellular infiltrates in the vessel wall (Fig. 39) secondary to an inflammatory process (specific and non-specific vasculitis, Eales disease, etc.) and to platelet emboli.

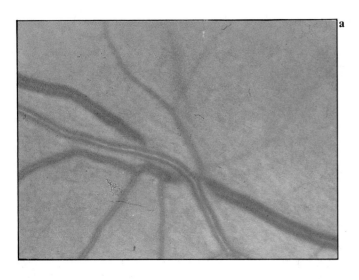
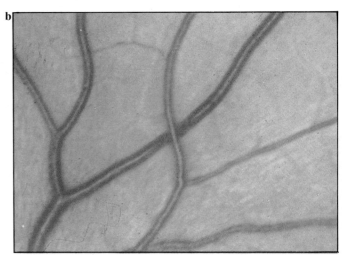
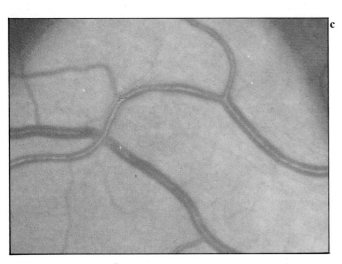
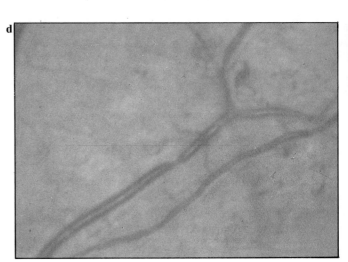

Fig. 34.   Pathologic reflexes and changes in vessel caliber.
a) and **b)** Copper wire reflex.
c) Silver wire reflex.
d) Attenuation of the arterial caliber.
e) Metallic vascular reflexes under high magnification.
f) Fluorescein angiogram of attenuated vessels.

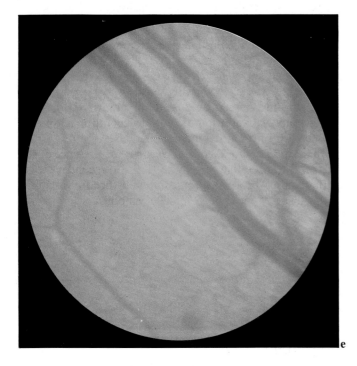
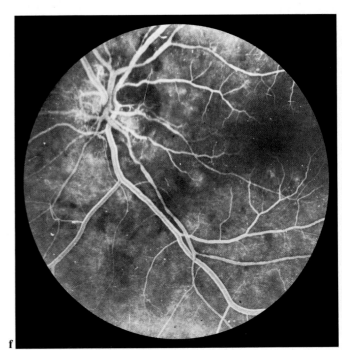

Fig. 35. Metallic reflexes and diffusely reduced vascular caliber.

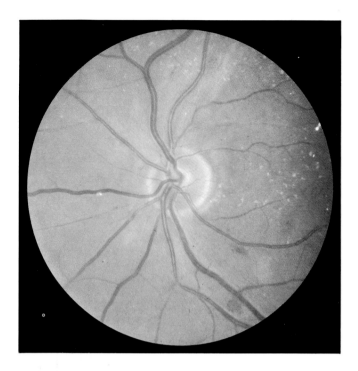

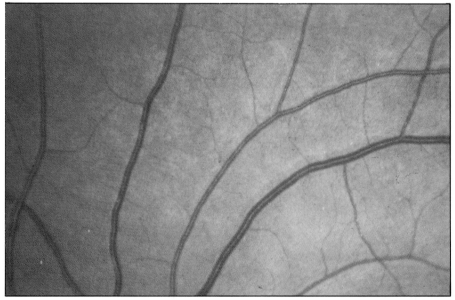

a

b

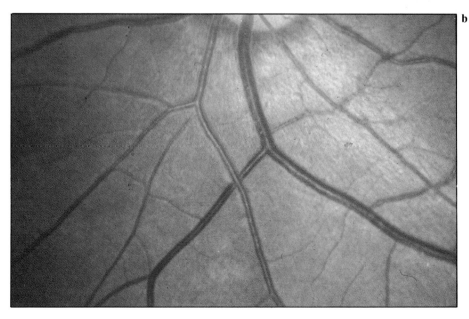

Fig. 36. Alteration in the transparency of the arterial wall.
a) Slight opacification.
b) Moderate degree of opacification.

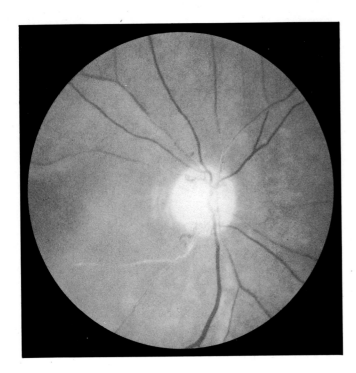

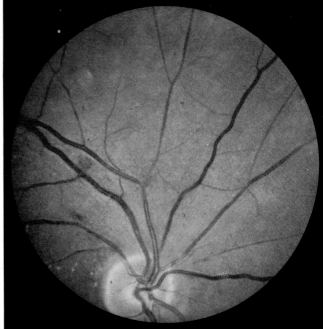

Fig. 37.   Opacification of an artery resembling a pipe stem (arteriolar hyalinosis).

Fig. 38.
a) Calcium deposits and reduction of vascular caliber.
b) Cholesterol crystal with reduction of vascular caliber.

a

b

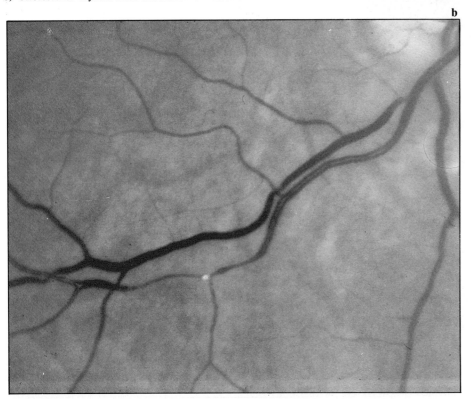

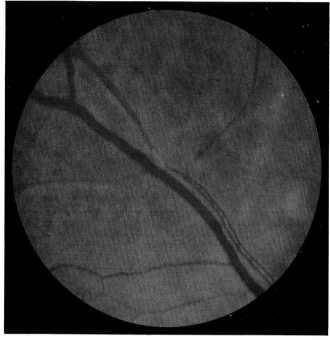

Fig. 39. Opacification due to cellular infiltration of the vessel walls.

ARTERIO-VENOUS CROSSINGS

We would like to reiterate that in a normal eye the retinal vessels cross each other apparently without that one influences the other; each vessel continues its previous course (Fig. 40).

In 70% of the crossings the artery lies on the vein (Figs. 40, 41 a) (arterio-venous or A-V crossing), in 30% (veno-arterial or V-A crossing) the vein lies more superficially (Figs. 40, 41 b).

It is always the vein which cedes to the artery deviating from the original retinal plane. The venous reflex disappears shortly before and after the crossing (Figs. 41 b, 42 a).

The crossing signs acquire a pathologic importance when morphologic and functional disorders develop in these areas, which we shall describe in order of progressing severity.

Gunn Sign

The venous vessel shows two pale zones in the area of the crossing. In general these lie at equal distance from the point of contact where the vascular reflex is lost. There is a more or less marked thinning of the two segments of the vein which seems to be interrupted (Figs. 41 c, 42 b).

This change is probale due to the transmission of pressure from the artery to the vein, as both vessels are enclosed into a common adventitial sheath; the vein deviates and dips into a retinal layer which has lost its trasparency. It then emerges again at a certain distance from the point of compression.

Salus Sign

The deviated vein disappears after its contact with the artery leaving a more or less abrupt gap. This shift assumes the form of a U if the two vessels cross each other perpendicularly, or of an S if the crossing is oblique (Figs. 41 d, 42 c). This phenomenon is also due to the common adventitial sheath of the two vessels.

Venous Engorgement

At the peak of the crossing the vein appears larger and tortuous, whereas at the trough of its course it is thinner and rectilinear (Figs. 43 a, b). This sign is typical for arterial hypertension and has a worse prognostic significance than the Gunn and Salus signs. This sign is due to decreased circulation. The increased pressure of the artery on the vein influences the venous backflow distal from the crossing producing turbulence in blood flow (Fig. 44) clearly demonstrable on fluorescein angiography (Fig. 45). The phenomenon of laminar flow during the early venous phase is a normal condition present in the main venous branches, both at the peak and in the valley of the arterio-venous crossing. It disappears, however, in the valley when the crossing becomes pathologic.

The Prethrombosis Sign of P. Bonnet

A few hemorrhages and small islands of hard exudates appear around the crossing point as if they were meant to identify this point better (Figs. 42 d; 43 c, d). This aspect must be considered a poor prognosis among crossing phenomena, often leading to a frank vascular occlusion.

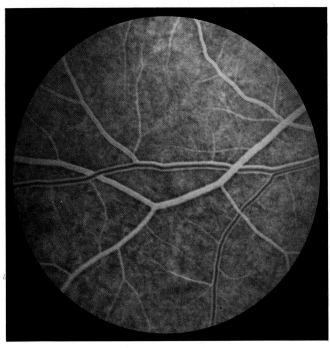

Fig. 40. Fluorescein angiogram of arterio-venous and veno-arterial crossings.

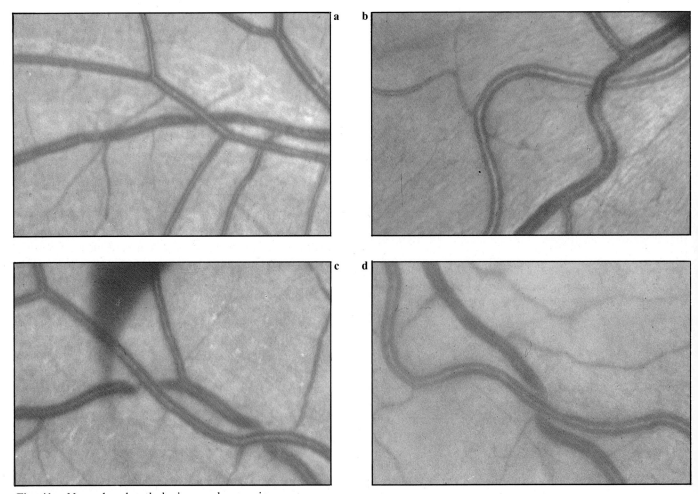

Fig. 41. Normal and pathologic vascular crossings.
a) Normal A-V crossing.
b) Normal V-A crossing (the venous reflex disappears in front and behind the crossings).
c) Gunn sign.
d) Salus sign.

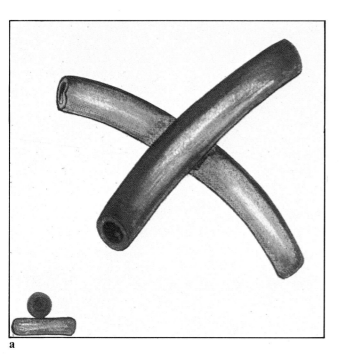

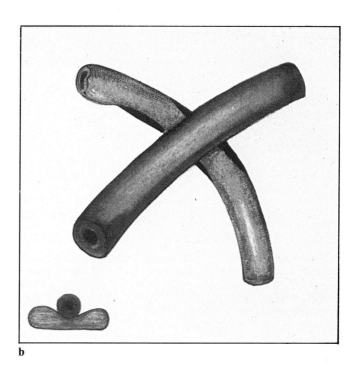

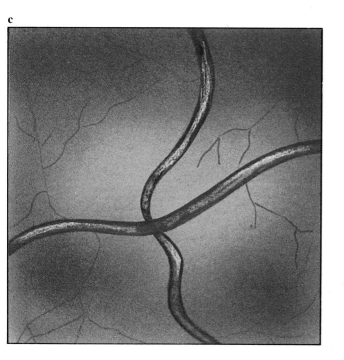

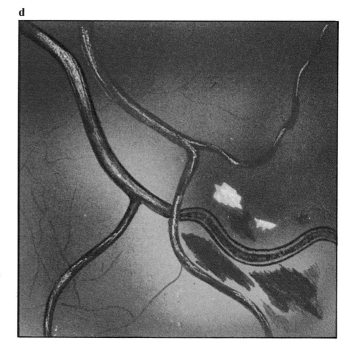

Fig. 42. Schematic drawing of normal and pathologic arterio-venous crossings.
a) Normal A-V crossing with disappearance of the venous reflex in the adjacent proximal and distal area of the crossing.
b) Gunn sign.
c) Salus sign.
d) Bonnet sign.

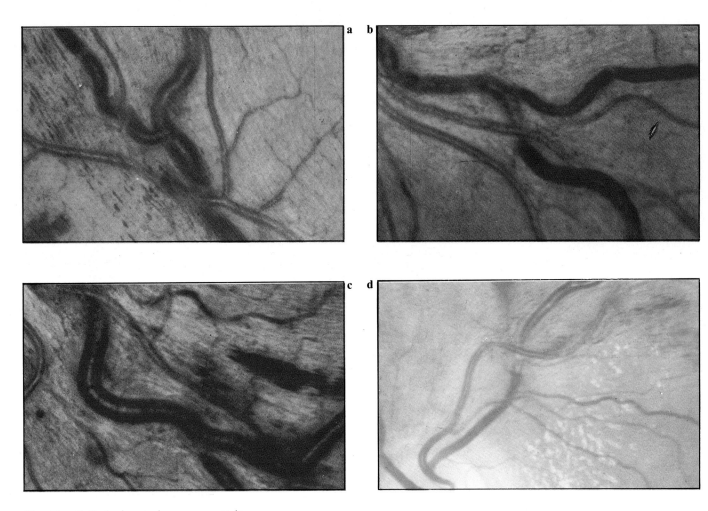

Fig. 43. Pathologic arterio-venous crossings.
a) and **b)** Engorgement of the vessels.
c) and **d)** Prethrombosis stage of Bonnet.

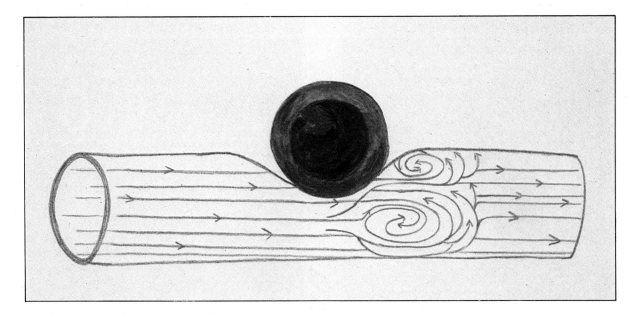

Fig. 44. Turbulence of blood flow due to a partial blockage of the circulation at the arterio-venous crossing.

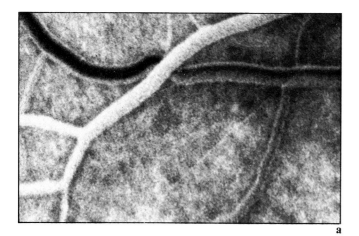

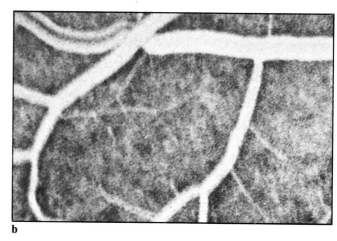

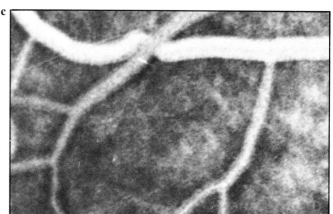

Fig. 45. Fluorescein angiogram of turbulence of flow due to partial blockage.
a) Early arteriovenous phase.
b) Late arteriovenous phase.
c) Venous phase.

VEINS

Dilatation

Some authors believe that the veins which do not possess a vasomotor control should be regarded as passive vessels. This could be a correct assumption because the most frequently seen change in the caliber of arterial vessels is a constriction, whereas in the vein it is practically exclusively a dilatation. This change follows a diminished arteriolar and capillary flow which can be seen in many chronic retinopathies, e.g., diabetes (Fig. 46), carotid insufficiency, blood dyscrasias, dysproteinemia (Fig. 47), leukemia, and occlusion of the central retinal vein.

Opacification

This is secondary to degenerative sclerotic and inflammatory changes of the venous vessel wall.

Phlebosclerosis: The sub-endothelial proliferation of collagen may lead to a hyaline, fatty degeneration producing a sheath around the vessel wall (Fig. 48 a).
This sheathing may assume characteristics forms:

— *pipe stem form* (Fig. 48 d): the sheath is due to an accumulation of fluid in the perivascular lymphatic spaces; this accumulation disappears in time and is replaced by an accumulation of degenerative material;

— *resembling snow on tree branches* (Fig. 49) the histologic correlate are large macrophages filled with lipid.

Retino-phlebitis: The lymphocytic infiltration of the vascular wall and of the perivenous spaces produces a thickening along the venous trunk or the vein passes through a small sleeve which encompasses the vessel for a more or less long interval (Fig. 50).

Blood infiltration of the vessel wall: Cellular elements of the blood may infiltrate the vessel wall and the spaces around it forming sheaths, as in leukemia, surrounding for a considerable stretch the ectatic and tortuous vein (Fig. 51).

Pigmented sheaths: In some pathologic conditions which also involve the retinal pigment epithelium (for example the classical retinitis pigmentosa) the pigment granules migrate along the glial cells of Müller and reach the walls of capillaries and veins surrounding them in a characteristic way (Fig. 52).

Tortuousity

A certain mild degree of venous tortuousity may be considered physiologic in infants, while it is nearly always an expression of a pathologic condition in adults.
It is a condition which may be produced by numerous etiologic factors: congenital (Figs. 53 a, b), angiomatosis (Fig. 54 a), degenerative, telangiectatic (Fig. 54 b) or due to changes in hemodynamics (Fig. 55).

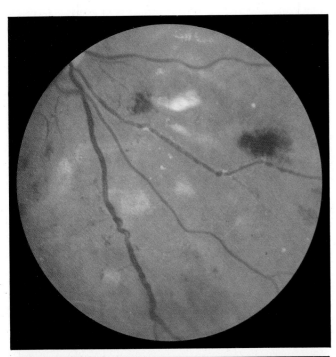

Fig. 46.   Predominantly segmental venous dilatation in diabetic retinopathy.

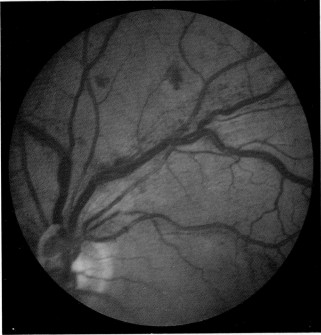

Fig. 47.   Diffuse dilatation in a case of macroglobulinemia (Waldenström), hemorrhage spreading by diapedesis along the vein.

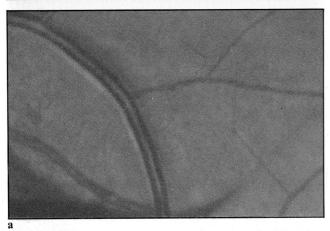

a

b

Fig. 48.   Venous sheathing.
a) Parallel sheathing.
b) Sheathing in the form of a pipe stem.

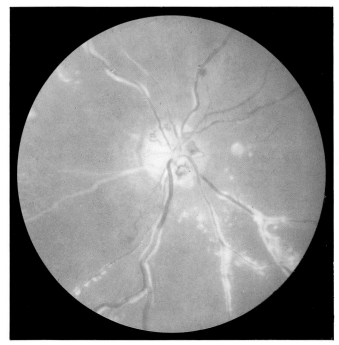

Fig. 49. Branches and pipe stem sheathing.

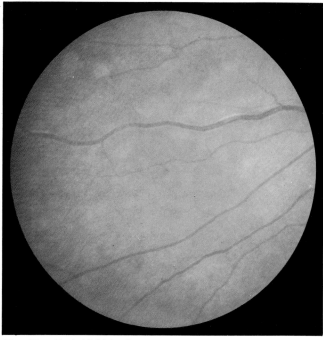

Fig. 50. Periphlebitic sleeve.

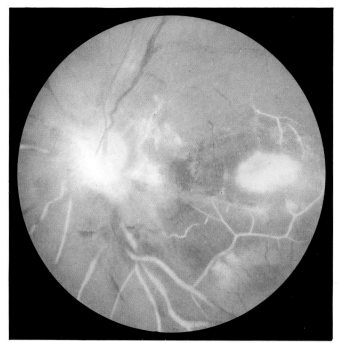

Fig. 51. Hemorrhagic infiltrates into the vessel wall in a case of leukemia.

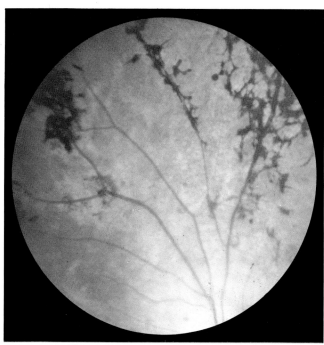

Fig. 52. Pigmented sleeves (retinitis pigmentosa).

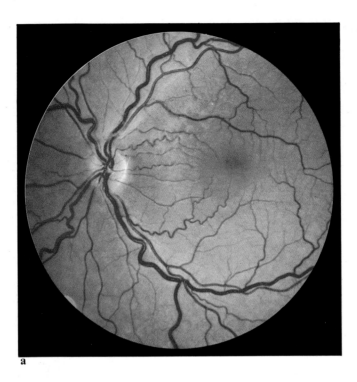

Fig. 53.
a) Congenital venous tortuousity.
b) Venous tortuousity in a case of retinal vasculitis of the retina
(Fluorescein angiogram).

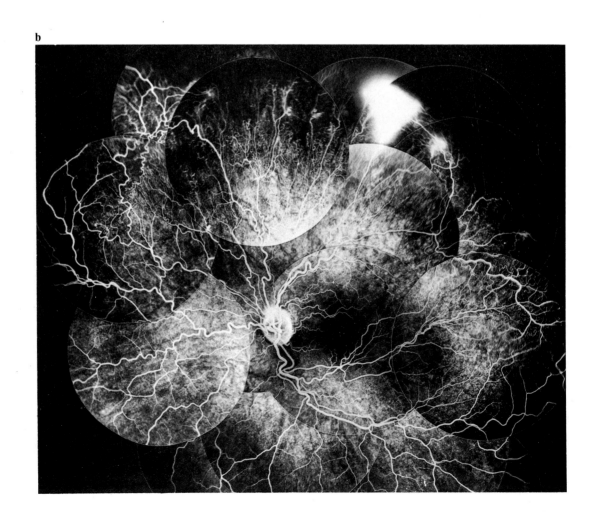

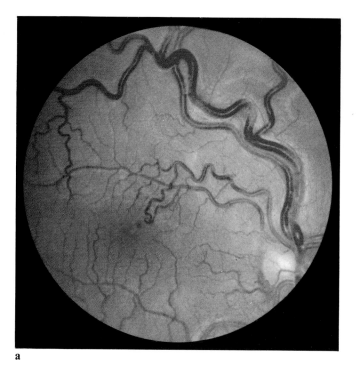
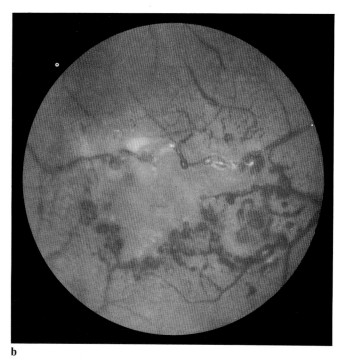

a

b

Fig. 54.
a) Angiomatosis retinae: arterio-venous anastomosis in the parafoveolar zone.
b) Telangiectasia.

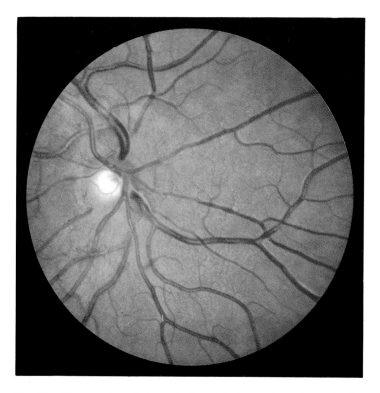

Fig. 55. Tortuousity of the retinal vessels due to hemodynamic disturbances (dysproteinemia).

NEOVASCULARIZATION

New-formed vessels are vascular elements which develop under pathologic conditions after the vascular system of the eye has already fully developed (or immediately before it) or it indicates vessel formation in normally avascular tissues. Such a definition implicitly excludes congenital vascular anomalies and anastomoses originating from a normal preexisting vascular network.

Two factors seem to constitute the pathogenic stimulus which produces neovascularization:

— metabolic products which form in the course of growth or with some pathologic conditions;
— local oxygen concentration.

In order to understand better the basic mechanisms which determine neovascularization it is perhaps useful to review briefly the embryology of angiogenesis.

The primitive capillaries develop from buds of endothelial columns sprouting from the central artery; other capillaries develop by a process of canalization within a network of mesenchymal undifferentiated cells.

The capillaries seem to prefer for their development a surrounding which is comparatively hypoxic. When an arterial trunk, as is frequently the case, accompanies a venous vessel the capillaries develop from the vein in a direction opposite to that of the location of the artery.

They therefore develop toward an area of relative oxygen deficit, perhaps with the aim to compensate and equalize the oxygen distribution over the entire retina.

This may explain the localization of the two layers of retinal capillaries which supply the inner half of the retina, i.e., the layers farthest away from the choriocapillaries. The latter supplies oxygen to the outer layers of the sensory retina. It is also intriguing to speculate that the perivascular capillary-free zone is arranged around the arterial trunks where the oxygen concentration is the highest. These remarks on the angiogenesis may serve as a model for an analogy in that the new-formed blood vessels also develop in situations where there is a lack of oxygen. In these cases of hypoxia the second pathogenetic factor (factor X of Michaelson and Weiss) would be activated; this factor would be liberated in hypoxic tissues which are not completely necrotic.

It is well known that new-formed blood vessels represent a characteristic sequel of retinal vein occlusions (where we have an infarct without necrosis of retinal tissue), but not after arterial occlusions (where there is total tissue necrosis with complete anoxia). The liberation of the factor X produces a histologic situation similar to that of embryogenesis in which across a mesodermal membrane a proliferation of endothelial cells leads to an exuberant proliferation of new-formed blood vessels.

The layers in which the neovascularization may occur can be divided into (Fig. 56):

— intravitreal,
— preretinal,
— intraretinal,
— subretinal,

— chorioretinal anastomoses,
— intramural,
— optic disc.

Intravitreal: These vessels originate from the retinal veins forming tufts which sprout in the form of a dense intravitreal network with numerous microaneurysms (Fig. 57 a). These networks may extend in the vitreous in all directions (caput medusae) until they reach the posterior surface of the lens (Fig. 57 b). At the level of the optic disc there is practically no barrier because the internal limiting membrane is absent. This area is therefore a site of predilection for neovascularization (Figs. 58 a, b). The new-formed blood vessels originate, however, from any retinal area. They perforate the internal limiting membrane and protrude into the vitreous (Fig. 58 c).

Preretinal: These vessels run on the surface of the retina (Fig. 59 a-d). They are enveloped into a matrix of primitive connective tissue (structurally similar to the gel of the umbilical chord) which constitutes a supportive membrane for the development of new-formed blood vessels. It is nevertheless possible to visualize such transparent membrane with the appropriate direction of the ophthalmoscopic light.

Retinal: The new-formed blood vessels develop at various levels within the sensory retina itself (Fig. 60).

Subretinal: These vessels are rare; they are usually tortuous and lack the characteristic axial reflex which constitutes a valuable differential diagnostic point when compared to the retinal vessels proper. These new-formed vessels originate from the choriocapillaries and constitute the end result of an evolution, e.g., of the age related disciform degeneration (Fig. 61 a-d).

Chorioretinal anastomoses: These vessels are usually associated with an area of atrophy or a coloboma. A retinal vessel traverses through these tissues to reach the underlying choroid (Figs. 62 a, b).

Intramural: These vessels develop within the intima (in contrast to the vasa vasorum which lie in the adventitia). They develop within the thickened wall of pathologic retinal vessels, e.g., in diabetes, hypertension and some types of vasculitis in young adults.

Optic disc: This is a clinical phenomenon without any specific etiologic cause. Such new-formed vessels can be found in a diverse group of pathologic conditions.
Ophthalmoscopically we can differentiate these vessels into:

— *on the optic disc:* lying between the disc surface and the vitreous; they usually do not extend beyond the disc margin (Fig. 63 a);
— *around the optic disc:* these extend in a frontal plane, centrifugally and parallel to the retrohyaloid plane up to 3-4 disc diameters from the disc margin (Fig. 63 b);
— *between the optic disc and the vitreous:* these vessels develop in an anterior/posterior plane (from the disc toward the vitreous) showing at their termination numerous microaneurysmatic dilatations; they are supported by a rete mirabile of glia (Fig. 63 c).

The fluorescein angiographic picture is frequently characteristic (Figs. 64 a, b) and the time interval between injection of the dye and filling of the vessel allows us to differentiate the afferent from the efferent branches. The diffusion of the dye becomes gradually more massive and is proportional to the degree of neovascularization. Three types of fluorescein angiographic pictures can be distinguished in the new-formed vessels:

— *early fluorescence:* the dye appears in the main afferent trunk before the retinal arteries are filled; it occurs soon after the deep laminar and prelaminar layers fluorescence, i.e., via the choroidal vessels. This type of disc neovascularization seems to be irrigated from the choroidal network.

— *Late fluorescence:* this appears in the main trunk of the new-formed blood vessels during the stage of laminar flow in the retinal vessels, at the same time as the superficial disc capillaries fill from the retina. We can therefore deduce that this second type of neovascularization is irrigated from the retinal vasculature.

— *Mixed form:* this is a combination of the two preceding types. It is however sometimes possible to distinguish two afferent trunks, one with an early fluorescence and the other one with a late one. The new-formed blood vessels on the disc show all three types of fluorescence. Those around the disc usually show late (retinal) fluorescence and those between the disc and the vitreous often have an early (choroidal) fluorescence.

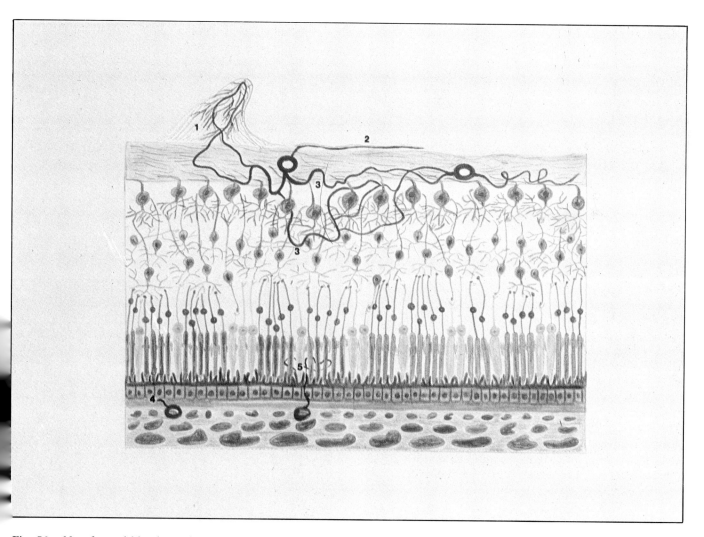

Fig. 56. New-formed blood vessels.
1 = Intravitreal new-formed blood vessels.
2 = Preretinal new-formed blood vessels.
3 = Superficial intraretinal new-formed blood vessels.
4 = Subretinal (subepithelial) new-formed blood vessels.
5 = Deep intraretinal new-formed blood vessels.

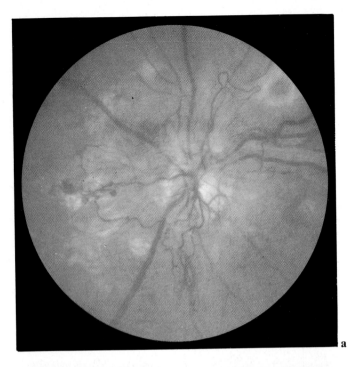 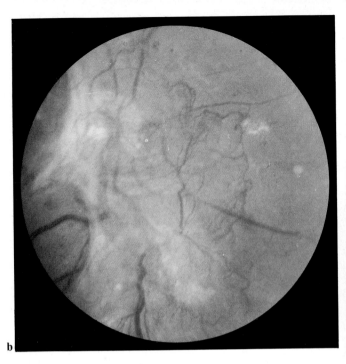

a   b

Fig. 57.
a) Intravitreal epipapillary new-formed blood vessels.
b) Intravitreal new-formed vessels with glial support tissue.

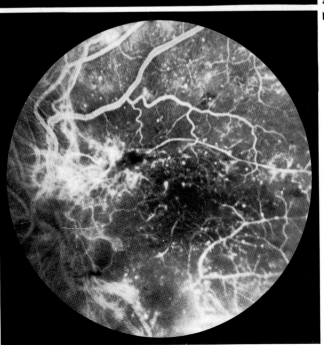

Fig. 58.
a) Intravitreal new-formed blood vessels coming from the disc (ophthalmoscopic appearance).
b) Early fluorescein angiogram of intravitreal new-formed blood vessels on the disc.
c) Intravitreal new-formed blood vessels sprouting from the retina.

a

b   c

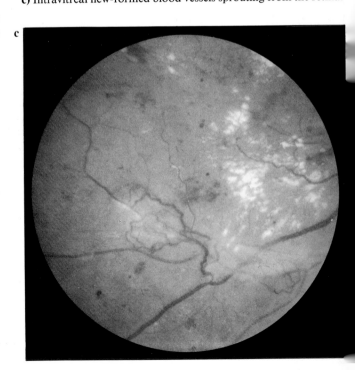

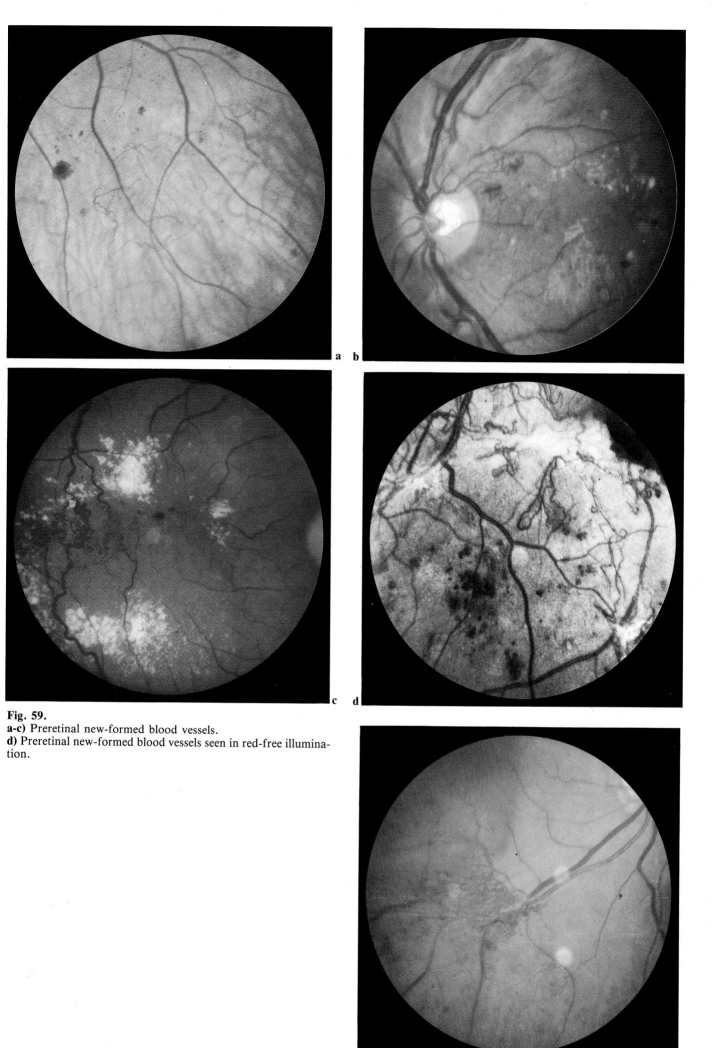

Fig. 59.
a-c) Preretinal new-formed blood vessels.
d) Preretinal new-formed blood vessels seen in red-free illumination.

Fig. 60. New-formed blood vessels in the retina.

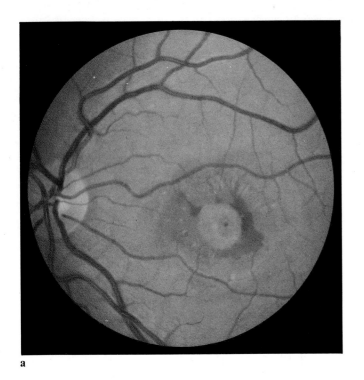
a

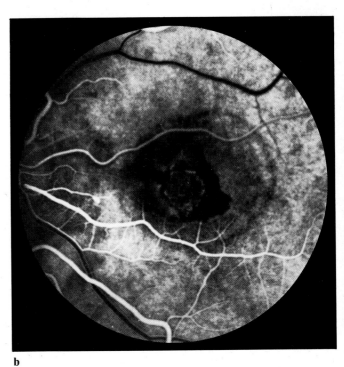
b

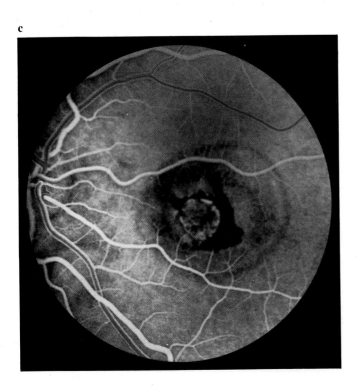
c

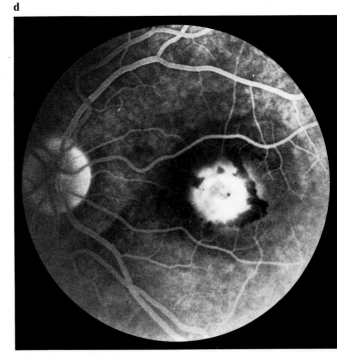
d

Fig. 61.   Subretinal neovascularization.
a) Ophthalmoscopic appearance.
b-d) Fluorescein angiogram: arterial phase (**b**); early venous phase (**c**) and late phase (**d**).

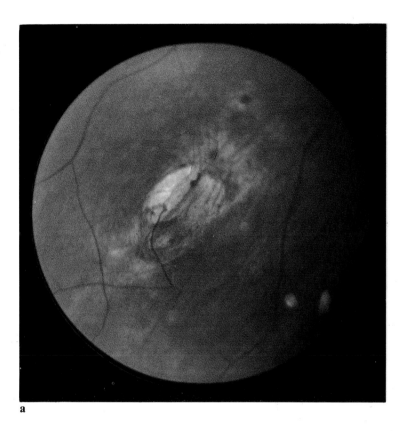

Fig. 62. Chorioretinal anastomosis.
a) Ophthalmoscopic picture.
b) Fluorescein angiogram.

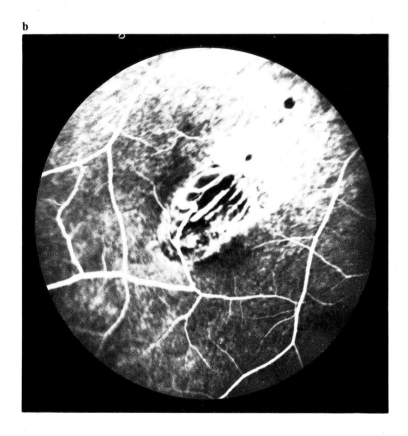

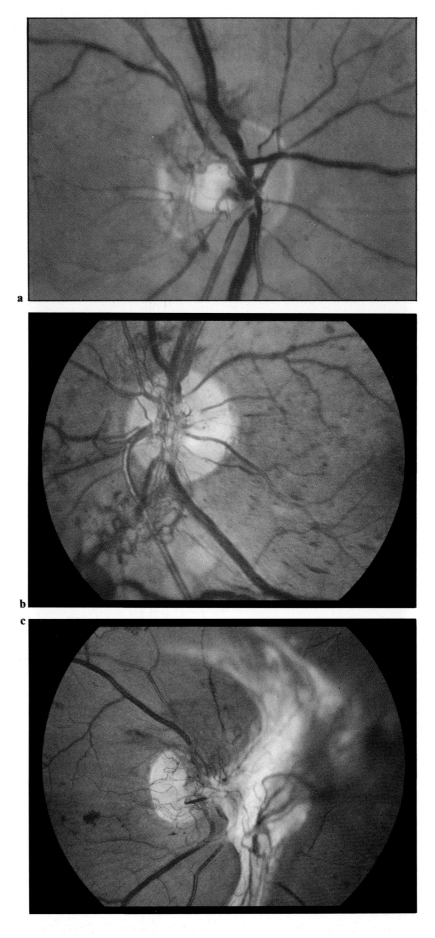

Fig. 63.
a) New-formed blood vessels on the disc.
b) New-formed blood vessels around the disc.
c) New-formed blood vessels extending from the disc into the vitreous.

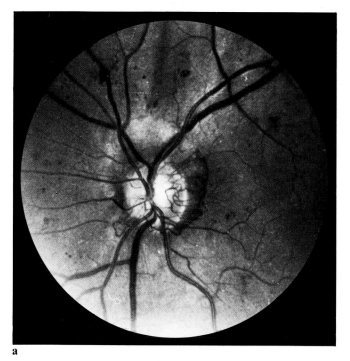

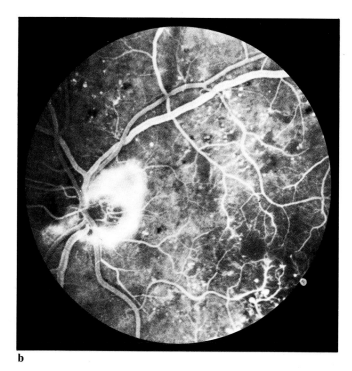

a
b

Fig. 64.
a) New-formed blood vessels on the disc in red-free illumination.
b) The same vessels in a late fluorescein angiogram.

MICROANEURYSMS

These are saccular, rarely fusiform, dilatations of the walls of small retinal vessels.

In general they represent a retinal manifestation of a generalized vascular disease. They usually develop from the venous side of the capillaries, though they may also occur on the veins and small arterioles. They have a diameter of 10-50 μ. We have to keep in mind that only microaneurysms larger than 30 μ will be visible with the ophthalmoscope. It is therefore understandable that the number of microaneurysms seen ophthalmoscopically is markedly smaller than the number made visible by fluorescein angiography.

The microaneurysms can be divided into two types:

— *small size:* from the size of a pinhead to a hardly perceptible small dot; vivid red in color, spherical with sharp borders, sometimes highlighted by a reflex; these small microaneurysms appear early around the fovea (Figs. 65 a, b) growing slowly in size, but they may also remain unchanged for years or they may disappear because of degenerative changes.

— *Large size* (Figs. 66 a-c): they appear frequently in groups, in chains or like a bunch of grapes (frequently close to an occluded vein) and are usually accompanied by hemorrhages and exudates.

These microaneurysms appear especially frequently in diabetic retinopathy, but they are certainly not pathognomonic for this condition. They may also be found in other diseases, e.g., arterial hypertension, blood dyscrasias, pulseless disease, etc. They may even occur in a normal subject, especially in the retinal periphery where the microcystoid degeneration leads to a lack of structural support for part of the vascular wall which then bulges laterally. The microaneurysms may also be found in various pathologic conditions of the eye, e.g., occlusion of the central retinal vein or its branches (Fig. 67 a), glaucoma, chronic uveitis, retinoblastoma, Eales' disease, Coats' disease (Fig. 67 b). Leber's telangiectasia, radiation retinopathy, parasitic infestations, disc edema (Fig. 67 c), age related and hereditary macular degenerations.

On flat sections (Figs. 68 a, b) and in histologic specimens the microaneurysms look like fruits on a branch; they are particularly well seen on flat preparations that are trypsin digested. The red blood cells appear packed into an endothelial sac. The thickened vessel wall may in the course of time undergo degenerative changes with hyalinization and lipid deposits. Calcium salts may also be deposited. The disappearance of pericytes does not always lead to the formation of microaneurysms; only in the diabetic retinopathy will the lack of pericytes lead to a disappearance of the intramural cells. In other pathologic conditions the microaneurysms develop in blood vessels which have normal pericytes.

Usually the aneurysms form at the border of an area of partial or complete obstruction of the capillary bed (Figs. 69; 70 a, b). Such microaneurysms have also been found around areas treated by photocoagulation.

From these findings one could deduce that the capillaries which surround ischemic areas have to endure a high hydrostatic pressure leading to a bulging and destruction of the vessel wall. Other authors, on the basis of the theory of Michaelson and Weiss, have put forward the hypothesis that the angiogenetic factor X is liberated from the non-perfused areas. This factor leads to the formation of new blood vessels and microaneurysms which some investigators consider an abortive form of neovascularization.

In diabetes the various factors favoring the formation of microthrombi also produce an increase in the hydrostatic pressure within the capillaries; this could provoke an alteration of the basement membrane and an endothelial defect caused by proteolytic enzymes.

The lack of pericytes then finally weakens the vessel wall exposed to an anomalous pressure head. In this first stage of the process the vessel wall becomes thin (Fig. 70 a); this is followed by a second stage in which the microaneurysm acquires a thick wall (Fig. 70 b). This is due to a reactive proliferation with increase in the basement membrane thickness due to an increased secretion from the endothelial and perivascular cells. Finally, the end result may be complete repair and restoration of the out-pouching of the vessel wall.

The microaneurysms may appear under different forms in the fluorescein angiograms:

— *They may not fluoresce at all:* the thrombosis within the cavity, packed with a mass of erythrocytes and surrounded by a cellular wall, does not allow any fluorescence. In this case the same microaneurysm may be seen ophthalmoscopically but not on fluorescein angiography.

— *There is transient fluorescence:* the fluorescence appears and disappears parallel with the dye in the blood vessels to which the microaneurysm is attached. The microaneurysm forms here a unit with the vessel of origin. It contains few erythrocytes and is surrounded by a hypercellular wall. This type of microaneurysm may dissolve, disappear or become fibrotic.

— *Prolonged fluorescence:* the fluorescence in the microaneurysm persists after the dye has disappeared in the blood vessels. The dye impregnates the thickened aneurysmatic wall which shows signs of hyalinization.

— *Prolonged fluorescence with a halo,* but without leakage into the retinal tissue. The intensity and the surface of the fluorescein area increases, but in a regular way; it remains round and well-delineated. This is usually seen in microaneurysms which have a strong tendency to grow, in contrast to old microaneurysms which are encapsulated by a layer of glia.

— *Fluorescence with leakage:* the diffusion into the retinal tissue proves a frank and anomalous permeability of the vessel wall, leading to perivascular retinal edema.

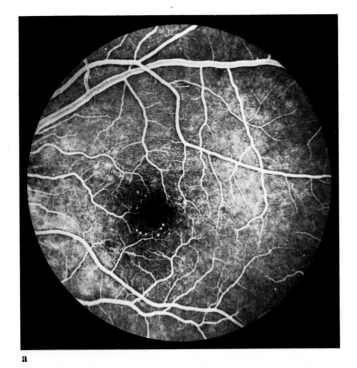

a

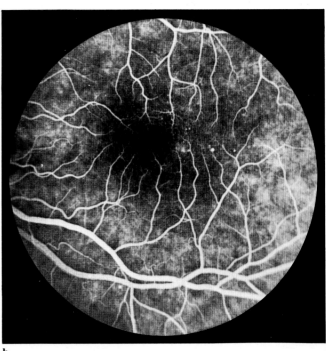

b

Fig. 65. **a** and **b)** String of small perifoveolar microaneurysms (fluorescein angiography).

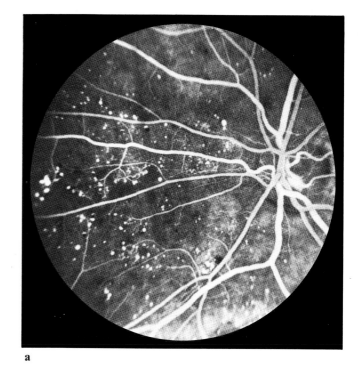

a

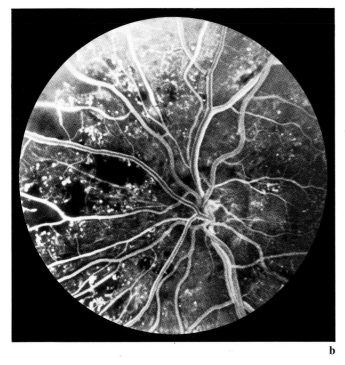

b

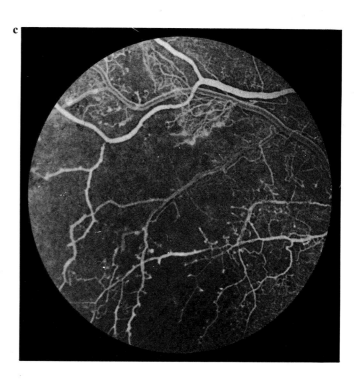

c

Fig. 66. **a-c)** Microaneurysms and telangiectasia (fluorescein angiography).

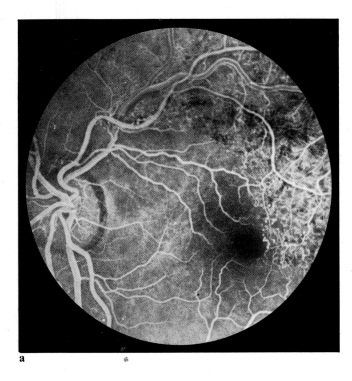

a

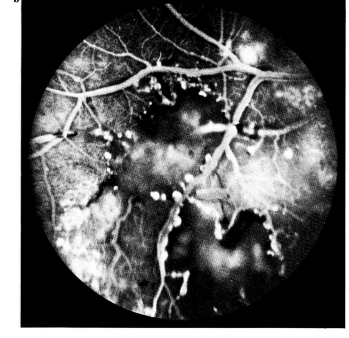

b

Fig. 67.
a) Microaneurysms in an eye with branch vein occlusion (fluorescein angiogram).
b) Microaneurysms and telangiectasia in Coats' disease (fluorescein angiogram).
c) Microaneurysms in disc edema (fluorescein angiogram).

c

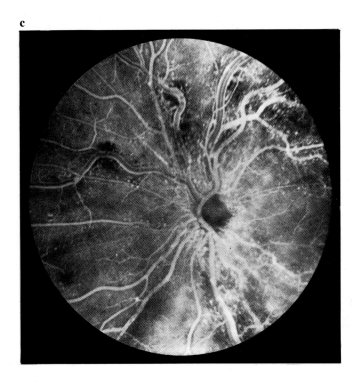

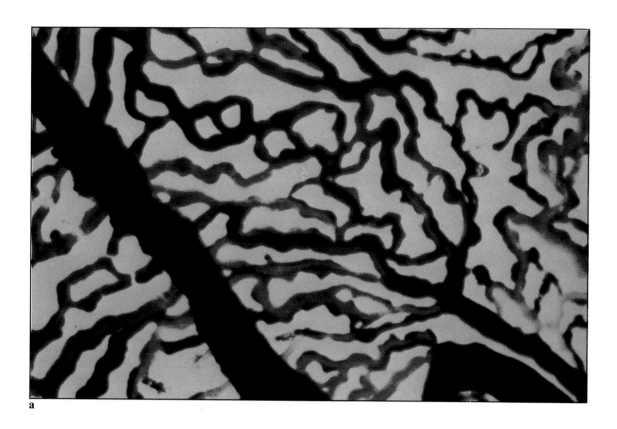

a

Fig. 68. **a)** and **b)** Histologic specimens of choroidal vessels injected with a polymer in a diabetic eye: numerous microaneurysms are visible.

b

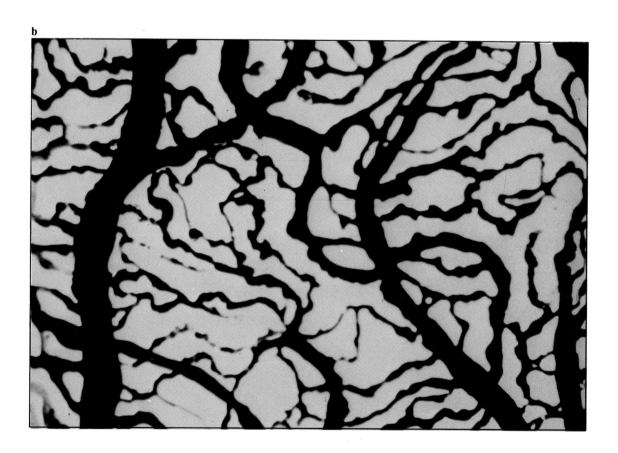

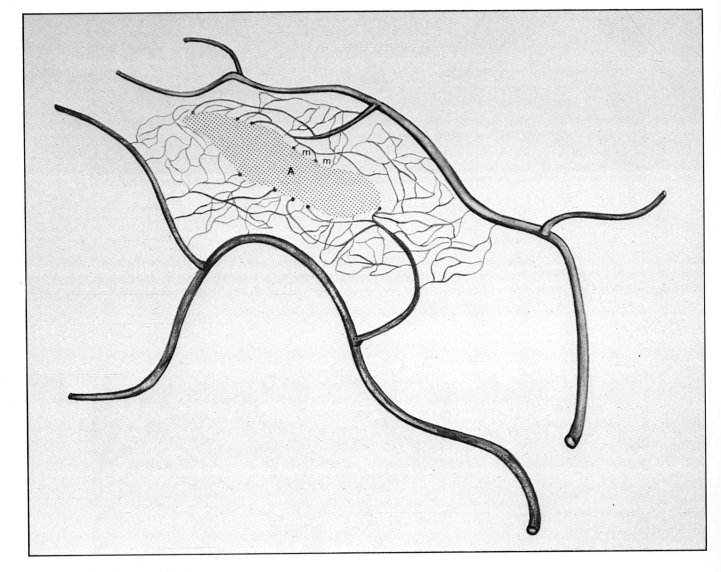

Fig. 69.   Ischemic area with microaneurysms.
A = ischemic area;
m = microaneurysms.

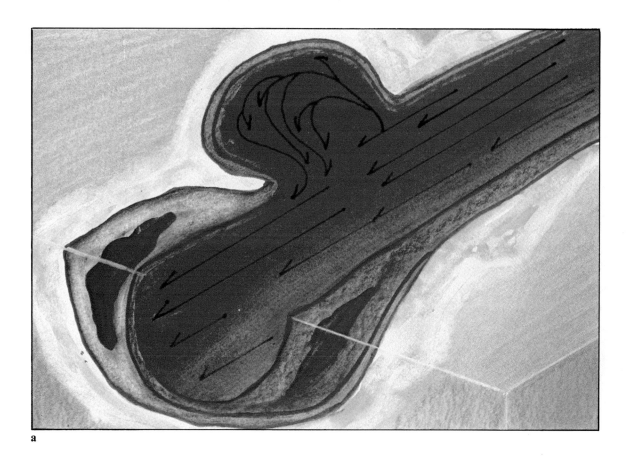

a

Fig. 70. Microaneurysms.
a) Thin walled microaneurysms.
b) Thick walled microaneurysms.

b

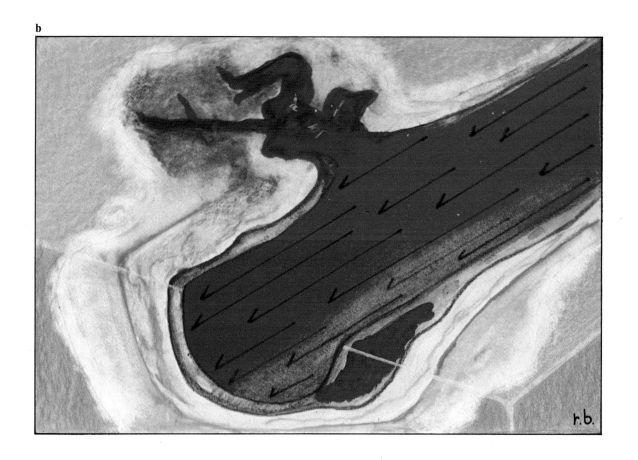

RETINAL AND CHOROIDAL HEMORRHAGES

Hemorrhages are probably the most frequent pathologic finding in the ocular fundus.

Observing the shape, color, brightness and outlines of a hemorrhage may give us valuable clues as to the etiology of the pathologic process.

In order to interpret hemorrhages correctly we have to keep in mind that there are three sources from which the blood could originate (retinal, choroidal and disc vessels) and that the shape of the hemmorrhage is closely connected to the cyto-architectonic in which the bleeding has occurred (Fig. 71). The blood either escapes the vessel by diapedesis or exits the vessel after a break in the vascular lining. The blood will then fill a potential preexisting space or will expand according to the histologic architecture molding itself according to the morphologic structure acquiring characteristic configurations which enable us to localize the site and the level of the bleeding. The following types of hemorrhage may be observed allowing a histo-topographic classification.

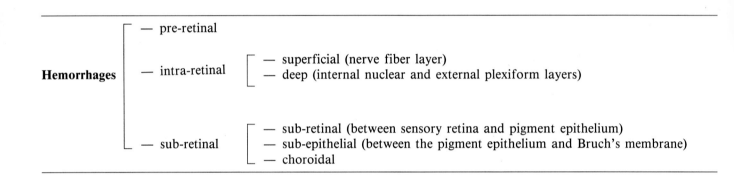

Hemorrhages
- pre-retinal
- intra-retinal
  - superficial (nerve fiber layer)
  - deep (internal nuclear and external plexiform layers)
- sub-retinal
  - sub-retinal (between sensory retina and pigment epithelium)
  - sub-epithelial (between the pigment epithelium and Bruch's membrane)
  - choroidal

Fig. 71. The appearance of pathologic deposits depends on the cytoarchitectonic of the retina and the choroid and on the layer in which these deposits appear.

1 = preretinal hemorrhage;
2 = superficial intraretinal hemorrhage (nerve fiber layer);
3 = deep intraretinal hemorrhage (inner nuclear and outer plexiform layers);
4 = subretinal hemorrhage (between sensory retina and pigment epithelium);
5 = subepithelial hemorrhage (between pigment epithelium and Bruch's membrane);
6 = choroidal hemorrhage;
7 = cotton-wool patches;
8 = hard exudates;
9 = accumulation of retinal pigment;
10 = accumulation of choroidal pigment.

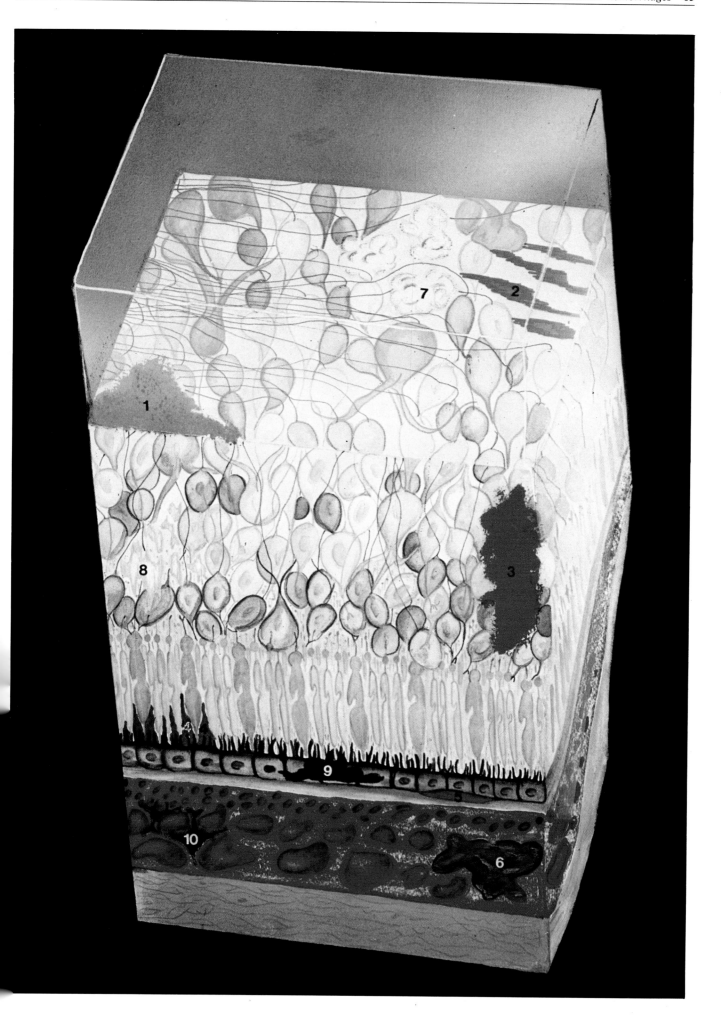

PRERETINAL HEMORRHAGES

According to some authors, the blood is here located in a virtual space between the posterior hyaloid and the internal limiting membrane; according to other authors it lies between the nerve fiber layer and the internal limiting membrane (and therefore would more correctly be called an intraretinal hemorrhage); these hemorrhages are in general of a definite extension, intensive red in color with a tendency for sharp borders (Figs. 72 a, b). The blood obscures completely the retinal vessels and the underlying fundus struc-tures. The sedimentation of the blood allows in time to divide the hemorrhage by a straight line demarcating exactly the inferior corpuscular part from the supernatant plasma (Fig. 72 c).

The periphery of the lesion then assumes a somewhat scalloped border, probably due to blood columns lying beneath the internal limiting membrane (Fig. 72 c). The hemorrhages generally are due to rupture of a large vessel in the nerve fiber layer or of capillaries in the superficial layers. Hypertension, diabetes, blood dyscrasias, trauma, as well as subarachnoidal and subdural (Terson syndrome) hemorrhages should be considered as etiologic factors.

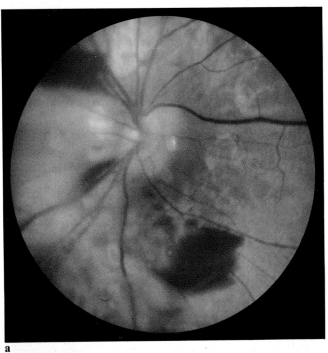

a

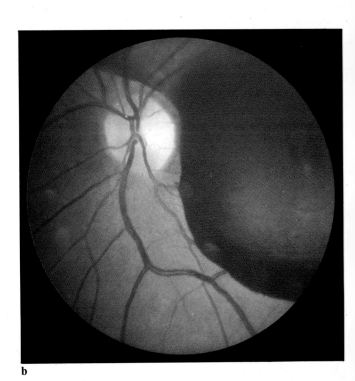

b

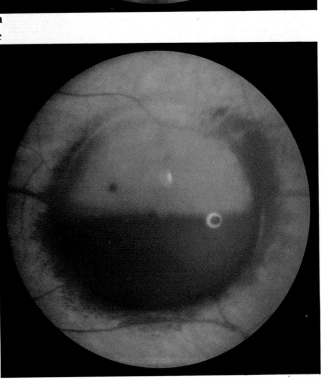

c

Fig. 72. a-c) Preretinal hemorrhages.

INTRARETINAL HEMORRHAGES

The nerve fiber layer of the retina also contains the large retinal vessels and the superficial capillary network, whereas the deep network lies at the border between the inner nuclear and the outer plexiform layers. The superficial retinal hemorrhages owe their flame shaped configuration to the parallel arrangement of the nerve fibers. These hemorrhages lie among these fibers which also surround and support them. This is especially evident in the para- and peripapillary areas (Figs. 73 a, b) (radial capillary network) and at the posterior pole (Fig. 73 c). Toward the periphery the superficial retinal hemorrhages become more oval as the nerve fibers lose their parallel arrangement and acquire lacunae in which the blood may accumulate.

The superficial hemorrhages are typically found in hypertensive retinopathy, in venous occlusions, in the various types of disc edema, in blood dyscrasias and with trauma.

The deep intraretinal hemorrhages (Figs. 73 d, e) stem from the deep capillary network and are therefore found between the inner nuclear and the outer plexiform layers. In these areas the cellular elements have a strong disposition for ver-

tical arrangement. Therefore the blood can accumulate there only in a more cylindrical shape and the cross section of these hemorrhages, as they appear in the fundus, acquire the shape of dots and blots.

In the macular area the external plexiform layer loses its usual vertical arrangement and the neurites and dendrites acquire an oblique, nearly horizontal arrangement (Henle fiber layer); the superficial hemorrhages therefore by necessity assume in this area a star like arrangement whereby the center of the star lies in the foveola. The shape and also the small size of the peripheral retinal hemorrhages are due to the crowding of retinal cells which does not leave much space for pathologic deposits. Such hemorrhages are found not only in diabetes and hypertension, but also in some blood dyscrasias, collagen diseases and in the hypotensive retinopathy.

White centered hemorrhages (Roth spots) may occur in the superficial and in the deep retinal layers (Fig. 74). This lesion was thought to be typical for subacute bacterial endocarditis; however, it may also be seen in leukemia, collagen diseases, mycoses and dysproteinemia. The white material which is found in the center of the hemorrhagic halo may consist of polymorpho-nuclear leukocytes, leukemic cells or fibrin.

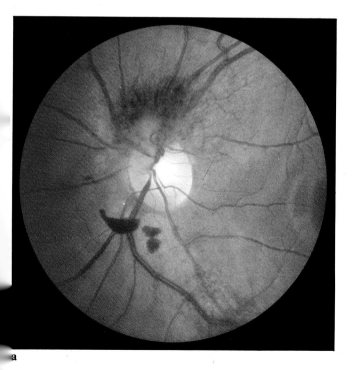

a

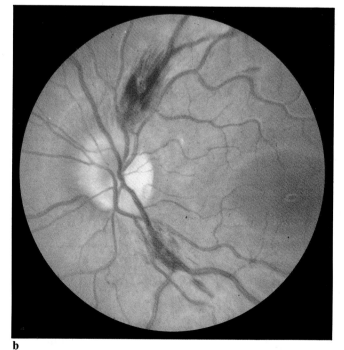

b

Fig. 73. Intraretinal hemorrhages.
a) and **b)** Superficial intraretinal hemorrhages near the disc.

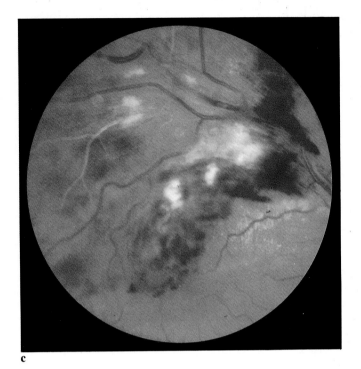

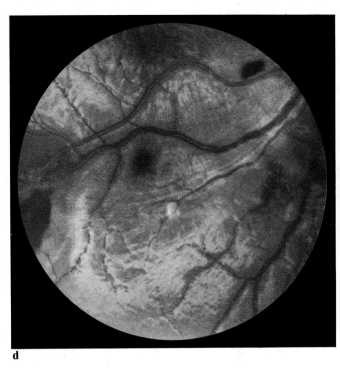

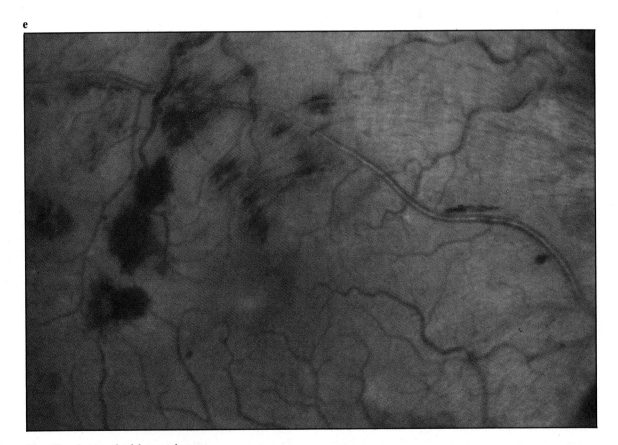

Fig. 73. Intraretinal hemorrhages.
c) Superficial intraretinal hemorrhages at the posterior pole.
d) Deep intraretinal hemorrhages.
e) Deep oval intraretinal hemorrhages.

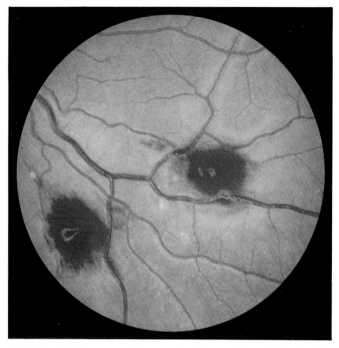

Fig. 74. White centered intraretinal hemorrhages in leukemia.

SUBRETINAL HEMORRHAGES

If the blood accumulates in the subretinal space (between sensory retina and pigment epithelium) (Figs. 75 a, b) its color is analogous to that of a deep intraretinal hemorrhage, but its dimensions are larger and the margins appear frayed because of the tenuous connection between the outer members of the photoreceptor cells and the pigment epithelium.

If, on the other hand, the blood accumulates beneath the pigment epithelium (between the pigment epithelium and Bruch's membrane) (Figs. 76 a, b) it appears more brown in color because of the effect of the overlying pigment epithelium.

In contrast to the subretinal space there is in the subepithelial area a dense adhesion between Bruch's membrane and the epithelium; the blood therefore has here a tendency to accumulate in definite, often circular spaces with sharply outlined borders.

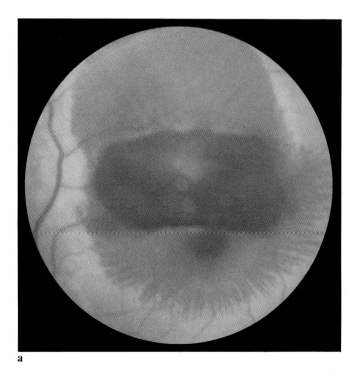

a

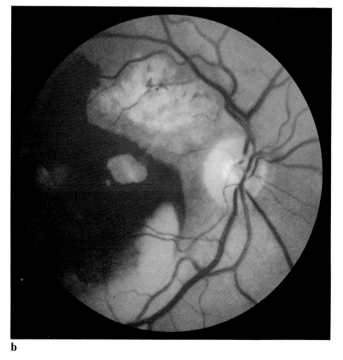

b

Fig. 75. **a)** and **b)** Subretinal hemorrhages (between sensory retina and retinal pigment epithelium).

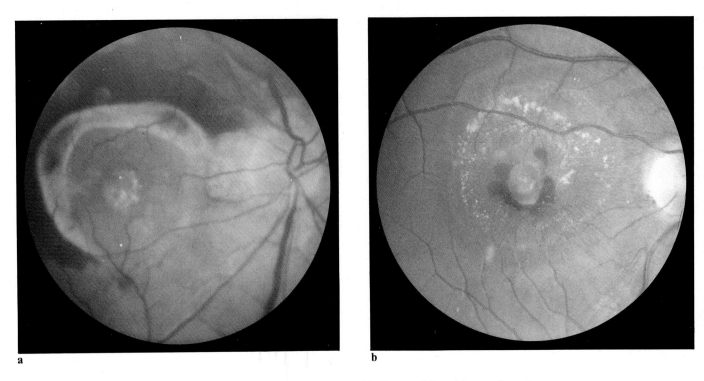

a
b

Fig. 76. **a)** and **b)** Subepithelial hemorrhages (between pigment epithelium and Bruch's membrane).

CHOROIDAL HEMORRHAGES

These hemorrhages have a geographic outline and a deep red color with superficial slate-grey reflexes (Figs. 77 a, b). The blood comes only from deep vessels (Fig. 77 c) and may be the sequel of new-formed blood vessels, trauma, tumor or choroidal inflammations.

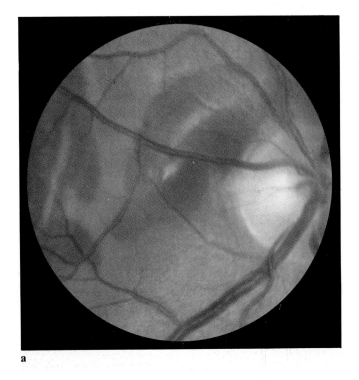
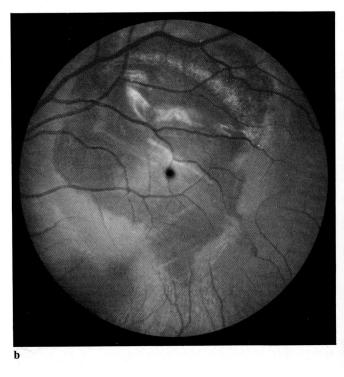

a
b

Fig. 77.
a) and **b)** Choroidal hemorrhages.

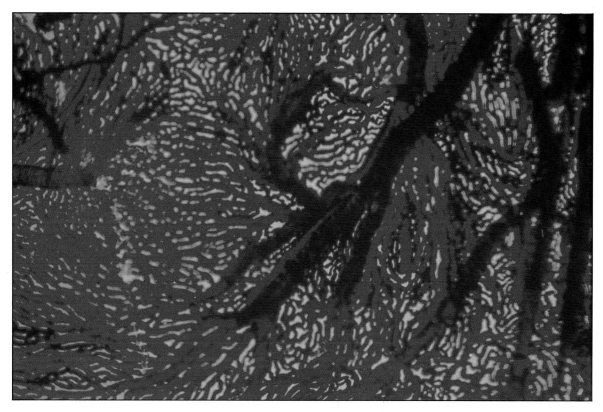

Fig. 77. **c)** Microscopic specimen showing the structures responsible for choroidal hemorrhages.

EDEMA AND EXUDATES

A breakdown in the blood retinal barrier will lead to an increase in the interstitial retinal fluid, enlarging the spaces among the cells and forming the *extracellular retinal edema* (Fig. 78, B). The break of this barrier implies a modification of capillary permeability by cellular changes which are found, for example, in the area of microaneurysms, capillary dilatations or new-formed blood vessels. This anomalous permeability is well documented on fluorescein angiography by the leakage of the dye (Fig. 79, a-b). The extracellular edema may occur in the superficial layers which gives the retina a dull appearance so that the physiologic reflexes disappear. The edema may also occur in deeper layers, e.g., the outer plexiform layer (Fig. 80, a-b). Here the fluid accumulates in multilobulated cystoid spaces which in the macular area give the characteristic fluorescein angiographic picture resembling the "petals of a flower" (Figs. 81 a, b). This is due to the peculiar arrangement of the cystoid spaces in the Henle fiber layer. The spaces may later coalesce and form one large central cyst. If the inner lamella breaks a macular pseudohole is formed.

The *intracellular edema* on the other hand (Fig. 78 A) consists of a swelling of the cells in the internal layers and of the nerve fibers. These cells imbibe water due to a sudden arrest in blood flow leading to acute state of anoxia. This condition will appear secondary to an occlusion of an artery, arteriole or precapillary as can be seen clearly on fluorescein angiography. The extent of this intracellular edema depends on the size of the occluded vessel: if it is the central retinal artery then the entire retina will be affected; if it is one of the main branches the edema will be limited to the area supplied by this branch (Fig. 82 a); if it is the precapillary arteriole the edema will be quite localized, irregular, floccular, usually called a cotton wool spot (Figs. 82 b-d).

The ischemic insult in the nerve fiber layer leads to a swelling of the neurites of the ganglion cells due to a blocked axoplasmis flow. Cytoid bodies are formed which histologically appear as round, oval or pear shaped formations, which are slightly eosinophilic and include a central area that stains more intensively. These cotton wool spots (incorrectedly called "*soft exudates*", but this pathologic material does not exude from a blood vessel) correspond exactly to non-perfused area on fluorescein angiography. The cotton wool spots are not characteristic for any specific pathologic condition and can be found in a variety of diseases, e.g., diabetic retinopathy, hypertension, pregnancy, Purtscher's retinopathy, septicemia and dysproteinemia, collagen diseases, venous occlusions, anemia and leukemia. In contrast to these soft lesions we find also *hard exudates*, which lie in the external plexiform layer, have a white-yellow color, vary in brightness, appear nearly waxy with sharp irregular outlines; they have a tendency to coalesce forming various and characteristic patterns, e.g., the macular star, a wreath, or resembling a group of islands in a sea (Figs. 83 a-d).

Many authors regard the hard exudates as extracellular deposits of lypoproteins, to a large extent taken up by macrophages; to others they represent hyaline degenerations due to colliquation and rupture of microaneurysms and subsequent hemorrhages together with chronic ischemic processes.

On fluorescein angiography these exudates do not stain and have a masking effect on the fluorescein flow beneath them. These hard exudates are also not specific for any definite pathologic entity but may be found in a diversity of condi- tions, e.g., diabetic retinopathy, hypertension, arteriosclero- sis, vasculitis, venous occlusion, and some types of vascular malformations.

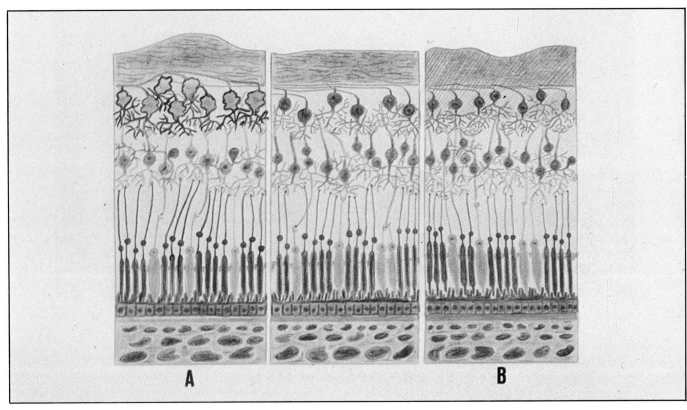

Fig. 78. Retinal edema.
A = Intracellular retinal edema.
B = Extracellular retinal edema.
  Between A and B = normal retina.

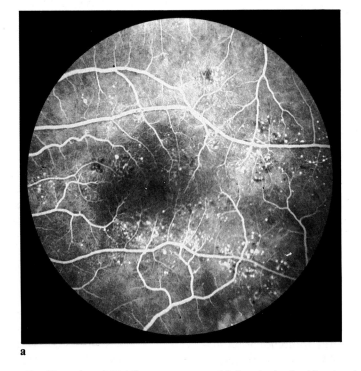

a

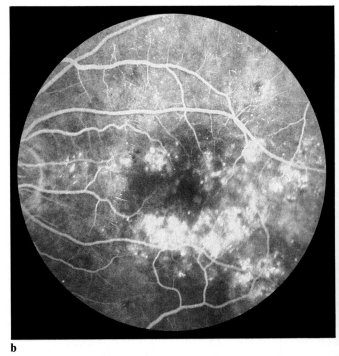

b

Fig. 79. **a)** and **b)** Microaneurysms with breaks in the blood retina barrier; fluorescein leakage.

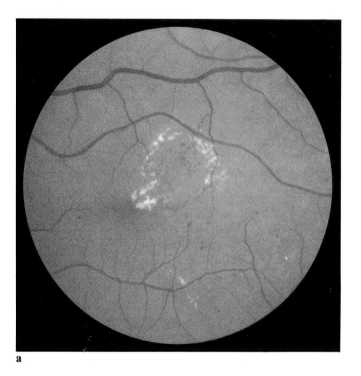 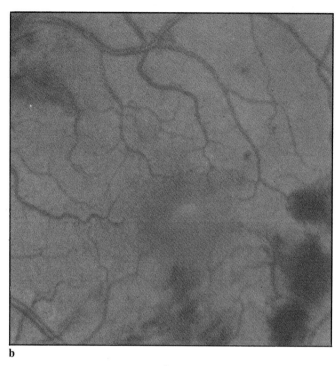

a

b

Fig. 80.
a) Extracellular edema: disappearance of the physiologic reflexes and half wreath of hard exudates.
b) Extracellular retinal edema in the macula.

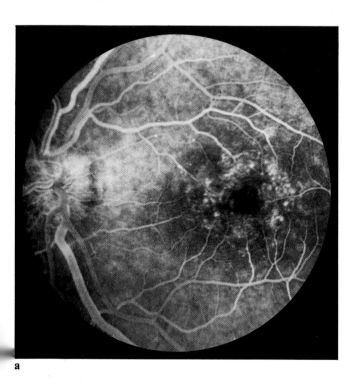 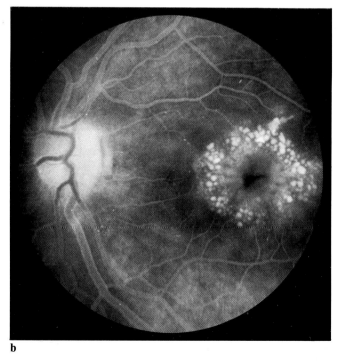

a

b

Fig. 81. **a)** and **b)** Fluorescein angiogram of deep extracellular retinal edema (external plexiform layer) with classical configuration of the cystoid spaces in the form of flower petals.

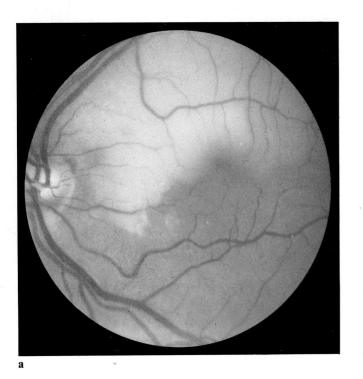

a

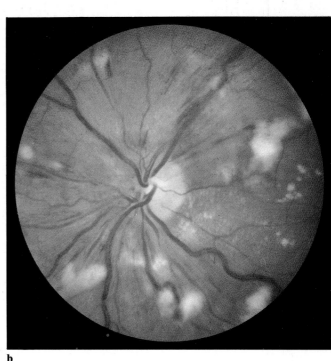

b

Fig. 82.   Intracellular retinal edema.
a) Intracellular edema with occlusion of a branch artery.
b-d) The so-called cotton wool patches.

c

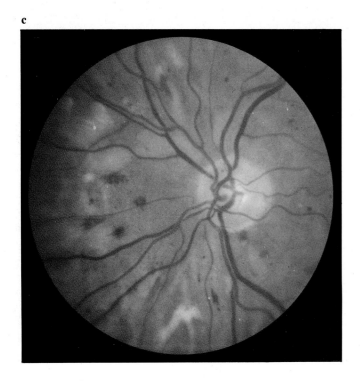

d

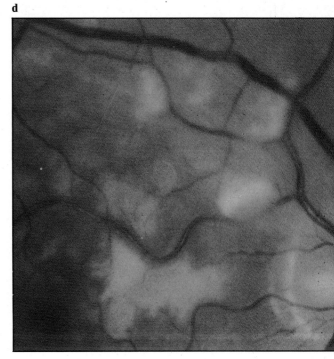

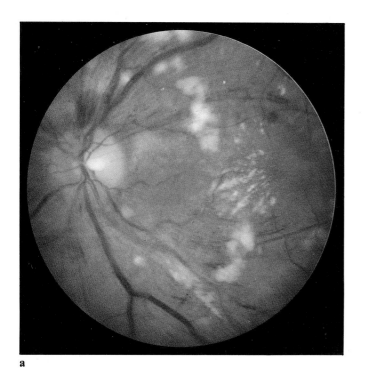

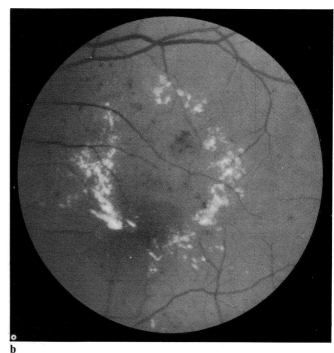

a

b

Fig. 83. Extracellular retinal edema.
a) Cotton wool patches and hard exudates arranged to a macular star.
b) Hard exudates arranged to a wreath.
c) Hard exudates distributed like islands in a sea.
d) Hard exudates forming a macular star.

c

d

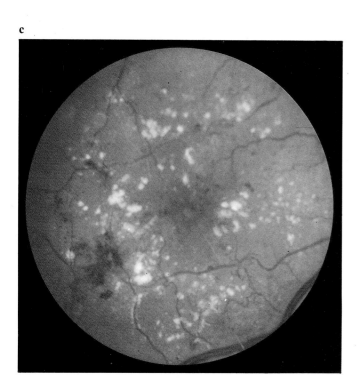

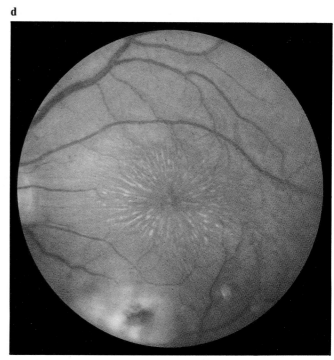

DRUSEN

This term is derived from German and signifies an accumulation of crystals. The drusen are nearly always found bilaterally, though the condition may be highly asymmetrical between the two eyes. These lesions are also called hyaline excrescences of Bruch's membrane or colloid bodies. Ophthalmoscopically (Figs. 84 a, c, d) they present themselves as white to yellow round spots with sharp outlines. Their size varies from 1/8 of a disc diameter to the diameter of one of the large veins (190-110 μ).

The individual spots may sometimes coalesce forming polygonal structures. Ophthalmoscopically they lie deep, beneath the retinal vessels. They have a certain predisposition for the posterior pole, but may be found in the periphery, especially in the equatorial area where they are often surrounded by a halo of pigment.

On a fluorescein angiogram (Fig. 84 b) they appear as hyperfluorescent spots which persist after the late venous stage. According to some this hyperfluorescence is due to a window effect caused by the changes in the pigment epithelium overlying the verrucosity; others believe that it is due to a staining of the drusen themselves.

The association of colloid bodies at the posterior pole with pigment deposits, loss of foveolar reflex, localized thickening of the retina and circinate deposits is the sign for the evolution of a detachment of the pigment epithelium or of an exudative macular degeneration.

The hyaline excrescences of Bruch's membrane can be classified as follows.

Primary:

— *Senile:* these occur in general among patients older than 60, but may be found in younger individuals.

— *Hereditary* (hereditary hyaline dystrophy): into this group belong the central guttate choroiditis of Hutchinson-Tay, the macular degeneration of Holthouse-Batten, the honeycomb degeneration of Doyne, etc.

Secondary:

— *To ocular conditions:* e.g., vascular processes, inflammations or degenerations of the retina or of the choroid; the secondary drusen are here an expression of a type of reaction from the pigment epithelium accompanying these pathologic intraocular changes.

— *To systemic conditions:* lypoproteinosis of Urbach-Wiethe, dysproteinemia, leukemia, scleroderma, pseudoxanthoma elasticum, ect.

The drusen develop on the internal surface of Bruch's membrane in the form of hyaline accumulations which histochemically consist of mucopolysaccharides (free sialic acid or bound to mucin) or of cerebrosides.

Initially the structure is granular, but later becomes homogenous. The drusen become slowly more prominent and cupuliform. In advanced age they are stratified and impregnated with calcium and lipids. In the advanced stage histopathologic examination shows that the outer members of the photoreceptors are damaged and there is a partial destruction of the choriocapillaries.

Some theories presume that the pathology of the drusen is an over-production of the cuticular part of Bruch's membrane and of the pigment epithelium. Other authors interpret these escrescences as a hyaline degeneration of the pigment epithelium secondary to autolysis of this layer determined by an abnormal lysosymal activity.

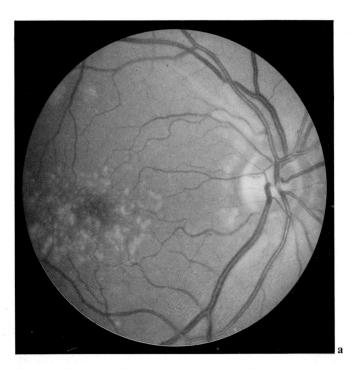 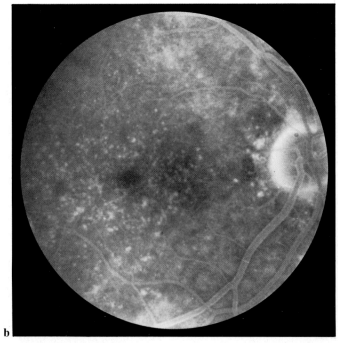

a b

Fig. 84. Drusen at the posterior pole. Ophthalmoscopic appearance (**a**) and fluorescein angiogram (**b**).

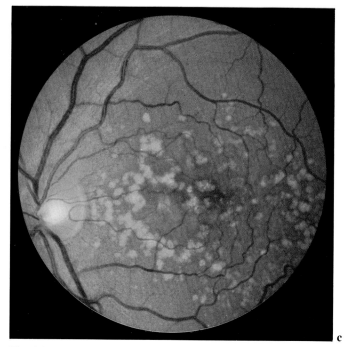 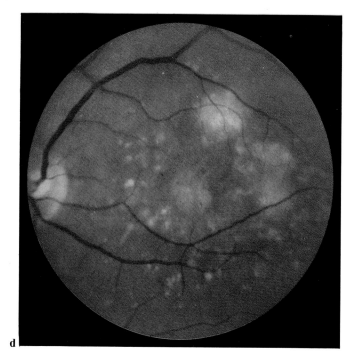

c d

Fig. 84. Drusen at the posterior pole.
c) Partly coalescing drusen at the posterior pole.
d) Drusen at the posterior pole with pigmentary deposits and age related macular degeneration (detachment of the pigment epithelium).

CHANGES IN PIGMENTATION

The pigment seen in the fundus has two sources of origin: the retinal pigment epithelium and the choroid.

The pigment appears in the pigment epithelium much earlier, around the sixth week of embryonal life. At birth the melanin granules are arranged at the base and at the borders of the pigment epithelium which is a cell of neuroectodermal origin.

The density of the pigmentation decreases from the posterior pole toward the retinal periphery. In the macula the cells are higher and more densely arranged.

The choroid becomes pigmented later in embryologic life. The granules appear during the sixth month and melanin can still be produced after birth.

The choroid contains two types of pigmented cells: the large melanocytes, which mainly lie subchoroidally, and the small melanocytes, which mainly lie in the stroma.

We also find melanophages with intense macrophage activity.

The retinal melanosome (specialized cell organelles of the melanocytes producing melanin) mature earlier than those of the choroid and this explains the pigmentary aspects of numerous pathologic conditions in the fundus of the embryo or shortly after birth.

We have already mentioned in the chapter dealing with the normal fundus that there is an indirect age relationship between the pigment content of the retina and that of the choroid: the pigment epithelium which early in life contains a great deal of pigment becomes progressively depigmented with age; the pigment content of the choroid increases on the other hand producing the typical tigroid appearance of the fundus in older individuals (Fig. 85).

This quantitative difference is accentuated by racial differences and by the specific zone of the fundus.

The optic nervehead is somewhat pale because in this area there is no retina nor choroid; the fovea on the other hand stands out by its red-brown color which is due to the rich pigmentation in that area. The fundus periphery becomes typically and progressively less pigmented compared to the posterior pole.

In order to recognize the physiologic variations of pigmentation it is necessary to familiarize oneself on a daily basis with the normal fundus. Pigmentary changes outside these limits are always an expression of a pathologic state of the retina, of the choroid or, which is frequently the case, of both of them. As far as the depth and localization of the pigment is concerned it is the rule that if the pigment appears dark black with sharp outlines it is probably located in the retina (Figs. 86 a, b), whereas if it is grey with blurred outlines it probably lies in the choroid (Fig. 87).

The outline of the lesion may also give us a valuable clue as to its location. The pigmentary lesion may solely or predominantly affect the posterior pole (Fig. 86 b), or only the periphery (Figs. 89-90). The pigmentation may appear distributed over the entire retinal area without any grouping or pattern (Fig. 89), or may be accumulated in definite areas (Fig. 90); it may more of less be arranged to a wreath surrounding an atrophic area (Fig. 88) or assume various branching or stellate figurations. Some pigmentations of the fundus are so characteristic that they constitute a nosologic entity (e.g., the bone corpuscle-like pigmentation in retinitis pigmentosa, the chorioretinal focus of congenital toxoplasmosis, certain types of syphilitic choroiditis, the chloroquine maculopathy, etc.). In any case the anomalous depigmentation, migration or regroupment of pigment represent often a common denominator of numerous chorioretinal diseases. To attribute certain morphologic aspects of the pigment to a specific pathologic entity may be arbitrary and even misleading as far as the correct diagnosis of the disease is concerned.

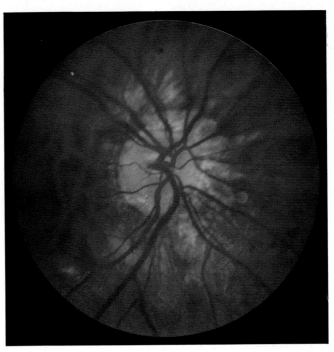

Fig. 85. Tigroid fundus in a patient of advanced age.

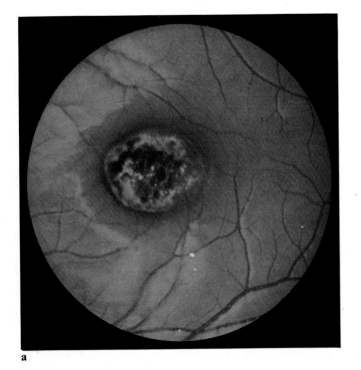

a

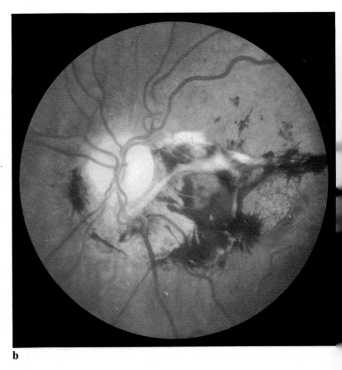

b

Fig. 86.
a) Changes of the retinal pigment epithelium in the macula (chorioretinal scar of congenital toxoplasmosis).
b) Marked post-traumatic changes of the retinal pigment epithelium at the posterior pole.

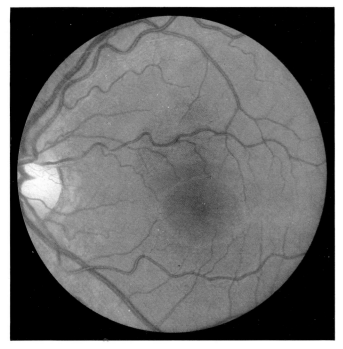

Fig. 87. Choroidal nevus.

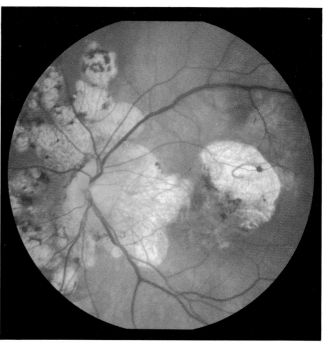

Fig. 88. Pigment accumulation around foci of chorioretinal scars.

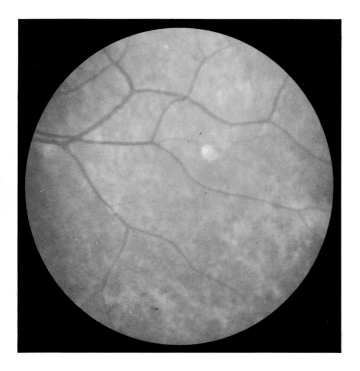

Fig. 89. Diffuse dissemination of pigment in the retinal periphery.

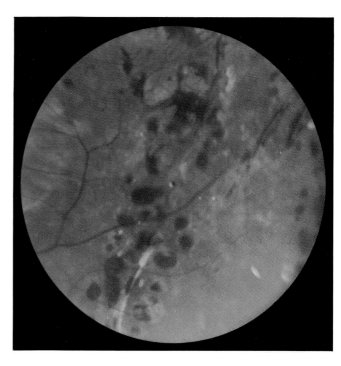

Fig. 90. Pigmented spots after photocoagulation with the argon laser.

Chapter 3

Congenital anomalies and malformations

ALBINISM

Albinism is the most important of the pigmentary ocular anomalies because of its grave associated functional defects. It is a recessive autosomal disease characterized by the congenital absence of melanin due to an inborn metabolic error (tyrosinase).

We distinguishe three types.

— The *complete form* with a generalized absence of melanin. It has a classical opthalmoscopic appearance: the retinal pigment epithelium seems to be absent causing an anomalous transparency so that the choroidal vessels become visible. There is pallor of the entire retina, especially of the macular area (Fig. 91).

The absence of a pigment screen gives at the level of the anterior segment the characteristic reddish appearance because the deep blood vessels shine through. The above described changes are usually associated with ametropia and with nystagmus and subsequent defective vision.

— The albinism may also occur in an *incomplete form* in which the melanin deficit is partial, or in an *isolated form* in which only the eye is involved.

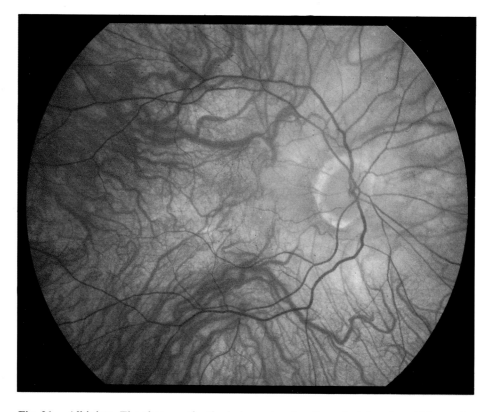

Fig. 91. Albinism. The absence of retinal pigment makes the underlying choroidal vascular network visible.

CHOROIDAL COLOBOMA

The coloboma may be caused by hereditary factors, by infectious diseases contracted by the mother during the first months of pregnancy and finally by chromosomal anomalies, e.g., trisomy.

The coloboma presents an incomplete closure of the embryonal fissure; the cleft should close during the fifth to sixth week of embryonal development. The coloboma is usually located in the inferior sector; its extent may vary: it may reach the disc margin and the fundus periphery continuing as a coloboma of the iris and the ciliary body. It may also be multiple, usuali occupying the inferiore portion of the eye.

This choroidal anomaly is always associated with a similar defect of the retinal pigment epithelium and of Bruch's membrane because these structures have a parallel embryonal development. The ophthalmoscopic picture is characterized by the visibility of the white sclera which becomes bared in the area of coloboma (Fig. 92); the margins of the coloboma are sharply delineated and sometimes hyperpigmented. Occasionally the large choroidal vessels are preserved, especially in narrow colobomas. There will be a visual field defect corresponding to the coloboma.

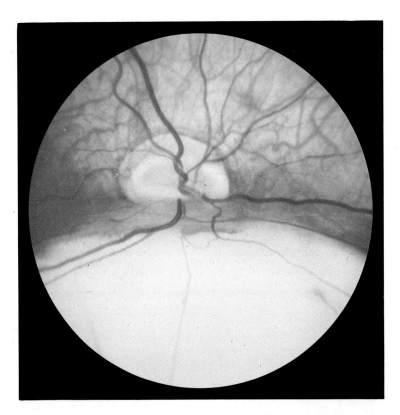

Fig. 92. Extensive choroidal coloboma in the inferior sector. The complete absence of the choroid and of the pigment epithelium makes the sclera visible.

MYELINATED NERVE FIBERS

The myelinated nerve fibers present a myelinization process of the optic nerve which instead of arresting at the lamina cribrosa extends into the area adjacent to the optic nervehead and into the retina.

The ophthalmoscopic picture is characterized by brilliant white formations of variable extension; they resemble elongated cotton balls and are usually continguous with the optic nervehead; they occur on the temporal or nasal side, but never in the papillo-macular bundle (Fig. 93). The myelinated nerve fibers may also occur at a distance from the nervehead, isolated in normal retinal tissue. In these areas the retinal vessels may be partly obscured. The diagnosis is easy, especially with fluorescein angiography which reveals a hypofluorescence due to the screening effect (Fig. 94). The visual disturbances are limited to scotomas in the visual fields, but these usually do not cause any symptoms.

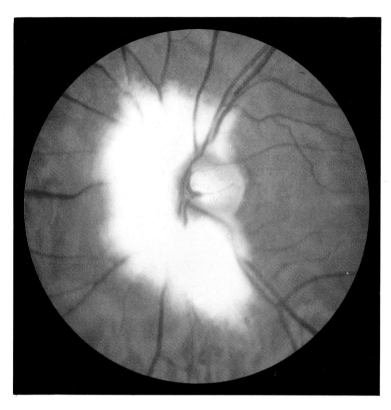

Fig. 93. Localized myelinated nerve fibers mainly on the nasal side of the optic nervehead. The retinal vessels seem surrounded and covered by these nerves.

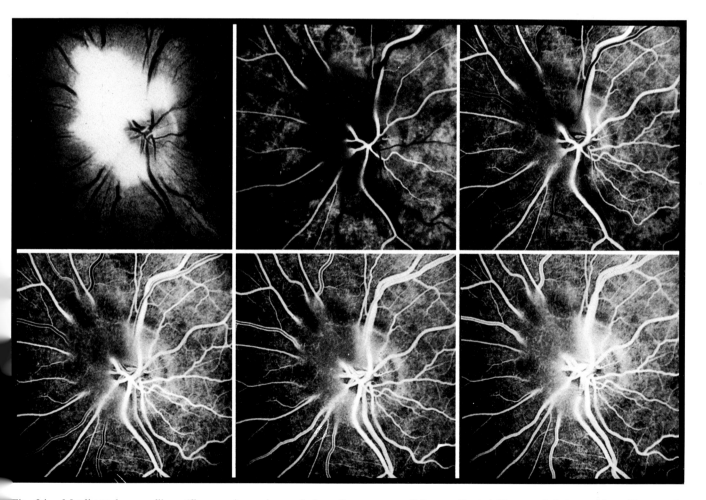

Fig. 94. Myelinated nerve fibers (fluorescein angiogram): hypofluorescence of the myelinated fibers and their masking effect on the fluorescence of the choroid and the retina.

HYPOPLASIA OF THE OPTIC NERVE

The uni- or bilateral hypoplasia of the optic nerve may be associated with aniridia or severe cerebral malformations, e.g., arhinencephaly or agenesis of the corpus callosum.

A hypoplastic optic nerve will cause conspicuous changes in the visual field because of the reduced number of nerve fibers entering the disc.

Ophthalmoscopically the optic nervehead appears oval with the long axis in the vertical meridian. The nervehead occupies only partially its place in the scleral canal (Fig. 95).

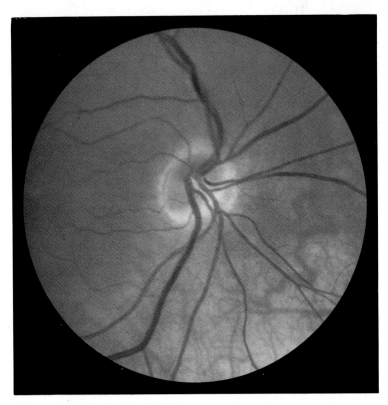

Fig. 95. Hypoplasia of the optic nervehead: the reduced size is clearly appreciated, mainly of the horizontal diameter.

COLOBOMA OF THE OPTIC NERVEHEAD

A coloboma of the optic nerve may appear in various clinical pictures. In the typical form the failure of closure in the area of the optic nervehead involves the inferior segment which then assumes an arcuate shape with the apperture downward. Such anomalies may be observed with a choroidal coloboma of varying extent. The blood vessels emerge from the margins of the disc and come from a deep excavation (Figs. 96-98).

The coloboma of the optic nerve may be quite small, but always and solely involve the inferior segment; it may not be accompanied by analogous changes in the choroid: these may only appear as a simple small zone of peripapillary dystrophy or may occasionally be absent altogether.

In some cases of coloboma there may be a differential diagnostic difficulty separating it from a physiologic excavation of unusual dimensions. The coloboma of the optic nerve causes a defect in the visual field corresponding to the anatomical deficit.

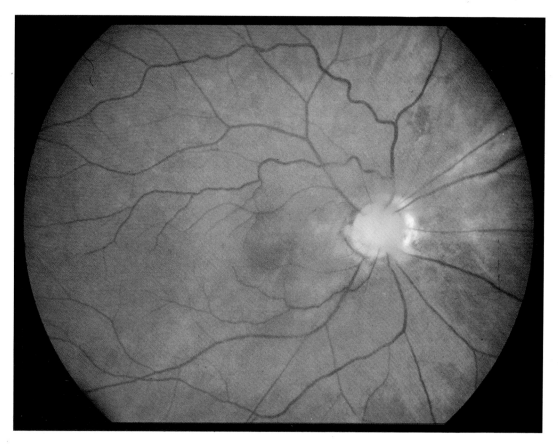

Fig. 96. Coloboma of the optic nervehead: the blood vessels seem to originate from the margin of the disc; there is a small zone of peripapillary distrophy.

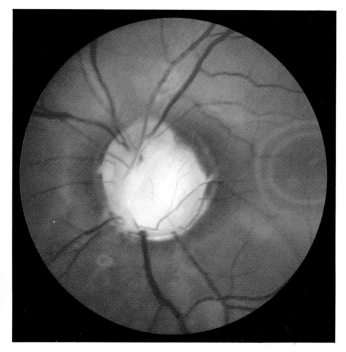

Fig. 97

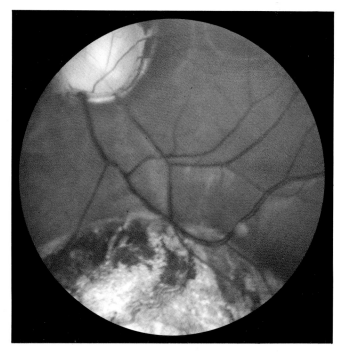

Fig. 98

Figs. 97 and **98.** Coloboma of the optic nervehead with the classical arcuate appearance and with the opening and slope downward. In Fig. 98 we see the associated choroidal coloboma.

PIT OF THE OPTIC NERVEHEAD

The colobomatous pits of the optic nervehead present themselves as round or oval excavations; they are small, white-grey and frequently located on the temporal side, rarely inferiorly (Figs. 99-100). They are usually isolated, but may occur multiple. They are asymptomatic, but may sometimes be complicated by a macular edema due to a serous detachment of the sensory retina extending from the pit. The subretinal fluid may come from the sheaths of the optic nerve. This edema may recur and may finally lead to a secondary macular hole and to severe changes of the pigment epithelium.

A colobomatous pit of the optic nervehead may also appear as an ophtalmoscopic picture which is similar to an occlusion of the central retinal vein.

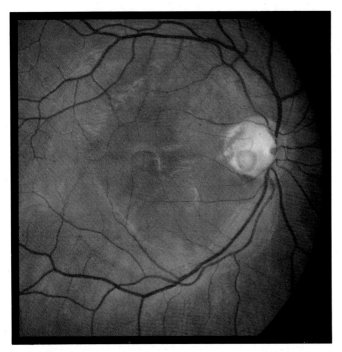

Fig. 99. Colobomatous pit of the optic nervehead localized on the temporal margin; the sensory retina is elevated in the area of the papillo-macular bundle.

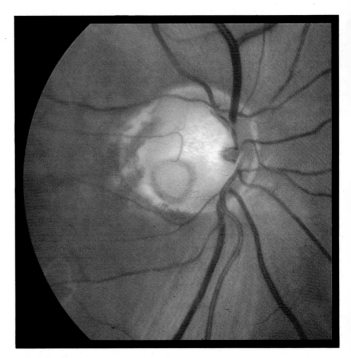

Fig. 100. Higher magnification of Fig. 99.

DRUSEN OF THE OPTIC NERVEHEAD

Drusen, sometimes also called hyaline bodies of the optic nervehead, are frequently hereditary and bilateral. They constitute cavities which lie in the fibers of the optic nervehead in front of the cribriform plate; these cavities are filled with a hyaline substance and may show calcification. Opthalmoscopically we differentiate between superficial and deep drusen. In the *superficial form*, which is typical for adults, we may see round, translucent, well-delineated structures (Figs. 101-103). In the *deep form*, typically appearing in young patients, the fibers of the optic nervehead seem to be elevated and the condition may be difficult to differentiate from a beginning papilledema (Figs. 104-106). In addition, the possible growth and the superficial location of these drusen may occasionally cause small hemorrhages.

Fluorescein angiography is in these cases decisive. The drusen show autofluorescence (Fig. 102) and stain during the late phase during which they appear as round, fluorescent structures in the area of the disc. The drusen may cause nerve fiber bundle defects in the visual field. The defects may slowly enlarge, rarely involving central vision.

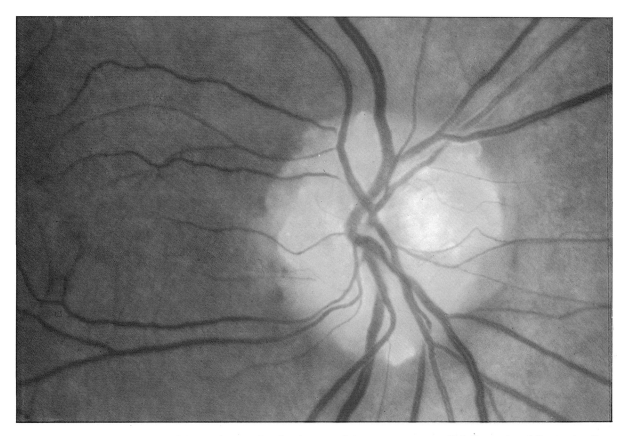

Fig. 101. Superficial drusen of the optic nervehead. The roundish structures are well delineated and lie on the disc.

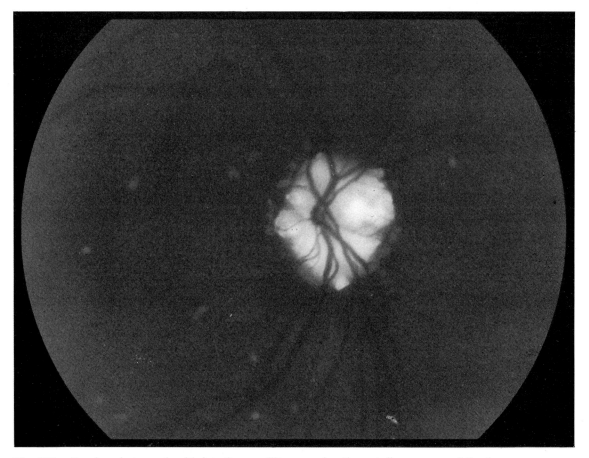

Fig. 102. Fundus photograph with interference filters proving the autofluorescence of the drusen.

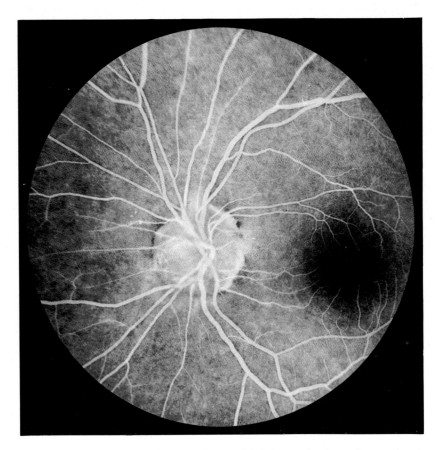

Fig. 103.   Fluorescein angiogram of superficial drusen in the optic nervehead.

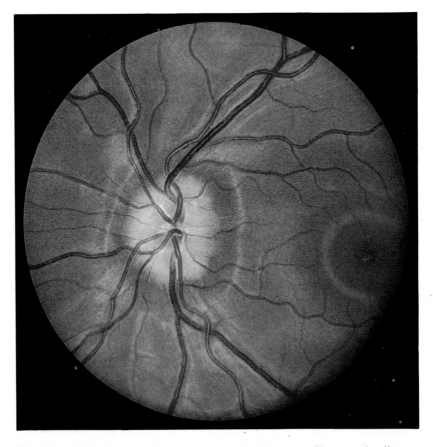

Fig. 104.   Deep drusen in the optic nervehead. The nerve fibers on the disc appear elevated.

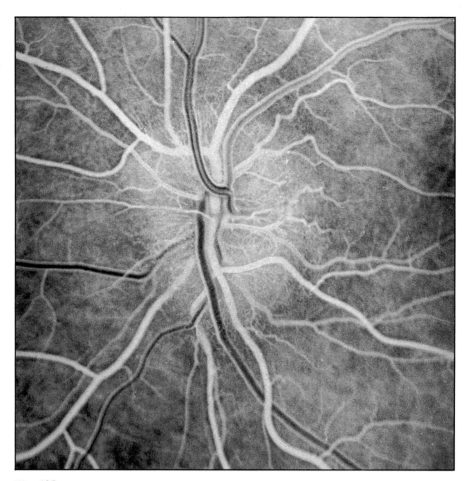

Fig. 105

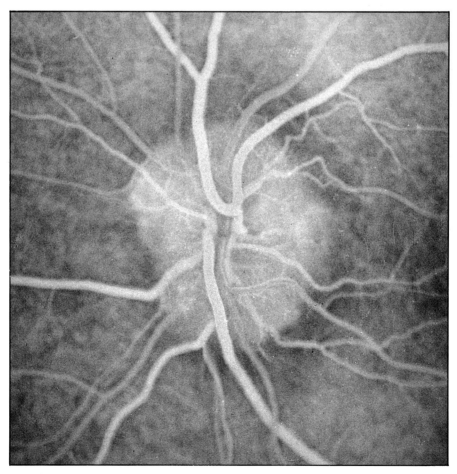

Fig. 106

Figs. 105 and **106.** A fluorescein angiogram of the drusen shows the characteristic features: during the late phase the drusen stain with the dye though there is no indication of the fluorescein leaking into adjacent tissues.

PERSISTENCE OF THE PRIMARY VITREOUS AND EPIPAPILLARY MEMBRANE

This anomaly is due to an incomplete absorption of the mesenchymal tissue which during normal development is replaced by the final vitreous.

The condition is nearly always unilateral.

The lens may show residuals of its vascular systems, but remains initially transparent. Behind it is a white tissue mass which pulls the ciliary processes toward it so that they assume the shape of spokes. Hemorrhages may occur and following the opacification of the lens there may be a secondary glaucoma, though more often the condition is associated with a microphthalmos. There are incomplete forms in which we only find residuals of the hyaloid artery in Cloquet canal and/or an avascular membrane which covers more or less completely the optic nervehead. This latter anomaly can be seen quite often and is secondary to a partial persistence of the glial sheaths of Bergmeister (Figs. 107 and 108).

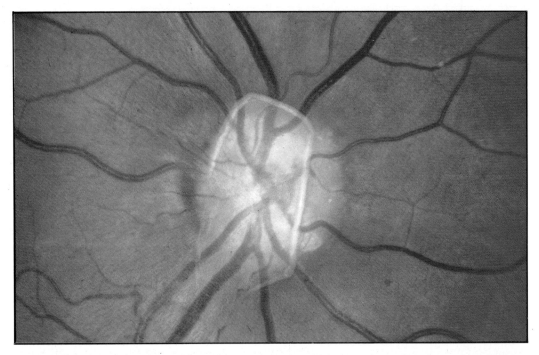

Fig. 107. Congenital epipapillary membrane. The retinal vessels are partly obscured.

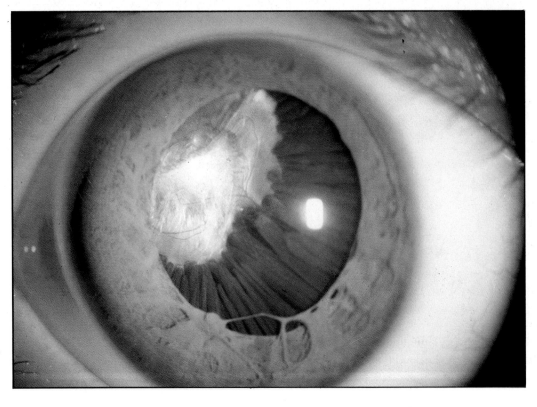

Fig. 108. Persistence and hyperplasia of the primary vitreous in a 7-year-old patient. The ciliary processes are pulled toward the fibro-vascular mass.

FALCIFORM RETINAL FOLD

This retinal malformation is often associated with vitreous anomalies. It is usually unilateral, but may be hereditary, transmitted as an autosomal recessive.

Ophthalmoscopically we see a retinal fold which is white, elevated, extending from the optic nervehead in a curvilinear fashion toward the periphery reaching the ciliary body and sometimes the lens. The fold constitutes a reduplication of the inner retinal layers. In this area the vessels appear tortuous or taut (Fig. 109).

The visual deficit depends upon the involvement of the macular area. The prognosis may be aggravated by the appearance of a peripheral retinal detachment.

In some instances there may be a difficult differential diagnosis with retinopathy of prematurity and with the familial dominant exudative vitreoretinopathy which may show similar clinical characteristics. The history may be helpful, especially in regards to the retinopathy of prematurity; the absence of severe changes of the vitreous will differentiate this condition from the exudative vitreoretinopathy.

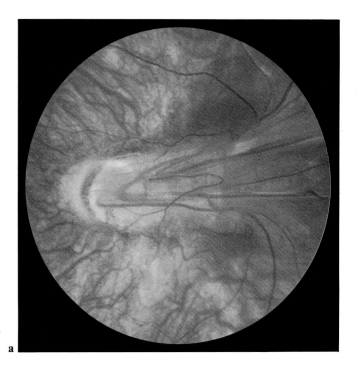

b

Fig. 109. **a)** Falciform retinal fold. The retinal fold extends from the optic nervehead toward the fundus periphery thereby dragging the retinal vessels.
b) In this case the falciform fold seems to be complicated by a peripheral retinal detachment.

Chapter 4

The ocular fundus in ametropia

Refractive errors of a certain degree will leave their imprints on the ocular fundus. This may produce morphologic changes which are quite characteristic and typical.

Hypermetropia, astigmatism, and myopia have their corresponding ophthalmoscopic picture which enables us often to make the identification and diagnosis before the refraction has been determined.

HYPERMETROPIA

All pathologic findings which have been described in this ametropia can be explained by changes in the size of the globe: early in infancy the retina tends to wrinkle probably due to the over-abundance of retinal tissue compared to the sclera; on ophtalmoscopy the retinal reflexes are particularly brilliant and frequently we see a certain tortuosity of the retinal vessels.

In high hypermetropia the optic nervehead is often red and elevated. This picture has been called "hypermetropic pseudopapillitis or the false optic neuritis of Spicer", also "pseudopapillary edema of Chamlin and Davidoff". The red discoloration of the disc, which is more evident in the center, is due to a crowding of the capillaries which seem to have increased in number per unit of surface (false hyperemia) (Fig. 100 a). The physiologic excavation is absent or extremely small. We frequently see radial striation in the peripapillary zone due to an accentuation of the nerve fiber pattern (Fig. 110 b). The disc borders seem blurred producing a greyish zone and simulating the appearance of an edema of the optic nervehead.

The changes of the optic nervehead are also due to the smallness of the globe: the stretching of the scleral canal forces the optic nerve fibers to crowd and to accumulate at the entrance of the scleral canal where they are bunched up and pass through a kind of bottleneck (papillary phimosis of Bregeat) which explains the characteristic appearance described above. The differential diagnosis against a true disc edema is established by determining the refractive error, perimetry, fluorescein angiography, electrophysiologic tests and observing the evolution of collateral vessels.

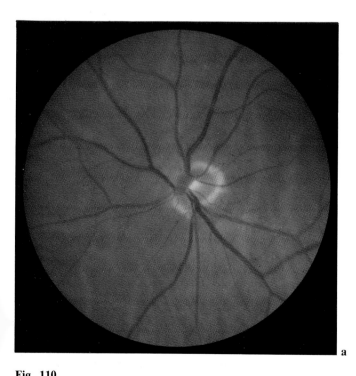 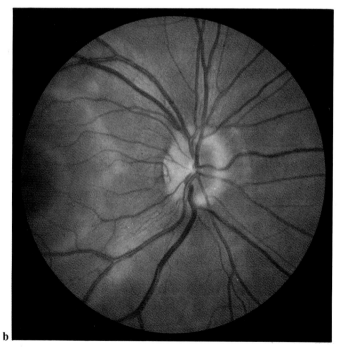

a b

Fig. 110.
a) Optic nervehead with a dark posterior pole in a hypermetropic eye.
b) Optic nervehead with conspicuous radial nerve fiber pattern in a hypermetropic eye.

ASTIGMATISM

In an eye with a high degree of astigmatism the ophthalmoscopic picture is that of a hypermetropic or myopic fundus.

The optic nervehead often appears ovoid whereby the long axis usually corresponds to the lesser degree of ametropia (Figs. 111 a, b).

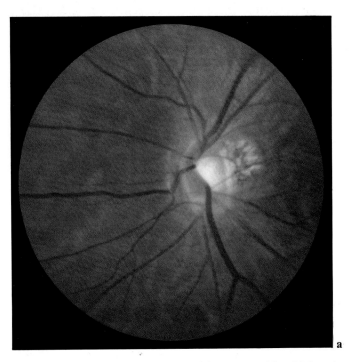 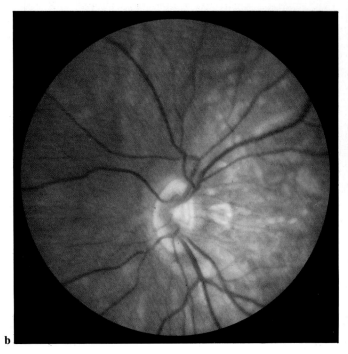

a b

Fig. 111. **a)** and **b)** Optic nervehead in an eye with a high astigmatism.

MYOPIA

We have to differentiate simple myopia which only influences the fundus picture to a moderate degree, from pathologic myopia which represents a true degenerative condition involving profoundly the various structures and various areas observable with the ophthalmoscope. In simple myopia, expecially of minor degree, the fundus may appear absolutely normal. On the other hand, the myopic crescent may be seen temporal to the optic nervehead and the choroidal vascular pattern is revealed in a usually pale fundus (Fig. 112). In pathologic myopia we distinguish from a didactic point of view changes in the *vitreous*, *optic nervehead*, *macula*, *extramacular area* and *retinal periphery*.

Vitreous

In a strict sense the alterations of the vitreous do not belong to the fundus changes and we would like to emphasize here only that the disorganization and depolymerization of the mucopolysaccharide framework is characteristic for the myopic eye. There is an upheaval in the relationship between the dispersing and dispersed part of the vitreous gel along the development of macro- and microfibrillar structures which form the base for the typical vitreous opacities of the myope. Another characteristic feature is the posterior vitreous detachment which frequently presents as ring shaped opacity corresponding to the disinsertion of the posterior hyaloid from the margin of the optic nervehead and which projects its shadow onto the underlying retinal surface.

Optic Nervehead

The most obvious change at the optic nervehead is the myopic (semilunar or sickle shaped) cone (Figs. 112 a, b; 113), sometimes present at birth; it frequently becomes paler during puberty. The cone may be small or white; it usually lies on the temporal side, but may occur at any place on the disc margin. Sometimes it is circular surrounding the entire disc. It may be of considerable size, even involving the macular area. The cone appears as a white, well-defined area in which we see the internal surface of the sclera. Quite often the margin toward the normal retina is pigmented; sometimes there is an area of transition in which the color is red-brown corresponding to a partially visible choroid.

The nerve fibers cross over the optic nervehead obliquely toward the nasal side while the choroid terminates at a certain distance from the disc border. It is partially or completely absent in the area of the cone.

The external retinal layers and the pigment epithelium may also be absent in that area so that only the internal retinal layers continue over the cone.

The way in which the myopic cone is formed is open to different interpretations: some authors believe that the scleral baring is due to the stretching of the posterior segment and to the subsequent traction on the choroid and pigment epithelium. Other authors assume that these tissues had a slower embryologic development than the sclera so that these structures could not merge at the disc margin. Another characteristic feature of the myopic disc is the super-traction of the retina (Figs. 114 a, b) which in contrast to the cone nearly always occurs on the nasal side of the optic disc. The retina seems to invade the superficial disc layers thereby obscuring its nasal margin; the blood vessels bend corresponding to the morphological relief.

Macula

Myopia induces in the macula a number of complex clinical pictures which for practical reasons are subdivided according to a system which seems most rational:

Myopic maculopathy with moderate or no ophthalmoscopic or fluorescein angiographic changes (Fig. 115). There is only a slight pigmentation of the macular area and the choroidal vascular network becomes visible. In contrast to the nearly normal ophthalmoscopic picture there may be considerable functional loss.

Degenerative atrophic maculopathy. The macular area shows pigmentary disturbances, white spots (Fig. 116 a) and ruptures of Bruch's membrane which may manifest themselves as whitish streaks traversing the macular area (Fig. 116 b).

Hemorrhagic maculopathy. This is typically seen in young individuals with a myopia exceeding 15 diopters (Fig. 117). The blood lies subretinal, has a dark red color and a round shape; it usualy lies in the foveola. Frequently we may still be able to see the foveolar reflex on top of the hemorrhage. The fluorescein angiogram shows a predictable masking effect; in rare cases the fluorescein angiogram may show an area of hyperfluorescence revealing the presence of a neovascular membrane. Histopatologically we find a rupture of the choriocapillaries associated with a discontinuity in Bruch's membrane. The final result may often be an atrophic or edematous maculopathy.

Degenerative, edematous and hemorrhagic maculopathy. Biomicroscopic examination and fluorescein angiography

have allowed us to subdivide the stages of this type of myopic maculopathy. It is probably the most frequent and most important one because of its implications on visual function.

— *Incipient stage* (Figs. 118 a-c). This stage is characterized by an association of a red spot with a slate grey area. The first is due to a hemorrhage which causes a slight elevation, the second to a serous detachment of the sensory retina itself. The fluorescein angiogram will prove the existence and outlines the extent of the neovascular membrane which breaking through the choriocapillaries and through Bruch's membrane determines by its hemorrhagic and exudative components the ophthalmoscopic picture.

— *The stage of Foster-Fuchs* (Fig. 119). This is characterized by pigment migration toward the area of the serous detachment presenting as a black ring which is frequently incomplete, has sharp outlines and may vary in shape, i.e., the classical Fuchs spot. Fluorescein angiography shows clearly also in this phase the neovascular membrane which seems to be encompassed within the pigment circle.

— *Stage of evolution.* The serous detachment extends beyond the Fuchs spot and there are numerous other hemorrhages. The posterior pole is covered by an extensive dark brown area. The Fuchs spot loses its color and appears on biomicroscopic examination flattened. The fluorescein angiogram shows a progressive evolution of the neovascular membrane.

The relative thinness of the myopic neovascular membrane, when compared to other neovascular membranes, is perhaps related to the choroidal circulatory handicap, which is typical for the myopic eye and limits the extension of such a pathologic membrane coming from the choroid.

A particular aspect of the myopic maculopathy is the presence of a central chorioretinal atrophy (Fig. 120).

Extramacular Area

Diffuse or circumscribed changes occur frequently in the extramacular area. The first appear ophthalmoscopically like a choroidal thinning associated with pigment disturbances. The smaller vessels seem to disappear and the larger ones become more prominent. This resembles a partial, purely ocular albinism (Fig. 121).

The atrophic changes may lead to the complete disappearance of certain tissues leaving only white areas of bare sclera. Adjacent areas may coalesce leading to polygonal configurations (Fig. 121 b). Histopathologically we find the choroid thin so that only Bruch's membrane and a slender supra-choroid remain. The choriocapillaries suffers early. There may be migration of pigment epithelium melanin into the choroid through discontinuities of the lamina vitrea. The increased permeability of the cuticular part of Bruch's membrane enhances the migration of pigmentary elements which then accumulates in the deep layers of the retina (Figs. 121 c, d).

Fundus Periphery

The changes in the periphery consist essentially of anomalies of pigmentation and of the typical cystoid degeneration. The pigmentary changes include more or less extensive areas of choroidal atrophy and coarse and widespread irregularities of the pigment epithelium. The cystoid degenerations (Blessing-Iwanoff) develop in the external plexiform and in the external nuclear layers. They are quite characteristic for the myopic retinal periphery. They may expand and coalesce so that in this area the retina may be reduced to the supporting structures only. This area may easily give way to vitreal pull thereby setting the stage for a retinal hole.

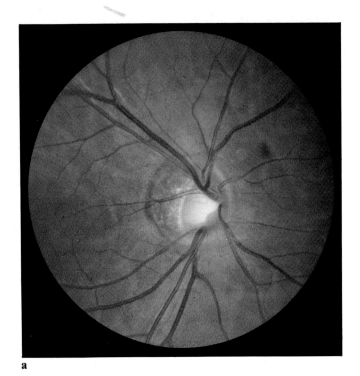

a

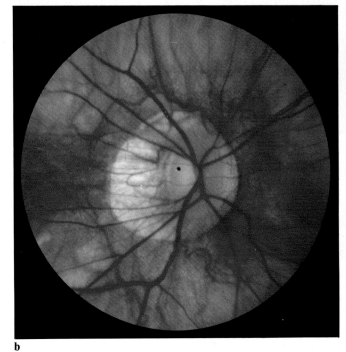

b

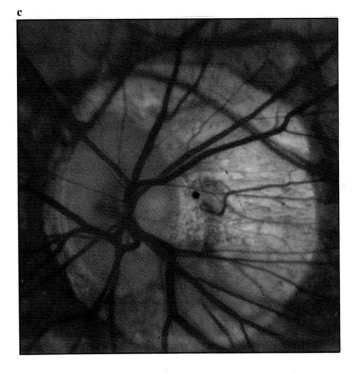

c

Fig. 112.   a-c) Myopic cone of various appearances and under varying magnifications.

Fig. 113.   The correlation of the ophthalmoscopic picture of a myopic cone and of the myopic retinal supertraction with the histologic appearance of the optic nervehead.

r   = retina;
s   = sclera;
Ch = choroid;
ep = pigment epithelium;
A   = central retinal artery;
V   = central retinal vein

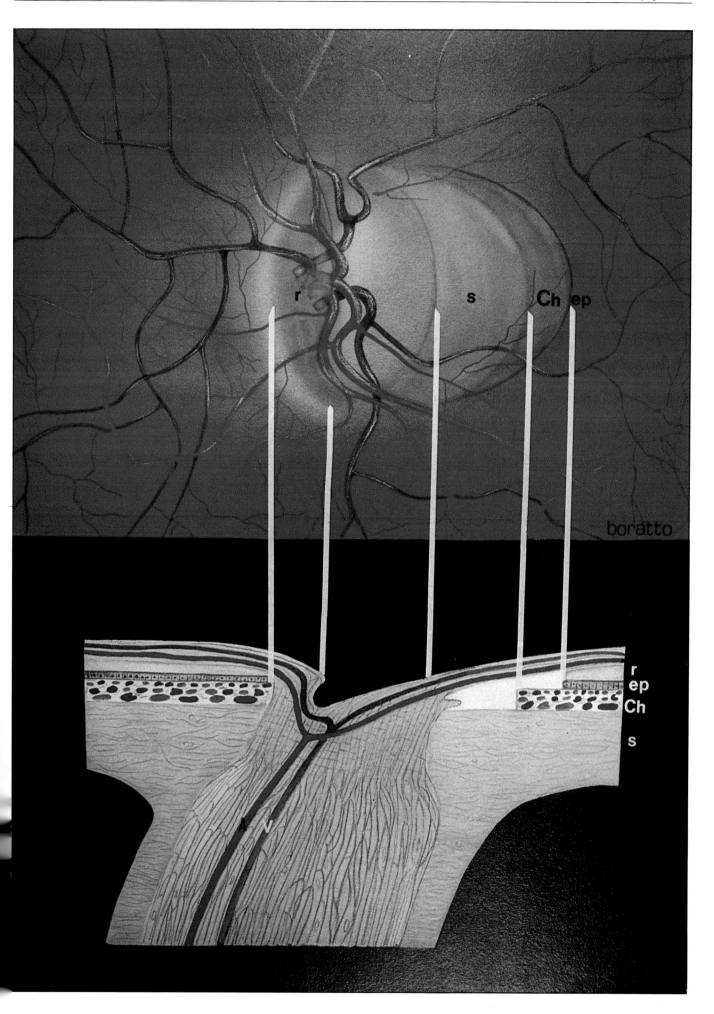

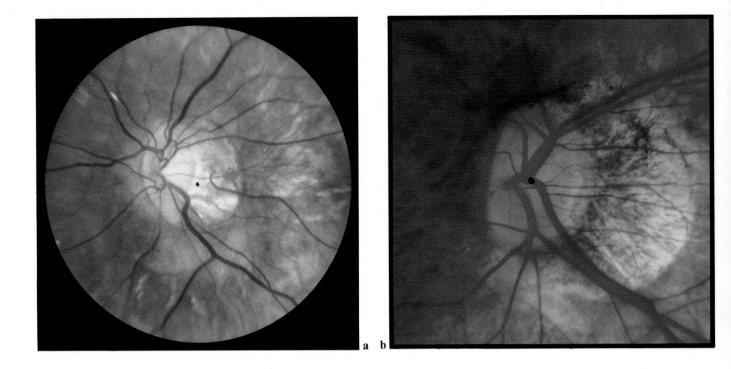

a   b

Fig. 114. **a)** and **b)** Retinal supertraction on the opposite side of the myopic cone.

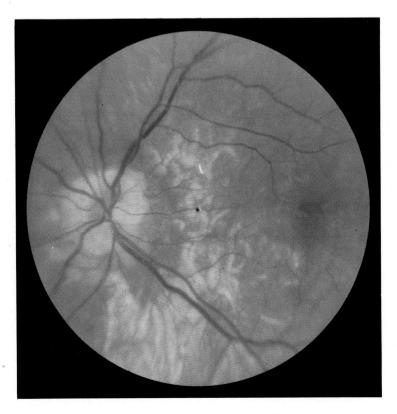

Fig. 115. Mild myopic maculopathy.

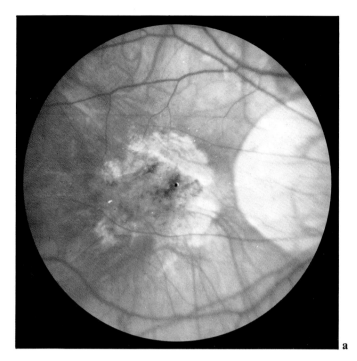 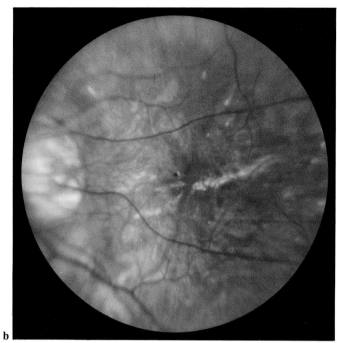

Fig. 116. Atrophic degenerative maculopathy.
a) Pigment accumulation in the atrophic areas.
b) Rupture of Bruch's membrane.

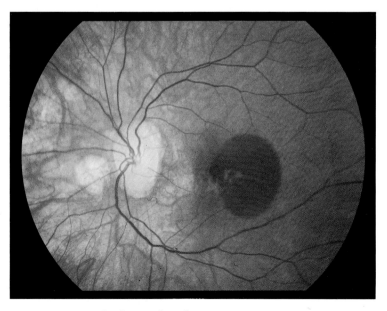

Fig. 117 Hemorrhagic maculopathy.

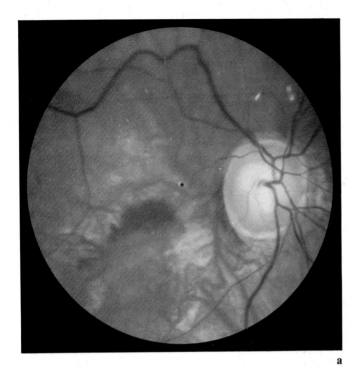

a

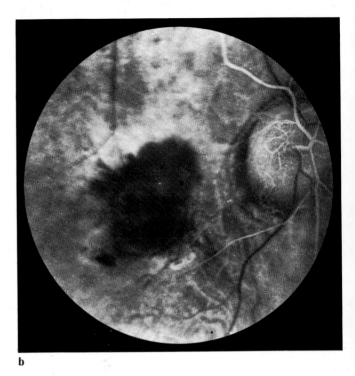

b

c

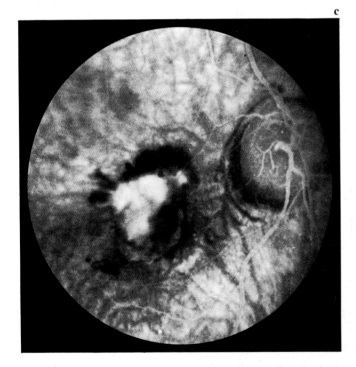

Fig. 118 Serous hemorrhagic maculopathy with a subretinal neovascular membrane.
a) Ophthalmoscopic picture.
b) and **c)** Fluorescein angiogram.

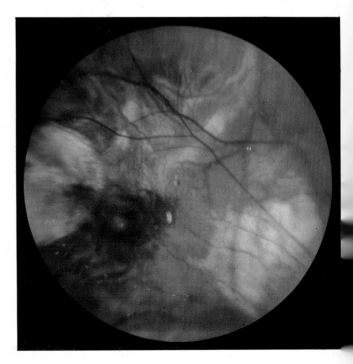

Fig. 119 Old hemorrhagic degenerative maculopathy.

Fig. 120 Central myopic atrophy.

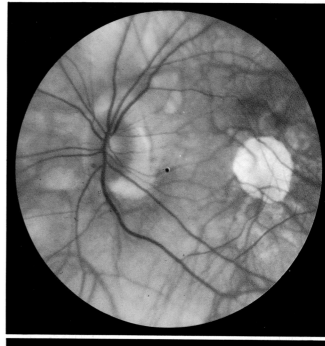

Fig. 121 Pathologic changes at the posterior pole in an eye with high myopia.
a) Partial myopic albinism.
b) Polymorph chorioretinal atrophy.
c) Loss of retinal pigment.
d) A black Fuchs spot.

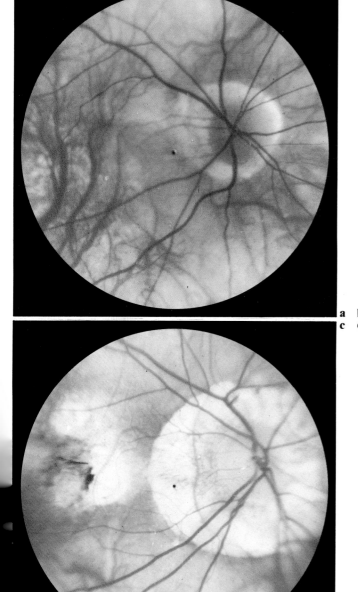

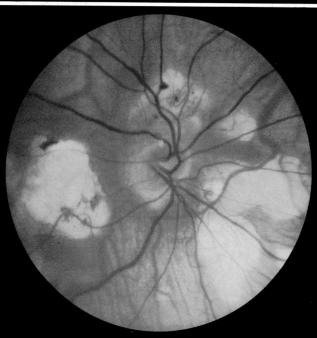

a	b
c	d

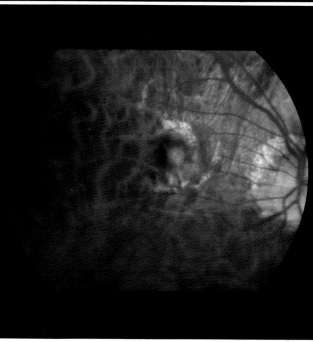

Chapter 5

Diseases of the optic nerve

It is necessary to realize certain characteristics of the second cranial nerve in order to understand better and interpret more correctly its pathologic changes. Actually this structure is erroneously called a nerve (Fig. 122). In fact, from an embryologic and anatomical point of view it is not a peripheral nerve, but a white cerebral commissure. The fibers are myelinated, but do not have a Schwann sheath; they are, however, covered by meninges. The vascular pattern of the optic nerve is somewhat similar to that of the brain; the vertebrocarotid system supplies the circle of Willis, like the ciliary system supplies the circle of Zinn-Haller.

The capillary network is similar to that of the brain, just as the nerve fibers are similar to the white brain substance. The optic nervehead is irrigated by a vascular system subdivided by Hayreh into a superficial capillary layer which is mainly supplied from the central retinal artery, and a prelaminar, laminar and retrolaminar layer mainly supplied by the posterior short ciliary arteries (Fig. 123).
The vascularization of the optic nervehead therefore derives from the retinal vessels on one and from the choroidal vessels on the other hand. All these characteristic features give the optic nerve a morphologic and functional peculiar aspect which explains the pathologic processes in these areas.

DISC EDEMA

This term signifies an accumulation of liquid within the optic nervehead expressing itself as an intrafascicular edema. Classically and from a didactic point of view we distinguish three types of disc edema:

— the pure or passive edema (stasis of the optic nervehead) (Fig. 124 a);
— the inflammatory or active edema (papillitis and neuroretinitis) (Fig. 124 b);
— the ischemic optic neuropathy (vascular pseudopapillitis) (Fig. 124 c, d).

These variations have different etiology, symptomatology and ophthalmoscopic pictures (Table 1), but the differential diagnosis is not always easy.

Pathogenesis

The disc edema resembles more a cerebral edema than an edema of the retina because of the particular structure of the capillary network causing a specific pathogenic mechanism which we would like to discuss briefly.
Inside the capillaries is an onkotic pressure which physiologically is in equilibrium with the hydrostatic pressure; the latter diminishes from the arterioles to the venules. This difference in the pressure level allows the

passage of liquids (water and small molecules) from the capillary lumen, into the interstitial space and the subsequent return from these spaces into the vessel with a constant exchange of fluid. All this depends upon the integrity of the endothelial wall of the capillaries.
These three factors, onkotic and hydrostatic pressure together with capillary permeability, are interdependent and in physiologic equilibrium. The alteration of one of these factors affects automatically the other two, inducing in this way a tissue edema.
The first stage is a congestive one. There is a hyperemia of the blood vessels with a round-cell infiltration around them. The interstitial spaces imbibe fluid thereby separating the nerve fiber bundles. This stage is followed by a degenerative one. The myelin is broken into small, vacuolar, degenerative spherules and the axons break down forming granular fibrils. The leukocytes which appeared during the congestive phase are now replaced by microglia (mesoglia with phagocytic faculties). The degeneration of the axons progresses in a central and peripheral direction until it reaches the ganglion cells. The degenerative phase is followed by a cicatricial one in which the neuroglia replaces the destroyed neural tissue. In some forms, at least initially, the axon may not be altered in its function while the conduction in the fibers is pathologically changed as of the earliest stages of the disease. The classical subdivision of

Bregeat is based on this premise: disc edema may be divided into the pure type (saving nerve conduction and function) and a secondary one (accompanied with functional deficits due to primary changes in the axon cylinders) as we see it in papillitis.

Symptomatology

We conventionally divided the natural evolution of disc edema into four stages; these have a purely didactic importance and from a practical point one stage may not always be clearly differentiated from another one.

Incipient stage (Fig. 125). The patient frequently experiences transitory obscurations; the ophthalmoscopic picture of the nervehead changes in a subtle and mild form. It is usually claimed that classically the disc edema begins in the nasal inferior segment; other authors believe that the center of the disc is initially most involved.
In this first stage the two biomicroscopic signs of Goldmann are of fundamental importance: the detachment of the prepapillary internal limiting membrane and the increased reflectivity of the disc margin.

The florid stage (Figs. 126, 127). The optic nervehead is elevated (up to 6-8 diopters). The disc tissue loses its transparency and the margins are obscured as the edema extends into the peripapillary retina. This also explains the concentric retinal folds which sometimes can be observed.
The optic nervehead is elevated and enlarged; the height is not always proportional to the enlargement; the congested vessels bend upward but then lose themselves into the edematous disc tissue.
The veins are dark, dilated, tortuous and without reflexes; the arteries are tortuous with diminished or absent reflexes. Their caliber is usually unchanged. The hemorrhages come from the capillaries and lie beneath the internal limiting membrane at the level of the nerve fibers and therefore assume a flame-shaped contour; rarely may they be localized in the outer plexiform layer and then appear as dot-blot hemorrhages. The dot-like exudates or dirty grey spots lie in the nerve fiber layer and occur usually in the papillary, juxtapapillary, or less frequently, in the zone between the disc and the macula.

Pre-atrophic stage (Fig. 128). The first ophthalmoscopic signs of an anatomical and functional damage to the optic nerve are the contractions of the retinal artery on the disc and the thickening of their sheaths. The optic nervehead loses tissue and the congestion is followed by pallor.

Atrophic stage (Fig. 129 a, b). The optic nervehead loses progressively its color and the edema disappears. The arteries are constricted and sheathed; the veins are somewhat dilated and tortuous. The physiologic excavation of the grey-white disc is filled with glial tissue. At the disc margin we find pigmentary remnants which are diagnostic characteristics of a past disc edema. The edema cannot occur in the atrophic nervehead because of the atrophy of the capillaries; the degenerated optic nerve fibers cannot take

up any fluid and the interseptal glial proliferation does not allow the separation of these nerve fibers.

It should be mentioned here that disc edema is less pronounced in an eye with high myopia or in a senile eye because of the changed condition of those tissues in which the edema would develop.

Classically disc edema produces from a functional point of view a triad of perimetric changes;

— enlargement of the blind spot,
— gradual slopes of the isopters around the blind spot,
— defects in spatial summation (photometric disharmony).

This triad is determined by the fluid imbibition of the disc tissue with accompanying separation of the nerve fibers. It can be found in the pure form of disc edema (stasis) or in the secondary form (inflammatory). In the latter form the primary affection of the axon cylinders explains the polymorph nerve fiber bundle defects and the deterioration of visual acuity.

Differential Diagnosis (Table 1)

Because of the grave prognostic and therapeutic implications we should always try to differentiate between the pure disc edema (passive edema or "Staungspapille" of the German authors, white edema) and the secondary edema (inflammatory edema, active or red edema, papillitis). The ophthalmoscopic picture is not always unequivocal, nor is the state of visual acuity which is usually normal in stasis and compromised in inflammatory edema, nor the various visual field defects which may differ markedly.
An attempt has been made to use the fluorescein angiographic findings for differential diagnoses: in pure edema (Figs. 130 a, d) we find a marked hyperemia of the optic nervehead during the arterial phase, while the deeper layers of the disc are poorly visible because of the overlying edema. During the venous phase the fluorescence of the disc increases slowly until it involves the entire optic nervehead; it is maximal at the late venous phase indicating a true local stasis.
Due to the stasis the capillaries can be recognized on the uniformly fluorescing background. The adjacent retina and choroid do not show any pathologic changes. In the inflammatory disc edema (papillitis) (Figs. 131 a, d) we see during the arterial phase only the central vessels filled with dye; the optic nervehead itself remains dark and no capillary stasis can be seen. The peripapillary retina obscures the circulation in the underlying choroid. The disc fluoresces diffusely during the venous phase and the capillaries are not visible any more.
In the differential diagnosis of disc edema it is absolutely indispensable to distinguish the true disc edema from a pseudopapilledema, especially in regard to the prognostic and therapeutic aspects which are often so important as far as the diagnosis of disc edema is concerned.
A blurring of the nasal disc margin may be physiologic and is due to the crowding of nerve fibres coming from the nasal half of the retina. These fibres are pushed together as they enter the scleral canal; they actually have only one-third o

Table 1. Differential diagnosis of disc edema.

	Pure form (passive stasis)	Inflammatory or Secondary	Pseudopapilledema	Anterior ischemic optic neuropathy (vascular pseudopapillitis)
Ophthalmoscopy	Considerable edema, dilated veins, hemorrhages and exudates, often bilateral.	Less marked edema, hyperemic nervehead, often vitreous opacities, usually unilateral.	Varying clinical picture, venous pulsation on the disc easy to provoke. No congestion or stasis of the optic nervehead.	Ischemic picture with hemorrhages.
Visual acuity	Preserved.	Reduced.	Preserved.	Reduced.
Visual field	Enlargement of the blind spot.	Nerve fiber bundle defects.	More or less normal.	Large defects.
Fluorescein	Hyperemia of the nervehead during the arterial phase, increased fluorescence during the venous phase.	During the venous phase only the central retinal vessels are filled; there is no capillary stasis. During the venous phase the optic disc shows diffuse fluorescence.	Normal fluorescence of the blood vessels.	The optic nervehead does not fluoresce, remains dark until the late venous phase when it acquires a blurred fluorescence.
ERG	Normal.	Normal.	Normal.	Normal.
Visually evoked potentials	Normal.	Pathologic.	Normal.	Pathologic.

the disc circumference available. The other two-thirds are ocupied by the papillomacular bundle and the fibres from temporal half of the retina. In an eye with high hypermetropia the reduced size of the eyeball and the constriction of the scleral canal may produce a kind of pseudopapilledema (papillary phimosis) with slight edema and hyperemia of the optic nervehead (see Chapter 4).

A pseudopapilledema may also occur with myelinated nerve fibers and with mesenchymal residues of embryonal tissue; the same applies to neoplasms, gumma, tuberculoma and disc drusen (hyaline bodies) (see Chapter 3).

A pseudopapilledema may also appear in an eye with subtotal occlusion of the central retinal vein and with foci of chorio-retinitis close to the disc (juxtapapillary chorioretinitis of Jensen) (see Chapter 6).

The evolution of the clinical ophthalmoscopic picture, biomicroscopic and fluorescein angiographic examination, as well as perimetry will furnish the necessary elements for a diagnosis.

Etiology

Numerous conditions can produce a disc edema.

Ocular causes. Hypotony of the globe secondary to a surgical procedure, contusion or uveitis; occlusion of the central retinal vein and tumors of the optic nerve or its sheaths; neuroretinitis, especially viral in nature, papillophlebitis, juxtapapillary retino-choroiditis, exudative retinopathy of Coats.

Orbital causes. Solid or fluid space occupying lesions in the orbit; tumors of the optic nerve, optic neuropathy in Graves' disease, cysts and vascular anomalies of the orbit.

Neurologic causes. Intracranial space occupying lesions, e.g., neoplasms, inflammation, cysts or hemorrhages which produce an endocranial hypertension, meningo-encephalitis, trauma to the skull, craniostenosis, thrombophlebitis of the cavernous sinus, pseudotumor cerebri, tumors of the medulla oblongata, subarachnoidal injections for anesthesia or other reasons.

In children when the cranial sutures are still open the disc edema may not develop, but an optic atrophy may develop without that the nervehead itself imbibes any fluid.

Cardiovascular causes. Congenital heart defects, systemic arterial hypertension.

Anterior ischemic optic neuropathy (vascular pseudopapillitis) is due to an acute ischemia of the optic nervehead which may involve all four layers of the nervehead as defined by Hayreh. It is usually due to an acute blockage of the arterial flow in the posterior ciliary arteries coursing to the nervehead. The main causes are arteriosclerosis, atherosclerosis, giant cell (temporal) arteritis (Horton), collagen diseases, diabetes mellitus, arterial hyper- or hypotension, increased intraocular pressure, carotid occlusion.

Hematologic causes. Leukemia, polycythemia, anemia, dysproteinemia.

Infectious causes. An infectious process may involve the optic nervehead from adjacent tissue, via the blood vessels or the nerve fibers. These may be focal infections, generalized (bacterial, viral, parasitic) infections, secondary inflammations (uveo-papillitis, neuropapillitis, uveo-meningoneuritis).

Fig. 122. Structure and vascularization of the optic nervehead and of the collar of the optic nerve.

1 = vitreous;
2 = nerve fiber layer;
3 = transparent retina;
4 = retinal photoreceptors;
5 = pigment epithelium;
6 = Bruch's membrane;
7 = choroid;
8 = sclera;

ZH = arterial circle of Zinn-Haller around the optic nerve;

A = central retinal artery;
V = central retinal vein;
acpb = short posterior ciliary artery;

a = branch for the circle of Zinn-Haller;
b = perforating branches of the first order;
c = anastomoses between the circle of Zinn-Haller and the choroid;
d = anastomoses between the choroid and the optic nervehead;
e = coaxial retrograde branches;
f = perforating branches of the second order;
LC = cribriform plate.

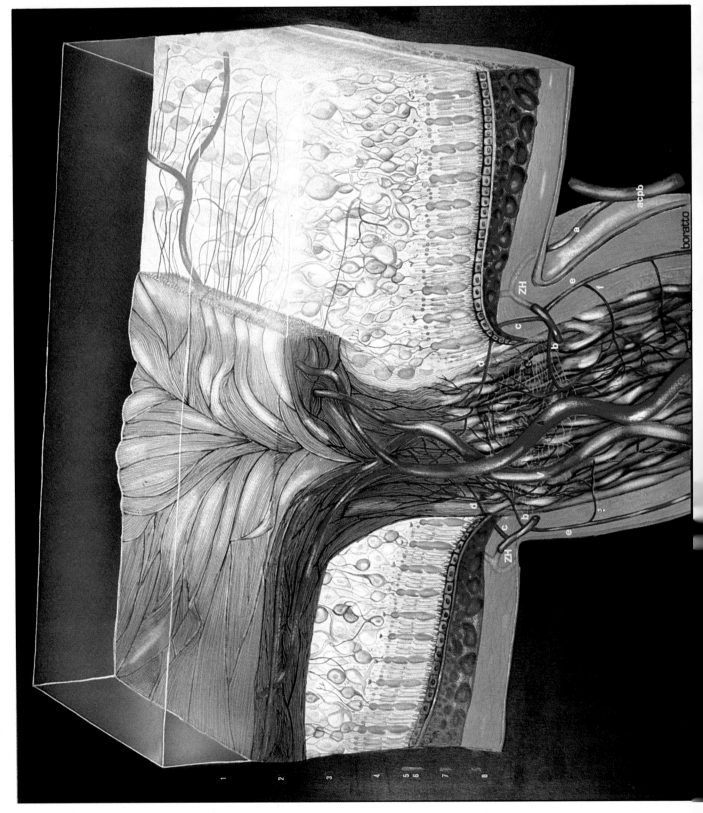

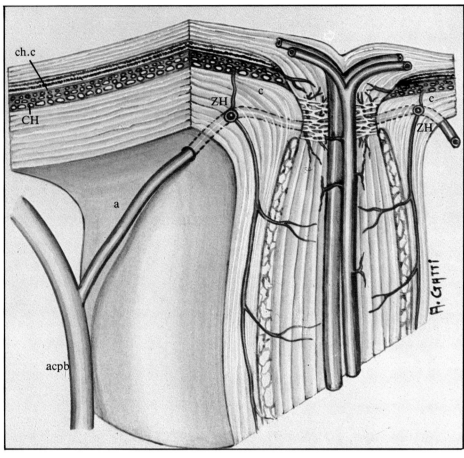

Fig. 123. The vascularization of the optic nervehead.
CH   = choroid;
ch.c. = choriocapillaries;
acpb = short posterior ciliary artery;
a   = the branch for the circle of Zinn-Haller;
ZH = circle of Zinn-Haller;
c   = choroidal branch of the circle of Zinn-Haller.

Endocrine causes. Addison disease, Graves' disease, hypoparathyroidism.

Toxic causes. Occupational or accidental intoxications (lead, methyl alcohol, benzoin derivates), medications (ethambutol, corticosteroids, vitamin A, phenothiazine derivatives).
These toxins usually cause a mild disc edema which is transitory and precedes an optic atrophy; these substances cause predominantly a retrobulbar neuritis.

The **Foster-Kennedy syndrome** consists of a triad of signs and is usually caused by space occupying lesions in the anterior part of the middle cerebral fossa:

— unilateral optic atrophy with an initial central scotoma, due to direct compression of the optic nerve (Fig. 132 a);
— anosmia on the same side on which the optic nerve is affected;
— disc edema on the opposite side due to intercranial hypertension (an atrophic optic nerve cannot be the seat of an edema because histologically there is absence of supporting tissue which would allow the imbibition with fluid (Fig. 132 b).

The term Foster-Kennedy syndrome is usually applied to an association of optic atrophy on one and disc edema on the opposite side (there is a pseudosyndrome of Foster-Kennedy due to vascular causes).

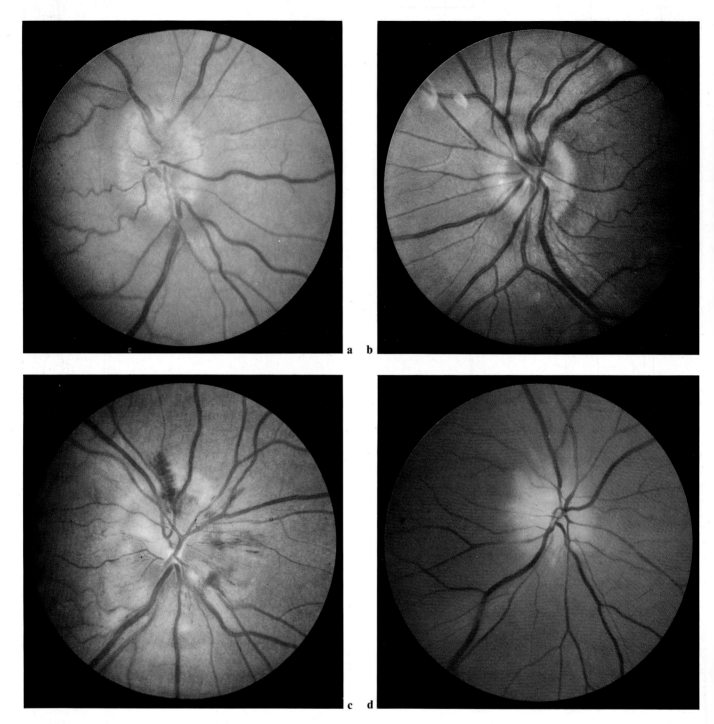

Fig. 124. Ophthalmoscopic picture of disc edema.
a) Ophthalmoscopic picture of a pure papilledema (stasis).
b) Ophthalmoscopic picture of an inflammatory papilledema (papillitis).
c) Ophthalmoscopic picture of a papilledema secondary to a benign vasculitis in the optic nervehead.
d) Ophthalmoscopic picture of disc edema in an anterior ischemic optic neuropathy (vascular pseudopapillitis).

Fig. 125. Pure disc edema (stasis): incipient stage.
Fig. 126. Disc edema: florid stage.
Fig. 127. Disc edema: florid stage.
Fig. 128. Disc edema: pre-atrophic stage.
Fig. 129. **a)** and **b)** Disc edema: atrophic stage.

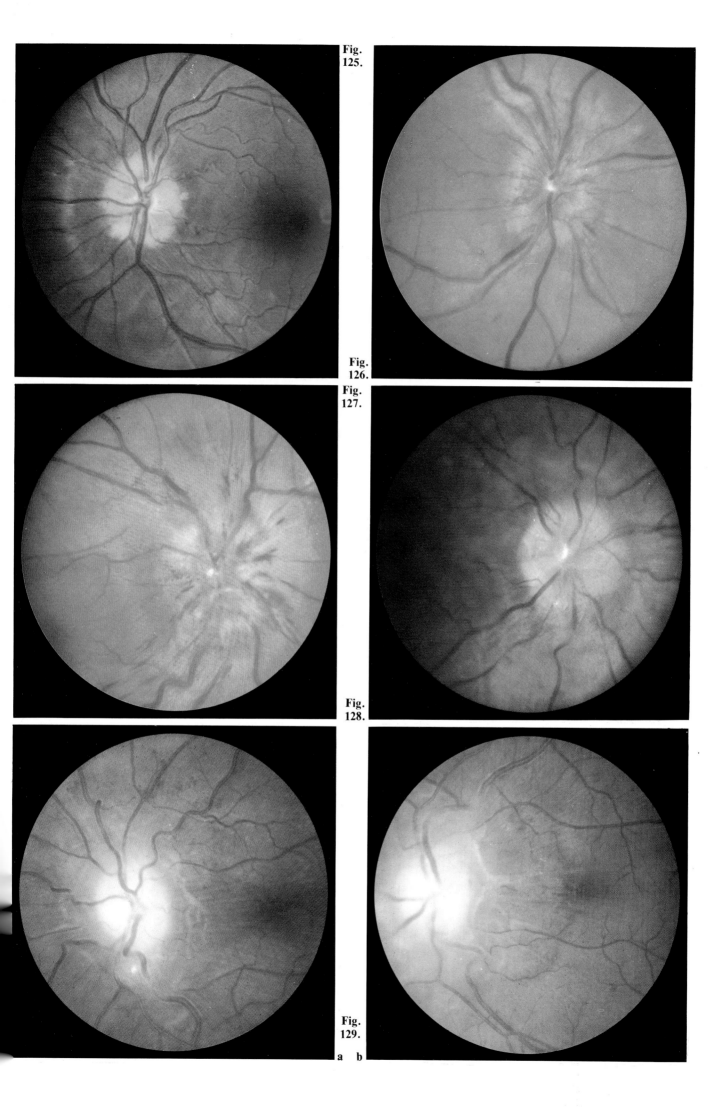

Fig.
125.

Fig.
126.

Fig.
127.

Fig.
128.

Fig.
129.

a   b

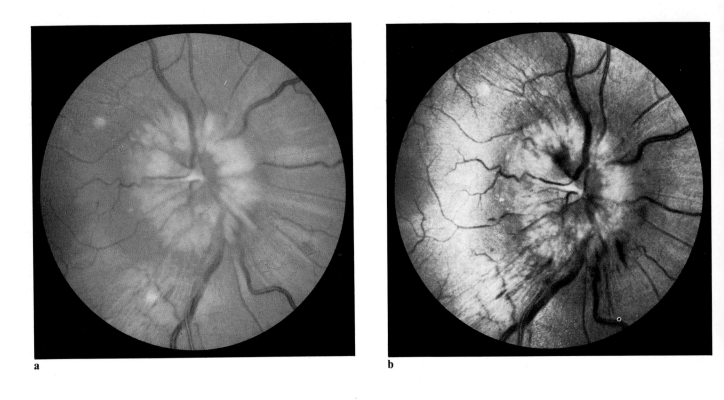

Fig. 130.
a) Ophthalmoscopic picture of pure disc edema or stasis of the nervehead.
b-d) Fluorescein angiograms of the same case: **b)** red free illumination; **c)** arterio-venous phase; **d)** venous phase.

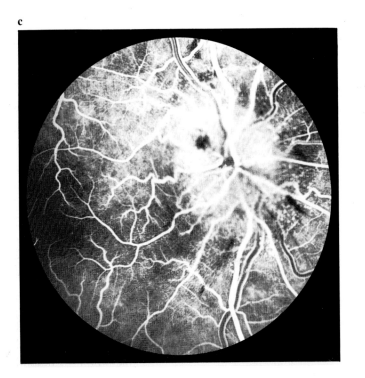

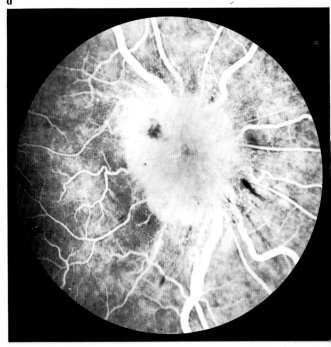

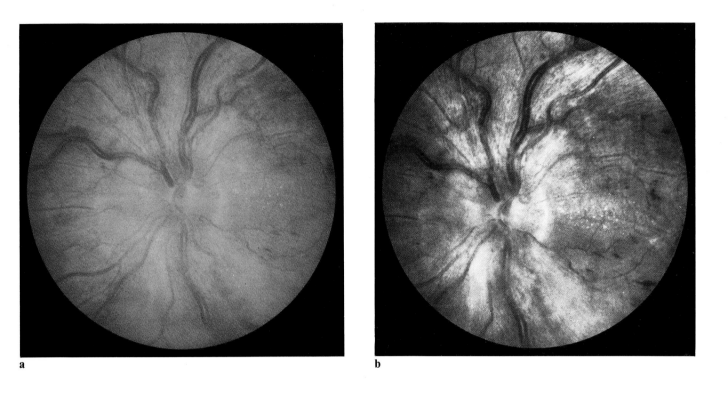

Fig. 131.
a) Ophthalmoscopic picture of an inflammatory disc edema (neuroretinitis).
b-d) Fluorescein angiograms of the same case: **b)** red free illumination; **c)** early arteriovenous phase; **d)** venous phase.

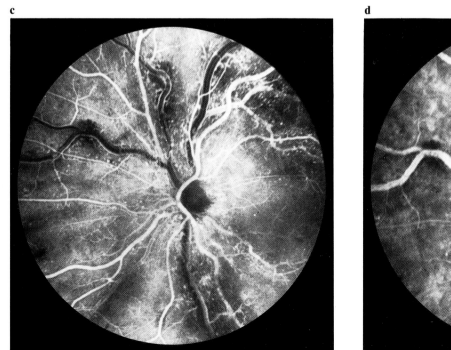

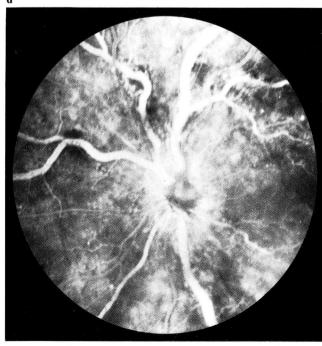

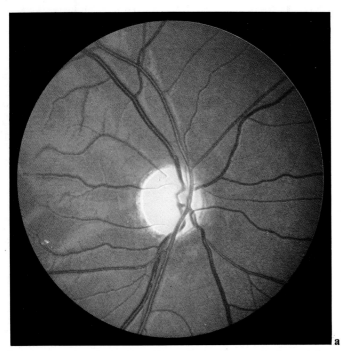 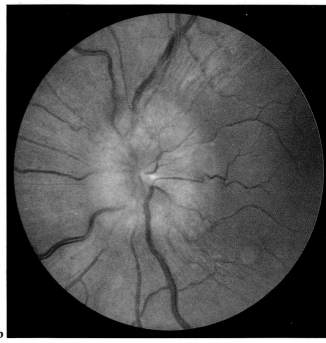

a b

Fig. 132. a) and **b)** Foster-Kennedy syndrome. Optic atrophy on the right **(a)** and disc edema on the left side **(b)**.

OPTIC ATROPHY

Optic atrophy means an ophthalmoscopic and functional degeneration of the optic nerve fibers in front of the lateral geniculate body.

The ophthalmoscopic picture of optic atrophy consists in a pallor of the optic nervehead, but atrophy and disc pallor are not synonymous. There are indeed eyes with pale discs, even advanced ones, without atrophy of nerve fibers and on the other hand there are atrophies of the optic nerve which do not express themselves as pallor of the disc. The discoloration of the optic nervehead may be total, partial or in one sector only. The papillomacular bundle is most vulnerable and therefore produces often initially a temporal pallor. The degeneration of the optic nerve fibers may be so severe that the cribriform plate becomes bared. On the other hand, the physiologic excavation may after an inflammation or a severe edema be filled with glial elements. The disc margins may be sharp (in primary atrophy) or blurred (in secondary atrophy). The retinal arteries may be normal, e.g., in cases of compression of the intercranial part of the optic nerve or of the chiasm; they may be constricted, e.g., in retinitis pigmentosa, or they may be thread-like, e.g., in an atrophy secondary to a central artery occlusion.

In the post-edematous optic atrophy the arteries are often surrounded by a sheath, while the veins are not markedly dilated.

From an ophthalmoscopic point of view and for a better understanding of the clinical course and the pathogenesis the optic atrophies may be classified into:

— with sharp disc margins (primary),
— with blurred disc margins (secondary),
— with a deep excavation.

Optic atrophy with sharp disc margins (primary) (Figs. 133 a, d). This is a total atrophy, e.g., in tabes or in generalized paralysis; the disc appears greyish-white with well defined margins and with an excavation at the bottom of which the cribriform plate may be visible. The capillaries are usually not visible; the atrophic process may involve only one sector. Most often involved is in these cases the temporal half of the disc indicating an isolated degeneration of the papillomacular bundle.

Optic atrophy with blurred disc margins (secondary) (Figs. 134 a, b). This is due to a pure disc edema (stasis) or to a secondary edema (papillitis). The optic nervehead appears grey-white, glial tissue fills the excavation and extends over the margins of the disc which thereby loses its sharp outline. There is frequently a rim of pigmentary disturbances indicating an alteration of the peripapillary choroid.

Optic atrophy with excavation (Figs. 135 a, b). This is classical and characteristic for glaucoma, though it is not pathognomonic for this disease; it may be found also in other conditions involving an insufficiency of the capillary network of the second layer (prelaminar) in the optic nervehead, e.g., arteriosclerosis (Fig. 136 a) and certain intoxications, e.g., methyl alcohol (Fig. 136 b) (pseudoglaucoma).

The nasal displacement of the vessels as they emerge from the optic nervehead, the characteristic bend which these vessels make in order to course around the disc margin, the size of the excavation (cup-disc ratio) and finally the disc pallor make up the classical ophthalmoscopic picture. In the hereditary optic atrophy of the recessive type the optic nervehead is also often excavated and pale. On the basis of our microscopic anatomical studies we found that the excavation of the optic nervehead is determined by a number of vascular factors, the pivotal one is the circle of Zinn-Haller. The pathogenesis of the excavation as it occurs in the last stage of glaucoma is intimately connected with the vascular network which supports and supplies these structures.

Like all other vascular systems, this one consists of (Fig. 137):

— an afferent system consisting of the branches of the short posterior ciliary arteries which form the above-mentioned circle of Zinn-Haller; these vessels surround the intraocular part of the optic nervehead (laminar part);
— the terminal branches consisting of:
  — the perforating branches of the first order which come from the circle of Zinn-Haller, penetrate radially into the interfibrillary spaces of the axon cylinders in the optic nervehead;
  — retrograde coaxial vessels which, numbering 10-12, may originate from the circle of Zinn-Haller, penetrate the nerve, run coaxial with it and then peter out about 4-5 mm from their origin;
  — perforating branches of the second order originating from the coaxial retrograde blood vessels penetrate perpendicularly the optic nervehead behind the globe between the head and the actual body of the optic nerve in an area which could be defined as the "collar" of the optic nerve.

When transilluminating a microscopic specimen of the optic nerve (Fig. 138 a) we can see the entire circle of Zinn-Haller and the afferent vessels consisting of the two temporal and nasal branches of the posterior ciliary arteries. Fig. 138 b shows the vascular circle around the optic nerve seen from the choroidal side; in the center of the transilluminated optic nerve is the central retinal artery, whereas in Figs. 139 a, b the terminal vessels around the optic nerve can be recognized. In the first case we see the perforating branches of the first order which course from the circle of Zinn-Haller within the optic nerve ending in a tight interfibrillary network; in the center of the nerve are the large trunks of the central artery and vein. In the second case the techniques of microdissection and injection show the retrograde coaxial vessels which course from the circle of Zinn-Haller posteriorly in the collar of the optic nerve; from these originate the perforating branches of the second order. Following this morphologic arrangement it is easy to comprehend what the consequences of an altered hemodynamic situation with increased intraocular pressure could mean: the increased pressure (Fig. 137) will be transferred through the choroidal layers to the short posterior ciliary arteries and from there via the appropriate branches to the circle of Zinn-Haller; from the circle the pressure is transmitted to the perforating branches of the first and second order, the terminal branches of nutrition to the nervous structures of the optic nervehead and of the retrolaminar area; the trophic damage to these structures will lead to an excavation of the disc (Figs. 140 a, c).

Symptomatology

There is no direct relation between the pallor of the optic nervehead and functional loss. The functional loss is an expression of the involvement of the anterior optic pathway, from the optic nervehead to the lateral geniculate body. Perimetric examinations are obviously relevant when the atrophic process progresses: there will be nerve fiber bundle defects when the optic nervehead is involved, heteronymous hemianopic lesions when the chiasma is involved and homonymous lesions when the tract is affected. In the end stage of optic atrophy we find a general constriction of all isopters as a sign that nearly all nerve fibers are involved.

The light sense may also be damaged: the threshold values will rise earlier in an atrophy secondary to papillitis than in an atrophy following pure disc edema. Color vision shows mainly changes in the green-red axis. The electrophysiologic tests show quite characteristic changes: the ERG is normal in cases of descending optic atrophy; it is diminished in ascending optic atrophy. The visually evoked potentials are altered corresponding to the functional deficit.

Fluorescein angiography gives in optic atrophy two rather distinct pictures:

— absence of staining of the optic nervehead during the entire angiography with a clear band of peripapillary fluorescence in the arteriovenous phase;
— normal staining of the nervehead and generalized atrophy of the retinal pigment epithelium.

The first picture is an expression of pathologic changes in the peripapillary choroidal vasculature; the second picture shows a selective affection of the cells and fibers of the neural tissue without vascular changes.

Differential diagnosis

The differential diagnosis of optic atrophy is mainly concerned with pseudo-atrophies of which the most important are: abnormal physiologic excavation, hypopigmentation of the optic nervehead in blonde individuals, myopia, the newborn, the aged patient, the aphakic eye; dysplasia, hypoplasis or retarded myelinization of the nerve; coloboma of the optic nervehead, pits or deep drusen of the disc.

Etiology

Examining the fundus will often give us a clue as to the etiology of the optic atrophy: occlusion of the central retinal artery or its branches, various maculopathies, foci of chorioretinitis, old juxtapapillary chorioretinitis, peripheral tapeto-retinal degenerations, etc.

A more complete and rational systematic classification distinguishes in principle two groups of atrophy:

— optic atrophy with excavation,
— optic atrophy without excavation.

With excavation. An irrigation deficit of the capillary network in the optic nervehead leads to a chronic decrease in blood flow with slow progression. There is progressive and irreversible decrease in the number of nerve fibers; Schnabel cavities form and enlarge; the tissue of the optic nervehead becomes atrophic and the lamina cribrosa becomes more and more visible. Such a deficit in blood flow can be produced by a change in the relationship between the intraocular pressure and the perfusion pressure of the capillaries (normative pressure), or may be secondary to a decrease in flow in the carotid or the ophthalmic arteries, or may be due to changes in the walls of the blood vessels (vascular sclerosis). Among the three optic atrophies with excavation are:

— *congenital glaucoma:* often in the form of a late excavation, in which the optic nervehead may become excavated while the scleral wall offers a certain resistance;
— *primary glaucomas of the adult;*
— *secondary glaucomas;*
— *low tension glaucoma of Von Graefe;*
— *pseudoglaucomas:*
    — methyl alcohol intoxication,
    — hereditary atrophy of the recessive type.

Without excavation

Hereditary optic atrophies

— Infantile hereditary optic atrophy transmitted as a dominant.
— Leber's optic atrophy, sex linked.
— Optic atrophy in lipid storage diseases (infantile form of Tay Sachs, juvenile peripheral form of Spielmeyer-Vogt, Hand-Schüller-Christian disease).

— Optic atrophy in hereditary demyelinating diseases (diffuse cerebral sclerosis, leukodystrophy).
— Optic atrophy in hereditary spinal ponto-cerebellar degenerations (optic atrophy of Behr, hereditary ataxia of Pierre-Marie).
— Optic atrophy in neuro-ectodermal dysplasias (incontinentia pigmenti).
— Optic atrophy in chondodystrophy or cranio-stenosis.
— Optic atrophy in tapeto-retinal degenerations.

Acquired

— Trauma to the orbit, cranium and face.
— Compression of the orbital, intracanalicular or intracranial part of the optic nerve including the chiasm and the optic tract. This may be due to solid tumors, fluid accumulation or vascular lesions.
— Intracranial hypertension.
— Meningitis.
— Malformations of the central nervous system.
— Vascular lesions: intracranial aneurysms of the anterior cerebral and anterior communicating arteries, thrombosis of the carotid (optic or pyramidal syndrome); severe hemorrhages; occlusion of the central retinal artery and its branches; vascular pseudopapillitis; aortic arch syndrome (Takayasu); systemic vasculitis and connective tissue diseases; secondary to surgical interventions on the teeth or the face with retrobulbar injection of a local anesthetic.
— Infections and inflammations: Opticochiasmatic arachnoiditis, systemic infectious diseases of the central nervous system (especially syphilis), meningitis secondary to a purulent sinusitis, etc. Optic neuritis in herpes zoster, Behçet disease, acquired viral pseudo-retinitis pigmentosa.
— Toxic conditions: always bilateral, atrophy secondary to various exogenous intoxications (alcohol, tobacco, lead, benzene, carbon sulphate, manganese, thallium, streptomycin, ethambutol, isoniazide, chloroquin, felix maris, methyl alcohol, and endogenous toxins [diabetes, gout, etc.]).

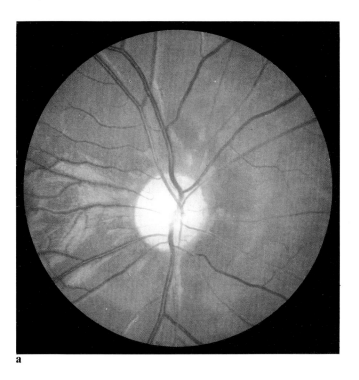

a

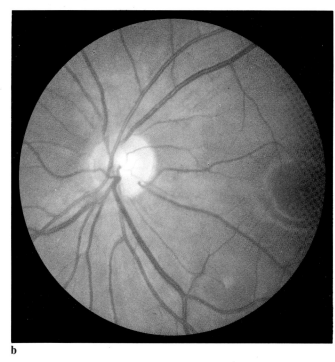

b

Fig. 133. Primary optic atrophy (with sharp disc margins).
a) Primary optic atrophy with sharp margins.
b) Primary optic atrophy occupying one sector.
c) Primary optic atrophy with sharp disc margins in a case of retinitis pigmentosa (the arteries are markedly attenuated).
d) Primary optic atrophy with sharp disc margins; the end result of an occlusion of the central retinal artery (thread-like arteries).

c

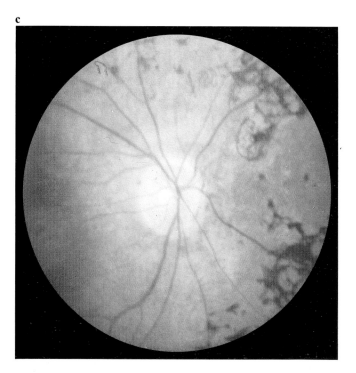

d

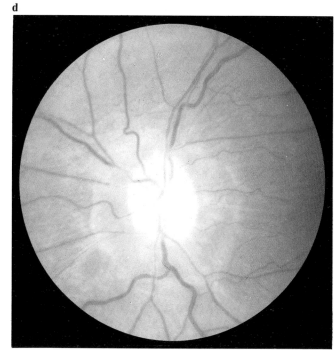

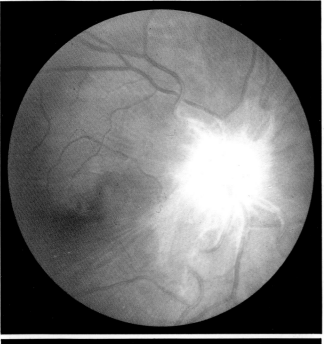

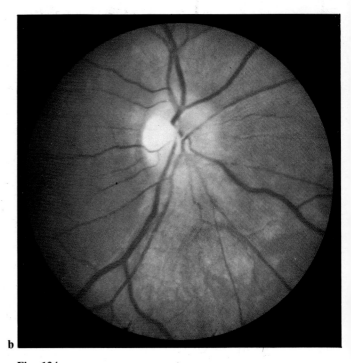

a   b

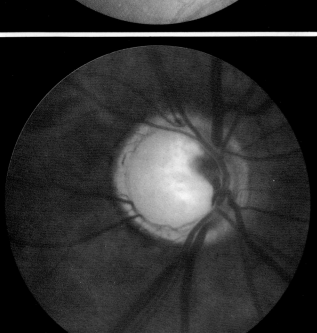

Fig. 134.
a) Optic atrophy with blurred disc margins secondary to disc edema.
b) Sector shaped optic atrophy with blurred disc margins secondary to papillitis.

Fig. 135.   **a)** and **b)** Glaucomatous optic atrophy with excavation.

a   b

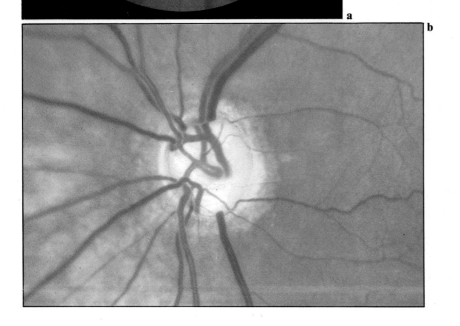

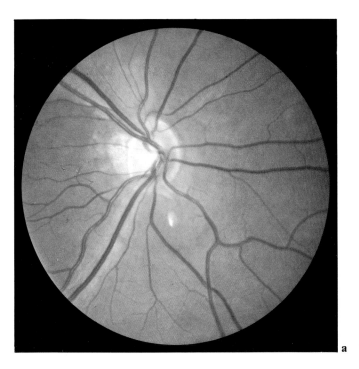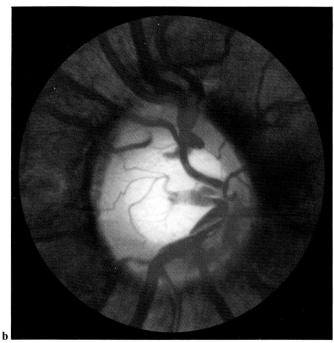

a   b

Fig. 136. Optic atrophy with non-glaucomatous excavation.
a) Optic atrophy due to arteriosclerosis.
b) Partial optic atrophy due to methyl alcohol poisoning.

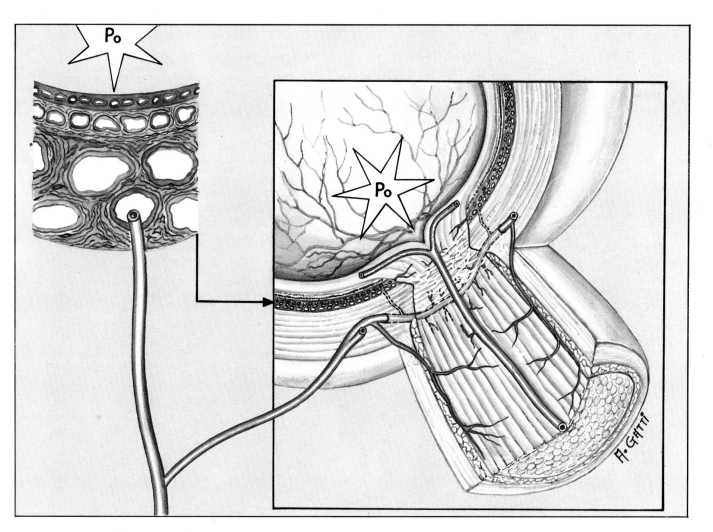

Fig. 137. Proposed hemodynamic pathogenesis of the disc excavation shown on the blood vessels around the optic nerve.
Po = intraocular pressure.

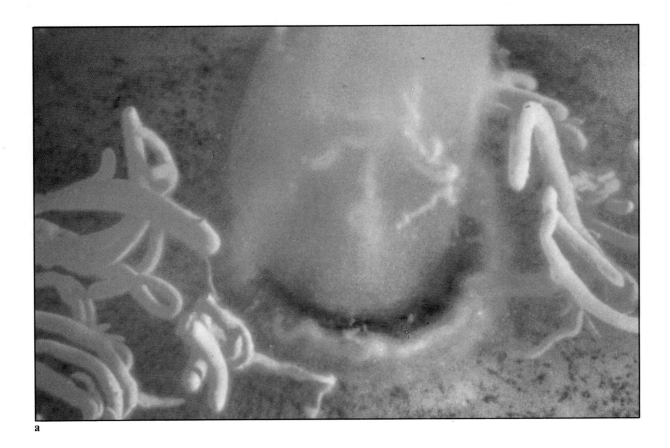

a

Fig. 138.   Microscopic specimens with injection of neoprene latex.
a) The vascular circle around the optic nerve which is being transilluminated; on both sides and contiguous the afferent nasal and temporal branches of the short posterior ciliary arteries.
b) Vascular circle around the optic nerve seen from the choroidal side; the trans-illumination of the nerve allows visualization of the central retinal artery.

b

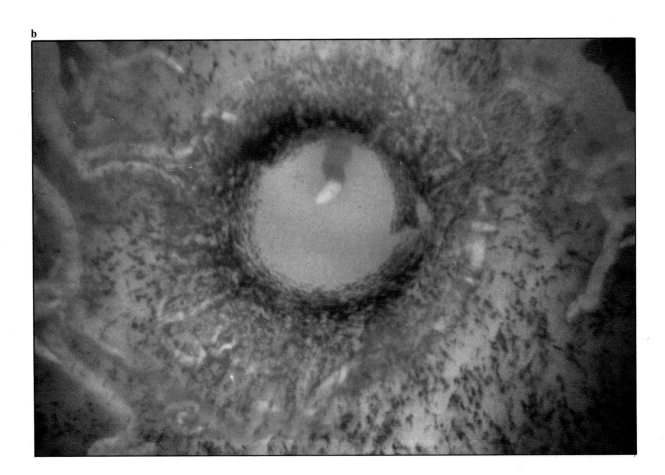

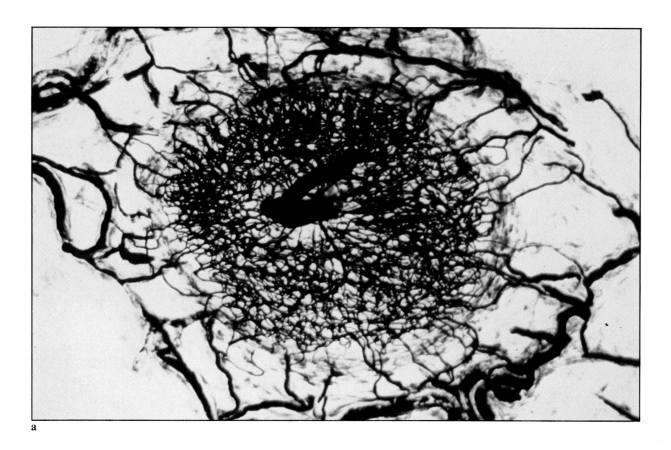

a

Fig. 139. Microscopic specimens after injection of indian ink.
a) The terminal branches from the perforating branches of the first order.
b) The coaxial retrograde vessels and the perforating branches of the second order.

b.

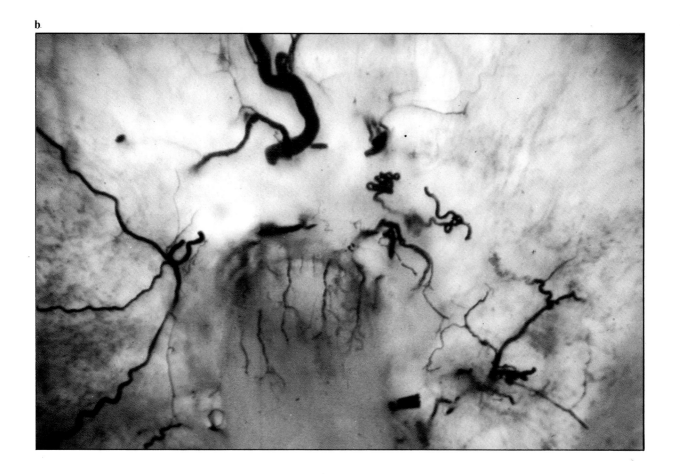

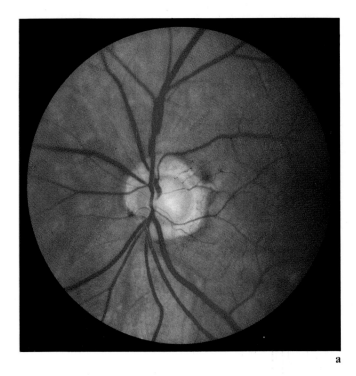

a

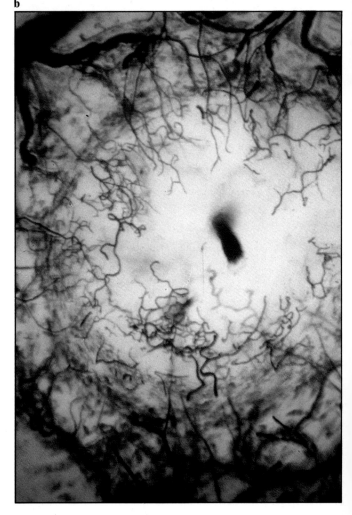

b

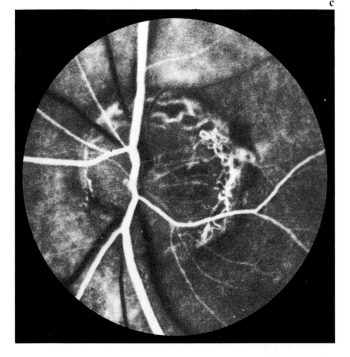

c

Fig. 140. Primary open angle glaucoma. The optic nervehead is nearly completely atrophic, excavated, resembling a pea-pot, disc-cup ratio = 1.0, mother of pearl appearance of the bottom of the excavation; marginal step is particularly evident on the vessels coming from the temporal side; glaucomatous peripapillary halo; the ophthalmoscopic picture (**a**) is corroborated by functional deficits and determined by the degree of hypertension, the function of the capillaries around the optic nerve demonstrated here in a microscopic specimen by the injection technique (**b**) and in a fluorescein angiogram (**c**).

Chapter 6

Retinal diseases

OCCLUSION OF THE CENTRAL RETINAL ARTERY AND ITS BRANCHES

The occlusion of the central retinal artery or one of its branches is nearly always due to a thrombus or an embolus. In young patients the cause is frequently a systemic disease, e.g., a mitral valve defect, which leads to embolization; in more advanced age the thrombotic process is usually secondary to an arterial hypertension or to arteriosclerosis. The emboli may also be septic, e.g., in subacute bacterial endocarditis; non-septic emboli may come from a prolapsed mitral valve, from calcifications at the cardiac valves and from atheromatous plaques. Occlusions of retinal vessels may also occur in a number of systemic diseases, e.g., atherosclerosis, arterial hypertension, collagen diseases (particularly lupus erythematosus, panarteritis nodosa and temporal arteritis), with oral contraceptives, sickle cell disease and polycythemia.

In young individuals the vascular occlusion may also be due to a prolonged angiospasm caused by neurovegetative imbalances or by paroxysms of hypertensive crises. In these instances the occlusion may be reversible (transitory ischemic attacks), but repeated spasms may in time lead to a progressive optic atrophy.

The *occlusion of the central retinal artery* leads to a sudden and total loss of vision. The ophthalmoscopic picture is characteristic; the entire fundus appears grey-yellow and milky because of the diffuse ischemic edema; at the posterior pole in the foveal area is the cherry red spot. The retinal arteries are thread-like with fragmentation of the blood flow which may also be seen in the veins. Occasionally we see peripapillary hemorrhages (Figs. 141, 142).
In about 20% of the eyes a cilio-retinal artery is present. This vessel derives from the choroidal circulation and permits preservation of central vision when the central retinal artery is occluded; ophthalmoscopically we see between the optic nervehead and the macula a zone of normal red retina. This zone has a triangular shape with the base toward the disc; it is sharply delineated from the greyish edema of the surrounding retina (Figs. 143, 144).
After about two weeks the edema absorbs completely and the atrophy of the optic nervehead becomes obvious. The retinal vessels show various degrees of sheathing due to degenerative processes in the vessel wall; in some cases white chords may replace the vessels (Fig. 145) (see Chapter 2).

In a *branch artery occlusion* the ophthalmoscopic changes and the loss of function are limited to the area supplied by the occluded vessel. The visual field may show an altitudinal hemianopia or quadrantanopia, whereas the ophthalmoscopic examination shows a retinal infarct distant from the occluded artery characterized by ischemic edema sharply demarcated from the surrounding healthy retina (Fig. 146). In these cases optic atrophy may also develop though it usually only involves one sector.
Therapy should be initiated as soon as possible consisting of vasodilators and anticoagulants in order to improve blood flow, and of corticosteroids in order to reduce the edema.
Hyperbaric therapy has recently been found to be useful.
Treating the underlying systemic disease is of the utmost importance in order to prevent further occlusive episodes in the other eye as it will frequently happen in connective tissue diseases.

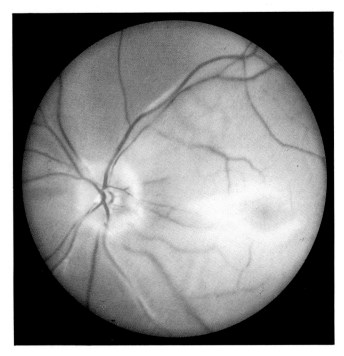

Fig. 141. Occlusion of the central retinal artery. Diffuse ischemic retinal edema, thread-like arteries with fragmented blood flow (box car phenomenon).

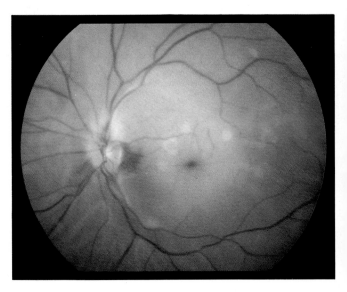

Fig. 142. Occlusion of the central retinal artery: cherry red spot in the macula and juxtapapillary hemorrhage.

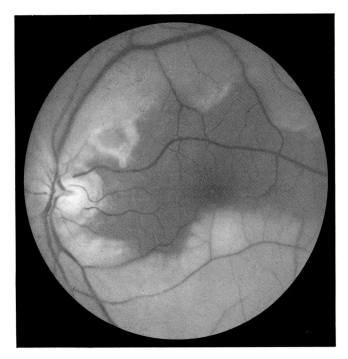

Fig. 143. Occlusion of the central retinal artery in the presence of an unaffected cilio-retinal artery.

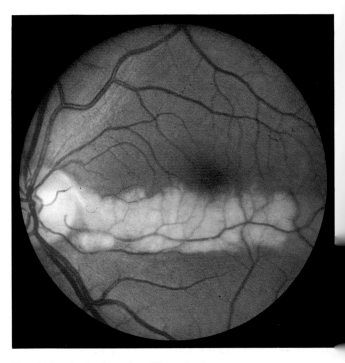

Fig. 144. Occlusion of a cilio-retinal artery.

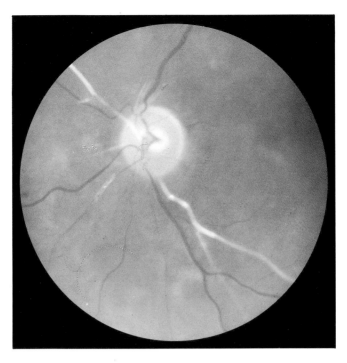

Fig. 145. Occlusion of the central retinal artery. End stage with white cords replacing the arterioles; optic atrophy (arterio-sclerotic).

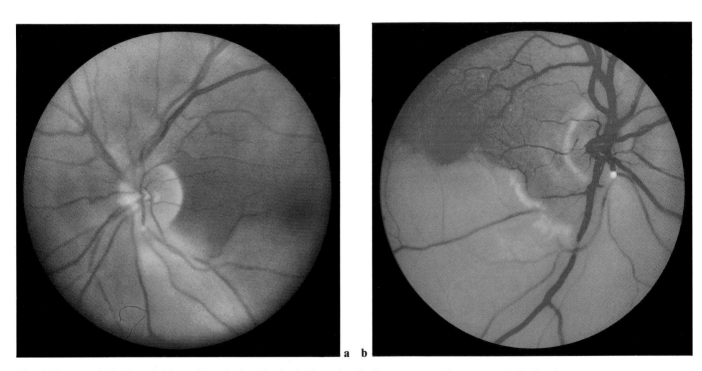

a b

Fig. 146. **a** and **b**). Arterial branch occlusion. Retinal edema in the lower temporal segment of the fundus.

OCCLUSION OF THE CENTRAL RETINAL VEIN AND ITS BRANCHES

Occlusion of the central vein and its branches is more frequently seen than an occlusion of the corresponding artery. The relationship is about 4:1.

This event may be encountered in arterial hypertension, arteriosclerosis, diabetes, in diseases characterized by thrombophlebitis, e.g., Behçet's disease, and in diseases associated with blood hyperviscosity, e.g., leukemia, polycythemia, and myeloma; in these conditions the vascular accident may be bilateral. Occasionally, especially in young patients, it may be possible to determine the cause.

Several factors contribute to the development of retinal thrombosis and often a number of them occur concommitantly, such as venous stasis due to local compression or, more rarely, systemic stasis, endothelial proliferations, blood hyperviscosity and increase of intraocular pressure. Branch vein occlusions are nearly always due to arterial hypertension and arteriosclerosis; they occur usually at the level of an arteriovenous crossing.

The *occlusion of the central retinal vein* manifests itself by sudden and severe loss of vision, but not with complete amaurosis as we see it in arterial occlusion. The ophthalmoscopic picture is characterized by severe hyperemia and edema of the optic nervehead; the veins are dilated, tortuous and dark (Figs. 147, 148). There are numerous flame-shaped hemorrhages, often arranged in rays on the disc area and along the retinal veins (as if ketchup had been thrown against the fundus (Figs. 149-151). In the retinal periphery the hemorrhages lose their flame-shaped appearance and become round, dark and blot-like. There are frequently polygonal white exudates, similar to cotton wool spots, distributed among the hemorrhages (Fig. 149). The evolution of a venous thrombosis is prolonged and insiduous; the absorption of the blood is slow and often incomplete. Sometimes there is also a hemorrhage into the vitreous.
Degenerative lesions in the vessel wall are frequent. The ischemia produces a vasoproliferative factor leading to newformed blood vessels in the retina and on the iris (rubeosis iridis); this may result in a neovascular glaucoma.

In *branch vein occlusions* the visual disturbances ar more variable and depend upon the involvement of the macular area. Ophthalmoscopically the affected area presents as a hemorrhagic triangle with the apex pointing to an arteriovenous crossing; the base lies toward the retinal periphery. The area consists of flame-shaped hemorrhages and occasionally also of white exudates, the cotton wool spots. Distal from the arteriovenous crossing the vein is extremely dilated and tortuous, whereas downstream of it is thread-like carrying practically no blood (Fig. 152). The cotton wool spots (or soft exudates) are a characteristic sign of a localized retinal infarct or, more frequently, the late stage of a hemorrhage.
The branch vein occlusion also develops slowly; the thrombosed vein is reduced to a whitish chord while the anastomoses between veins and capillaries appear to compensate for the blocked circulation.
If the superior temporal vein is involved the prognosis is serious because the hemorrhages and the edema are localized in the macular area producing frequently irreversible degenerative changes (disciform degeneration, macular hole). The treatment of a central vein occlusion consists mainly in the treatment of the underlying systemic disease. Laser therapy may be useful in the prevention of complications, e.g., the neovascular glaucoma.

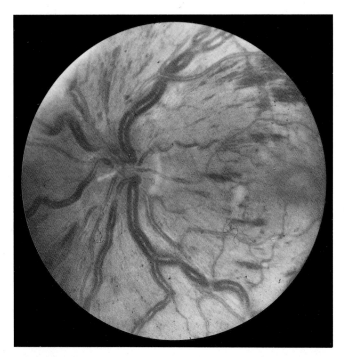

Fig. 147. Occlusion of the central retinal vein: venous congestion, dilatation and tortuousity; numerous peripapillary flame-shaped hemorrhages and hyperemia of the disc in a patient with macroglobulinemia of Waldenström.

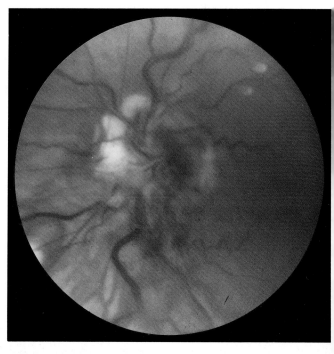

Fig. 148. Early stage of a central retinal vein occlusion in a myopic patient with arteriosclerosis: hyperemia, congestion and hemorrhages of the optic nervehead.

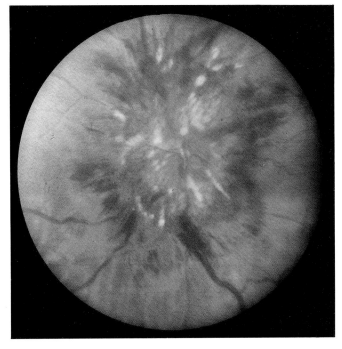

Fig. 149

Figs. 149-151. Central retinal vein occlusion: numerous hemorrhages splashed over the posterior pole; cotton-wool patches in various sizes; the disc is obscured by edema, hyperemia and hemorrhages.

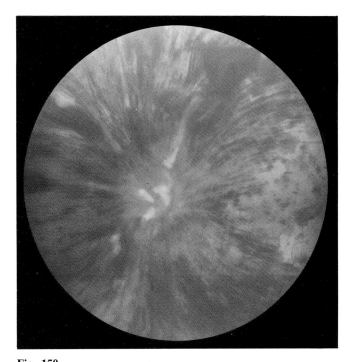

Fig. 150

Fig. 151

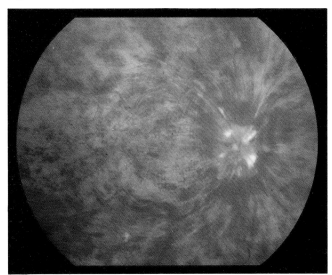

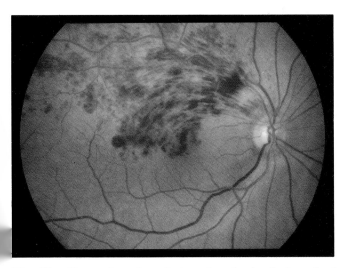

Fig. 152. Venous branch occlusion: thrombosis of a branch of the upper temporal vein, flame-shaped hemorrhages in a triangular arrangement.

RETINOPATHIES
IN SYSTEMIC DISEASES

DIABETIC RETINOPATHY

The retinopathy is one of the most important ocular manifestations of diabetes and is an expression of the generalized angiopathy found in this disease.

During the last fifty years diabetic retinopathy has increased in frequency to an astonishing degree. In fact, with the introduction of insulin and of oral hypoglycemic medications the natural history of diabetes has been modified resulting in a considerable increase in life expectancy. The modern therapeutic measures have, however, not influenced the vascular damages, especially the retinopathy. The incidence of this latter complication has progressively increased from 14-15% during the years 1930-1935 to 45-50% at the present time. The frequency of retinopathy is especially high in juvenile diabetes, but has increased in all age groups corresponding to the increase in the duration of diabetes. This means that after 10-15 years of diabetes 50% of the patients will be affected; after 20-25 years 80% of

diabetes. In addition to the metabolic control it seems that in insulin dependent patients genetic factors also influence the susceptibility to the retinopathy; in these patients a relation between the retinopathy and the histocompatibility antigens HLA-DR4 has been found.

The retinal lesions and their natural course are followed with the ophthalmoscope and with fluorescein angiography. The latter method allows us to observe the smallest details of retinal circulation and enables us to make an early diagnosis of the retinopathy and to come to a more objective evaluation of the retinal lesions over the course of time (Table 2). Classically, diabetic retinopathy is divided into a **non-proliferative** (background) and a **proliferative** retinopathy. Among all the classifications proposed the system of Scuderi (Table 3) follows essentially anatomical clinical principles which consider the characteristics of the basic lesions as well as the stage of the disease. This classification distinguishes three different clinical forms: 1) the pure form; 2) the mixed form; 3) the proliferative retinopathy. The pure form can be subdivided into a mild, marked and severe vasculopathy.

Table 2.   The evolution of diabetic retinopathy (Brancato).

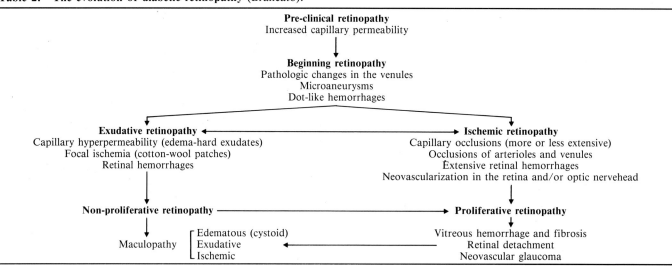

the patients or more will be involved. As a matter of fact, in the industrialized nations with the increase in life expectancy for diabetic patients this retinopathy has become one of the most frequent causes of blindness in middle age persons (20%). A well-regulated diabetes in metabolic equilibrium will decrease the incidence of the retinopathy as it will smoothen the natural course of the disease. The frequency is in relation to the duration of the disease and to the efficacy of the treatment, especially during the first years of the disease; it is independent from the severity of the

The mixed form includes the diabetic-arteriosclerotic retinopathy in which we find in the fundus not only the typical diabetic lesions, but also signs of an arteriosclerosis, as well as diabetic hypertensive (nephropathic) retinopathy in which the diabetic manifestations are seen together with those caused by renal damage in malignant hypertension. The proliferative retinopathy finally is a class by itself; it has an ominous course with a characteristic propensity for the formation of vascular and connective tissue; it may develop also from the mild or the mixed vasculopathy;

Table 3. Classification of retinal changes in diabetics (Scuderi).

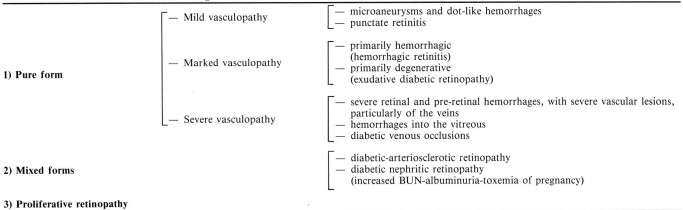

1) Pure form	— Mild vasculopathy	— microaneurysms and dot-like hemorrhages — punctate retinitis
	— Marked vasculopathy	— primarily hemorrhagic (hemorrhagic retinitis) — primarily degenerative (exudative diabetic retinopathy)
	— Severe vasculopathy	— severe retinal and pre-retinal hemorrhages, with severe vascular lesions, particularly of the veins — hemorrhages into the vitreous — diabetic venous occlusions
2) Mixed forms		— diabetic-arteriosclerotic retinopathy — diabetic nephritic retinopathy (increased BUN-albuminuria-toxemia of pregnancy)
3) Proliferative retinopathy		

once established it can develop in a completely independent fashion.

Mild vasculopathy. The first changes noticeable ophthalmoscopically and the first signs of a beginning retinopathy are the capillary microaneurysm, i.e., small circumscribed ectasias of the post-capillary venules; there may also be some small hemorrhages at the posterior pole. These hemorrhages may be due to breaks in the capillary wall, to diapedesis or stem from the adjacent microaneurysms. The *microaneurysms* appear as red dots, are usually spherical (Fig. 153), and lie in a plane that is deeper than the retinal vessels, close to the perimacular veins which appear congested. The aneurysms remain unchanged for many months, sometimes years, and with fluorescein angiography we can study their evolution, their thrombosis and hyalinization. On the angiogram the microaneurysms appear as dot-like fluorescent specks directly in contact with the capillaries. They are more numerous than one would expect from the ophthalmoscopic examination in redfree light (Fig. 154); we may also see microaneurysms that measure less than 30 μ deriving from saccular extension of a small part of the capillary wall (see Chapter 2).

Dot-like hemorrhages can be distinguished from the microaneurysms by their larger size (Figs. 155 a, b), by their darker red color and by their tendency to absorb within a few days or weeks. The differential diagnosis is better made with a fluorescein angiogram. The hemorrhages usually lie at the posterior pole and are histologically located in the inner nuclear and outer plexiform layers. They originate by diapedesis through the walls of the microaneurysms (sometimes they form a wreath around such aneurysms) and of capillaries which show congestion and stasis.

In the first stage of retinopathy we frequently also see pigmentary changes in the macula (*diabetic macular pigmentopathy*), characterized by lesions which may show hypo- and hyperpigmentation due to a dystrophic damage to the pigment epithelium and to the external retinal layers secondary to functional changes of the choriocapillaries.

The *punctate retinopathy* (Fig. 156) is in addition to microaneurysms and to dot or granular, round or irregular hemorrhages characterized by small glistening, white and well-outlined irregular deposits which over time assume a more yellowish color. They somewhat resemble bread crumbs or candle droppings. These are the *hard exudates* which occur mainly at the posterior pole, but can be found in any retinal area. Initially they constitute isolated deposits, but they have a tendency to coalesce and form large masses consisting of deposition of hyalin, lipoprotein, and lipids within the internal retinal layers (Scuderi). On fluorescein angiography these "hard exudates" appear as dark spots on the fluorescent background.

Marked vasculopathy. With the passage of time, especially in juvenile diabetics and in those that are poorly controlled, the "hard exudates" become more numerous and coalesce so that they finally occupy all or part of the macular and paramacular area (Figs. 157 a, b); they are accompanied by more or less diffuse hemorrhages, progressive vascular changes, especially of the venous part, and occlusions of the capillary network showing ophtalmoscopically the white blurred patches, the so-called "cotton-wool spots". These changes are frequently accompanied by a more or less extensive retinal edema which is usually also localized at the posterior pole.

In the *hemorrhagic form* (Fig. 158) we find flame-shaped hemorrhages, peripapillary and along the veins; these vessels show diffuse varicosities with tortuousity, loops and nodular, circumscribed and segmental ectasias. We may also see new-formed blood vessels sprouting in a brush- or tuft-like fashion from venous branchings; there may also be venous new-formations (shunts) corresponding to the occluded veins. They rejoin peripherally the original vessel. Histologically we find in these areas degenerative changes and endothelial proliferation in the veins together with hyalin and glycoprotein deposits (Figs. 159, 160).

In the *exudative form* (Fig. 162) there are in addition to the above described vascular changes and "hard exudates" —

which may coalesce and may produce the clinical picture of a circinate retinopathy — also white fluffy lesions, nodular or oval, the cotton-wool patches or *"soft exudates"*. These patches may be found anywhere in the retina and are usually less numerous than the "hard exudates". Their size varies and they may appear within a few days, disappearing rather rapidly within a few months; they may also remain unchanged for months or years. On fluorescein angiography they appear as non-fluorescent, greyish spots, usually small, but occasionally large. These lesions are the signs of a micro-infarct due to the occlusion of small arterioles in the nerve fiber layer of the retina and correspond histologically to the "cytoid bodies", the bulb-like degenerations of the interrupted axons from the retinal ganglion cells. These are round or oval structures with a "pseudonucleus", actually an accumulation of material caused by the interruption of axoplasmic flow. The vascular occlusions create ischemic retinal areas of varying sizes from which new-formed blood vessels of irregular caliber sprout. These vessels are flat or club-shaped, branching and with a rather irregular pattern of distribution and course; they break easily and may cause new hemorrhages.

Severe vasculopathy. In this stage the vascular changes increase markedly: the large veins become ectatic and ribbon-like showing varicosities. They demonstrate endo- or perivasculitis and assume the shape of a "rosary" with numerous ectasias and alternating constrictions. The capillary new-formations occur mainly at the posterior pole and are in connection with arteriovenous crossings or the bifurcations of large veins. Hemorrhages are always present, either as multiple dots at the posterior pole or as large hemorrhagic pools invading more or less extensive retinal areas. The new-formed blood vessels usually take an irregular course and extend either in the retina itself or into the virtual space between the retinal surface and the hyaloid membrane. They may advance somewhat into the vitreous. Their fragility contributes to further hemorrhages with subsequent opacification of the vitreous, organization, neovascularization and general aggravation of the pathologic process (Figs. 161; 163 a, b; 164 a, b). All these changes may be accompanied by another severe complication: the venous occlusion. This may affect a peripheral branch or the central retinal vein itself (Fig. 165). Frequently seen are preretinal hemorrhages and blood seeping into the vitreous. This does not absorb in a short period of time, but may have a tendency for organization with connective tissue proliferation in the vitreous body. In the mixed forms (diabetic-arteriosclerotic) we see in addition to these characteristic signs of a severe vasculopathy the changes caused by arteriosclerosis, hypertension or renal dysfunction (Figs. 166-168).

Proliferative Retinopathy

Proliferative retinopathy, occlusion of the central retinal vein, secondary retinal detachment and neovascular glaucoma are the most important causes of blindness in diabetics. Proliferative retinopathy can be found in 14-16% of diabetic patients with retinopathy. This condition is not pathognomonic for diabetes, but may also be seen in Eales disease, in some blood dyscrasias, in the aortic arch syndrome (Takayasu), in retinopathy of prematurity and in other conditions which cause a marked hypoxemia in one or several retinal areas. Proliferative retinopathy should not be considered as a final end-stage in the evolution of diabetic retinopathy; the development and gravity of proliferative retinopathy are independent from the type (mild, marked, severe or mixed) of the retinopathy, as well as (in part) from the state of the retinal vascular tree.

Proliferative retinopathy is characterized by capillary and connective tissue proliferations which originate in the retinal vessels and which invade the outer and inner retinal layers as well as the vitreous. This process usually begins at the disc and along the large veins; ophthalmoscopically it appears as a subtle veil with few blood vessels covering the disc and part of the posterior pole. It soon extends toward the vitreous (Figs. 169, 170). We also see linear tufts or whitish strands containing the new-formed capillaries and extending from one point to another covering one retinal quadrant, thereby pulling and elevating the retina in several areas (Figs. 171-173).

The appearance of new-formed blood vessels in front of the retina is accompanied by the production of connective tissue and by vitreo-retinal adhesions causing syneresis, disorganization and contraction of the vitreous framework. The new-formed blood vessels, stretched by the detached vitreous, may break and cause new hemorrhages while the traction on the adjacent retina may produce a detachment (Figs. 174; 175 a, b).

Recently the progression and therefore the prognosis of diabetic retinopathy have improved because of the treatment with photocoagulation, using either the xenon light or the argon laser (Figs. 163 and 164).

The aim of photocoagulation is to arrest or at least delay the progression of the retinopathy and to prevent more advanced stages with grave complications, e.g., macular edema, vitreous hemorrhage, retinal detachment and neovascular glaucoma. The objective of photocoagulation in the exudative type of diabetic retinopathy is to destroy the abnormal and leaky vessels which are often found in the center of retinal exudates. Photocoagulation of an ischemic retinopathy is aimed at the ischemic retinal periphery and attempts to prevent neovascularization with subsequent proliferative retinopathy and neovascular glaucoma.

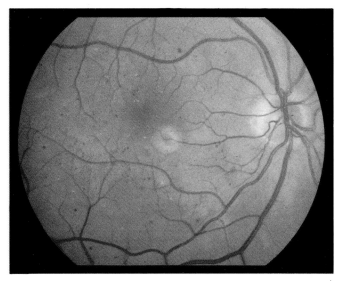

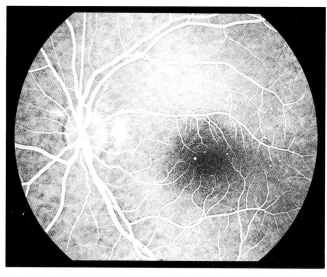

Fig. 153. Mild diabetic retinopathy. A few aneurysms, dot-like hemorrhages and small hard exudates at the posterior pole.

Fig. 154. Mild diabetic retinopathy. The fluorescein angiogram shows microaneurysms at the posterior pole. They are here more numerous than seen with the ophthalmoscope; ectasia of the perifoveal capillaries (the fundus photo of this eye did not show any noteworthy changes).

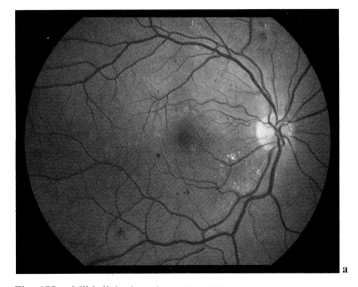

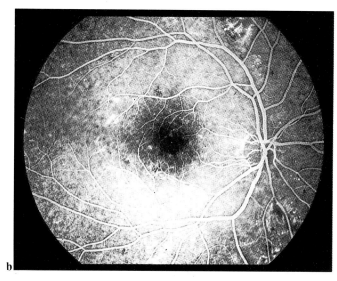

a b

Fig. 155. Mild diabetic retinopathy. Microaneurysms and dot-like hemorrhages, more numerous at the posterior pole and along the large vessels. A few hard exudates, slight macular and perimacular edema.
a) Fundus photo.
b) Fluorescein angiogram: two areas of non-profusion next to the nasal lower and temporal upper branch are visible.

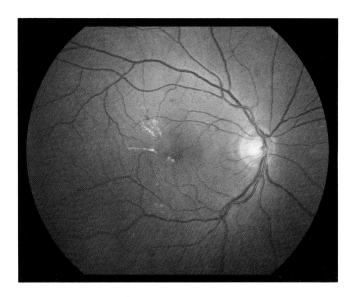

Fig. 156. Mild diabetic retinopathy (punctate retinitis). Microaneurysms, small hemorrhages of various forms and size, various hard deposits.

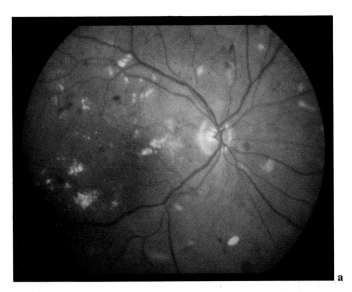 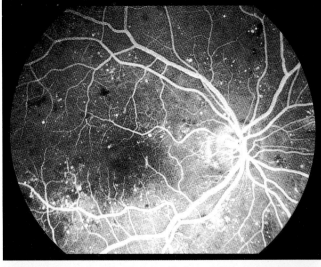

Fig. 157. Severe diabetic retinopathy. Numerous hemorrhages, microaneurysms and degenerative deposits ("hard exudates") at the posterior pole and along the vascular arcades; the retinal edema is more pronounced at the posterior pole.
a) Fundus photo.
b) Fluorescein angiogram.

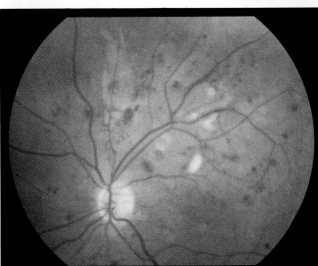

Fig. 158. Severe diabetic retinopathy, primarily hemorrhagic. Numerous hemorrhages of various forms and size; a few cotton-wool patches around the upper temporal arcade and at the posterior pole; moderate macular edema.

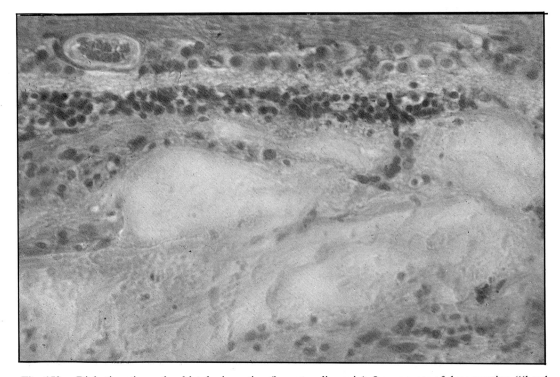

Fig. 159. Diabetic retinopathy; histologic section (hematoxylin eosin). Large areas of degeneration ("hard exudates") in the external retinal layers; an aneurysmatic thrombosed vessel is seen in the ganglion cell layer.

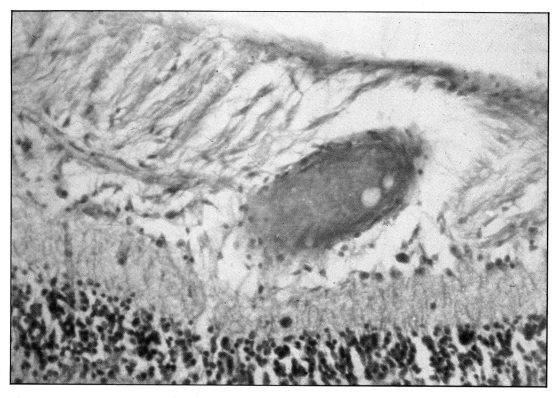

Fig. 160. Diabetic retinopathy, histologic section (hematoxylin-PAS). A thrombosed aneurysm is transformed into an amorphous mass of hyalin; the afferent capillary is still visible; considerable edema and atrophic changes in the ganglion cell and nerve fiber layers.

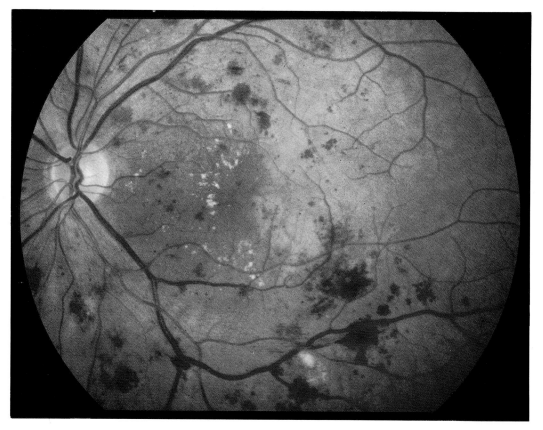

Fig. 161. Severe diabetic retinopathy. Marked congestion and irregular caliber of the veins, especially in the lower segment; numerous and diffuse hemorrhages of various size and extension; hard exudates at the posterior pole; a cotton-wool patch in the lower segment.

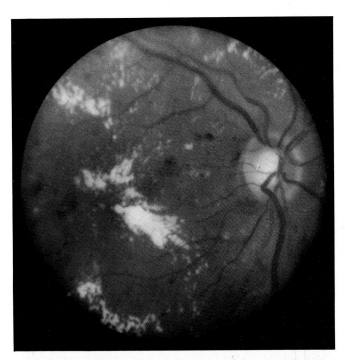

Fig. 162. Marked diabetic retinopathy, primarily degenerative. Numerous yellowish degenerative deposits resembling "old wax" (hard exudates) especially at the posterior pole; diffuse dot-like hemorrhages; congested and tortuous veins.

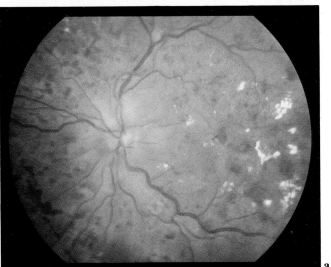 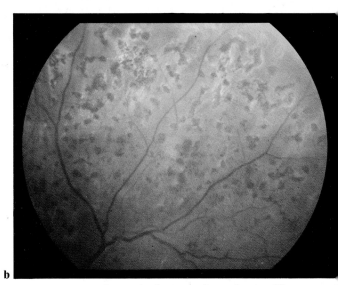

a   b

Fig. 163. Severe diabetic retinopathy: result of panretinal coagulation with the argon laser. At the posterior pole are still numerous hemorrhages and several hard exudates.
a) Posterior pole. **b)** Upper temporal quadrant.

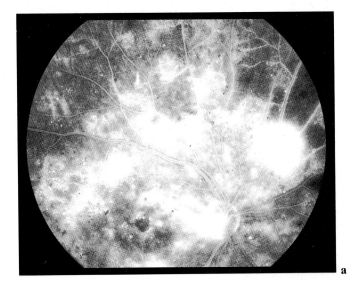 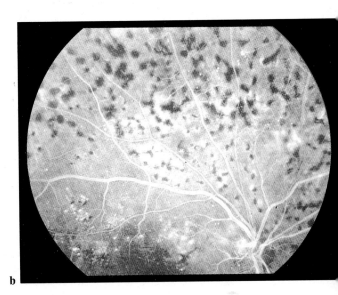

a   b

Fig. 164. Severe diabetic retinopathy. Fluorescein angiograms.
a) Microaneurysms and small hemorrhages at the posterior pole; edema of the posterior pole with large areas of non-perfusion in the mid-periphery; epiretinal neovascularization along the upper temporal arcade. **b)** After panretinal photocoagulation with the argon laser the retinal edema is reduced and there is complete regression of the epiretinal neovascularization.

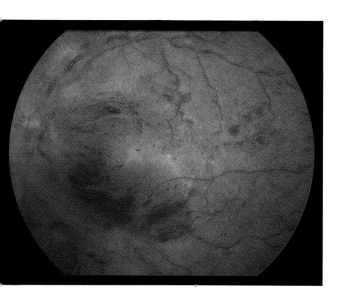

Fig. 165.   Severe diabetic retinopathy. Acute central retinal vein occlusion.

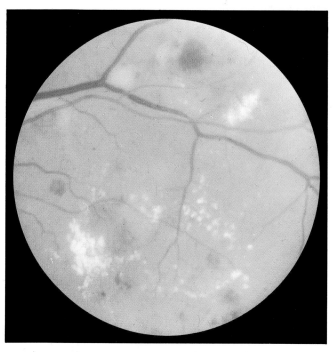

Fig. 166.   Mixed diabetic retinopathy (diabetic-arteriosclerotic-hypertensive). Thin and spastic arterioles change the arterio-venous relation (1 to 3); crossing phenomena; numerous hard exudates at the posterior pole and hemorrhages of various forms and size.

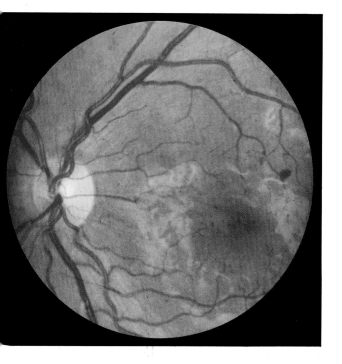

Fig. 167.   Mixed diabetic retinopathy (diabetic-uremic). Considerable macular and perimacular edema; venous congestion; small hemorrhages and perimacular microaneurysms.

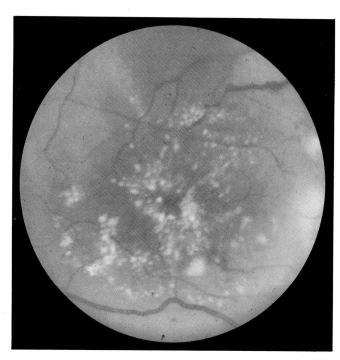

Fig. 168.   Mixed diabetic retinopathy (diabetic-uremic). The exudates have a tendency to assume a star-like arrangement around the macula; above a ribbon-like vein contains no blood.

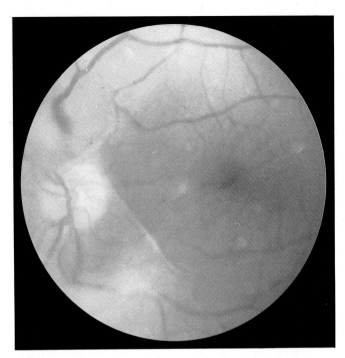

Fig. 169.   Proliferative retinopathy. A poorly vascularized proliferative veil obscures the optic nervehead and part of the surrounding retina; a few exudates at the posterior pole.

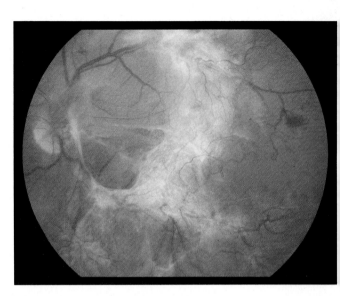

Fig. 170.   Proliferative retinopathy. An abundantly vascularized proliferative veil extends from the optic nervehead along the vascular arcade (especially above).

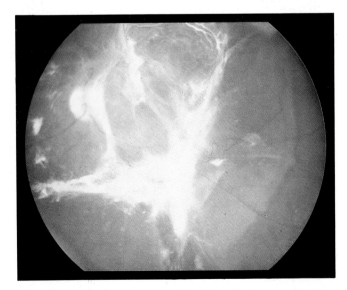

Fig. 171.   Proliferative retinopathy. Extensively sprouting area of white tendinous proliferative retinopathy covering a good part of the posterior pole.

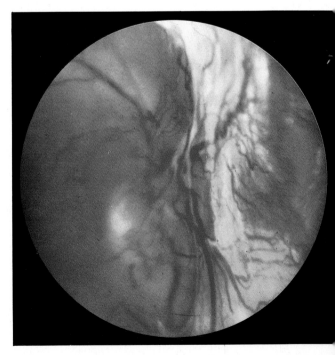

Fig. 172.   Proliferative retinopathy. Large sprouts of proliferative peripapillary retinopathy. Neovascularization at the optic nervehead.

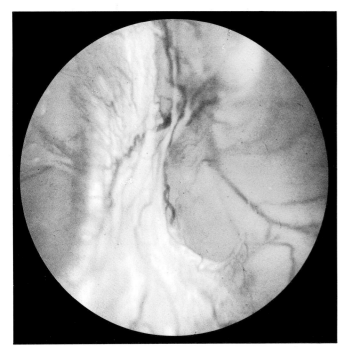

Fig. 173. Proliferative retinopathy. Large sprout of prolifcrati-ve tissue pulling and detaching the retina in several areas.

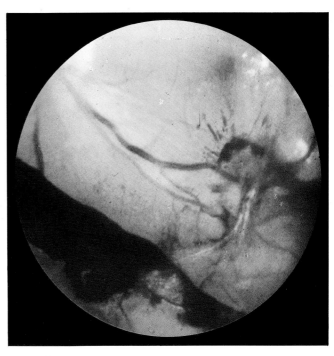

Fig. 174. Prolifcrativc rctinopathy. Ncw-formcd vcsscls and con-nective tissue in the area of the lower temporal vessels; vitreoreti-nal traction and surrounding retinal hemorrhages; large prereti-nal hemorrhage and secondary inferior retinal detachment.

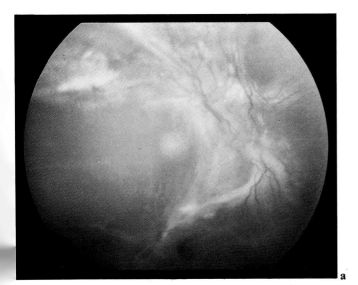
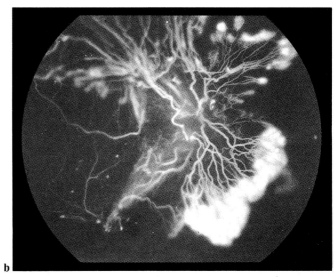

a   b

Fig. 175. Proliferative retinopathy. Marked vascular and connective tissue proliferation into the vitreous obscuring the optic nervehead and the vascular arcades.
a) Fundus photo.   **b)** Fluorescein angiogram.

HYPERTENSIVE RETINOPATHY

The retinal changes secondary to systemic hypertension represent frequently the first signs of this disease. The per chance detection of such a retinopathy permits us to establish the diagnosis and with it initiate a rapid treatment; studying the evolution of the retinopathy gives us valuable clues as to the efficacy of the antihypertensive treatment and the gravity of the systemic disease.

The effects of arterial hypertension on the retinal structure are related to the duration of the disease and the height of the arterial blood pressure. They also vary according to the pre-existing state of the retinal vessels.

According to the classification of Keith, Wagener and Barker hypertensive retinopathy can be clinically subdivided into four stages:

First stage. This is characterized by a moderate attenuation and beginning sclerosis of the retinal vessels, most conspicuous in the peripheral arterioles. These changes are mainly seen in young individuals and during the first phases of systemic hypertension (Fig. 176), i.e., before the degenerative sclerosis sets in.

Second stage. Here we find a more severe degree of vascular changes leading to arteriolar sclerosis with localized or generalized attenuation of the vessels, accompanied by arteriovenous crossing phenomena. Ophthalmoscopically the retinal arteries appear thin, rigid, taught, with irregular caliber, sometimes thread-like and with an axial reflex resembling a copper wire and later a silver wire; the veins are tortuous and slightly congested. Characteristic are the arteriovenous crossing signs with bending, dislocation and dilatation of the vein (Figs. 177, 178) (see Chapter 2).

Stage III. This stage is characterized by perivascular changes, e.g., edema, hemorrhages and retinal exudates. The retinal edema may be a barely perceptible variation of the light reflex from the ocular fundus, or it may involve vast retinal areas finally going over into an exudative retinal detachment. The hemorrhages come from the capillaries and the venules; they have a tendency to remain in the superficial retinal arteries and have the typical flame-shaped appearance. The cotton-wool patches ("soft exudates") are characteristic for this retinopathy; they appear as white-grey, superficial spots of varying size and are fluffy with blurred borders. They correspond to a focal micro-infarct in the nerve fiber layer (Fig. 179). The so-called "hard exudates" are deposited in the external plexiform layer and have a predilection for the macular area where they assume a radial arrangement (macular star) (see Chapter 2). The vascular changes progress and lead to dilatation, capillary anastomoses and venous branch occlusions. In the malignant juvenile type of hypertension signs of arterial angiospasm predominate. The disc and the retinal edema sometimes acquire extraordinary dimensions; the exudates, primarily the cotton-wool patches, become numerous and disseminated. They may coalesce and form snow banks (Fig. 180), whereas diffuse flame-shaped and dot-like hemorrhages inundate the retina.

Stage IV. In addition to the signs of the third stage we find here also stasis of the optic nervehead due to the accompanying intracranial hypertension.

The *nephritic retinopathy* is a particular type of hypertensive retinopathy; it is connected with increased BUN or albuminuria (Figs. 181, 182). In the *retinopathy of toxemia of pregnancy* the severe vascular changes in the retina also involve the uveal vessels and may cause a bilateral exudative retinal detachment which may resolve spontaneously after delivery leaving typical pigmented scars surrounded by a yellow halo and arranged along the sclerotic white choroidal vessels (Elschnig and Siegrist spots).

The treatment of hypertensive retinopathy consists in treating the underlying disease.

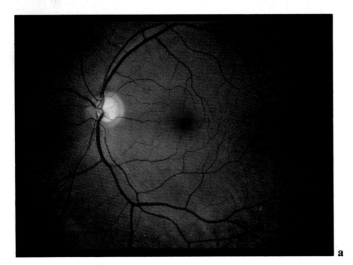 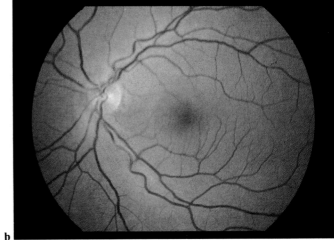

a b

Fig. 176. a) and **b)** Initial stage of hypertensive retinopathy: the arterioles are attenuated and rectilinear; the veins are congested.

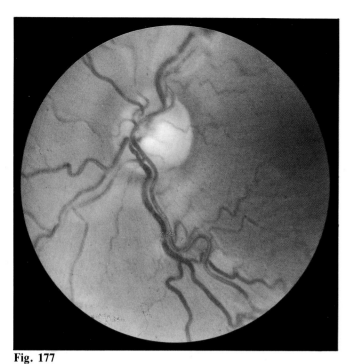

Fig. 177

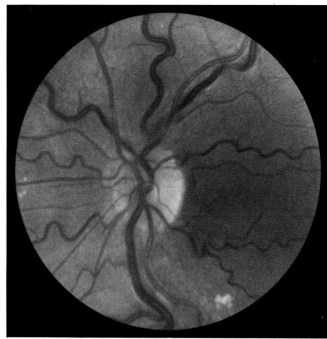

Fig. 178

Fig. 177 and **178.** Hypertensive retinopathy: copper wire arteries, venous tortuousity and congestion, early arterio-venous crossing signs, perivascular retinal edema and a few hard exudates.

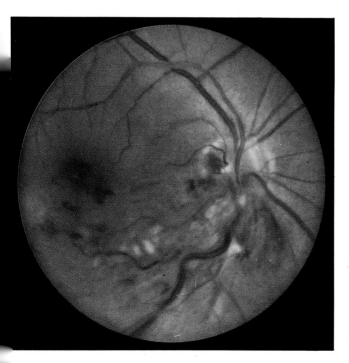

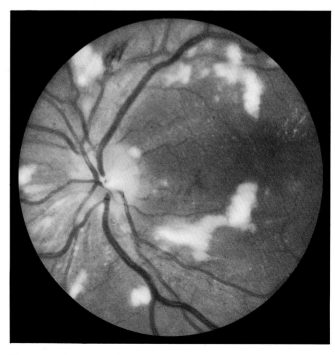

Fig. 179. Hypertensive retinopathy: arterio-venous crossing signs, flame-shaped and prepapillary hemorrhages, a few cotton-wool patches and retinal edema.

Fig. 180. Malignant hypertensive retinopathy: Numerous cotton-wool patches which coalesce to large geographic formations, arterial angiospasm and venous congestion.

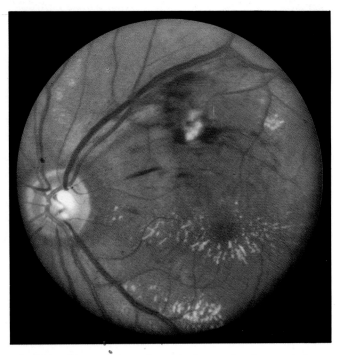

Fig. 181. Hypertensive retinopathy in uremia: characteristic macular star of hard exudates, cotton-wool patches and flameshaped hemorrhages.

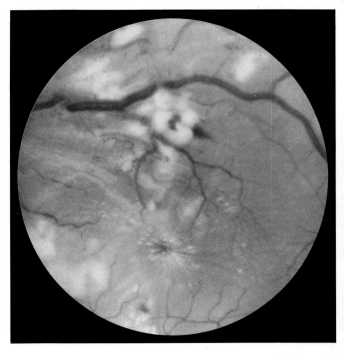

Fig. 182. Diabetic-hypertensive retinopathy: cotton-wool patches, hard exudates arranged to a macular star, venous congestion and flameshaped hemorrhages in the upper temporal quadrant.

ARTERIOSCLEROTIC RETINOPATHY

Degenerative sclerotic changes of the retinal vessels occur with advancing age and do not necessarily represent a retinopathy; the arteriolar sclerosis represents a reactive change of the middle sized arteries and arterioles to arterial hypertension. This will, at least initially, not interfere with the blood supply to the retina.

The arteriosclerotic retinopathy will develop with progression of the sclerotic degenerations and/or with arterial hypertension; the blood flow in the retinal capillaries becomes insufficient and there is subsequent anoxia of the tissues. If, however, the arteriolar sclerosis is complicated by a marked hypertension the ophthalmoscopic picture is dominated by those features which characterize hypertensive retinopathy (see page 136).

In general, the simple arteriosclerotic retinopathy progresses slowly.

The sclerotic vascular changes are nearly always bilateral, but the retinopathy may remain unilateral for a long period of time.

Ophthalmoscopically we see the classical signs of a degenerative vascular sclerosis with the typical attenuation of the arteries, which show a rectilinear course, un uneven caliber and the axial reflexes of a copper or silver wire; there is dilatation and tortuousity of the veins (Figs. 183) and finally the Gunn and Salus signs of the arteriovenous crossings appear (Fig. 184) (see Chapter 2).

With the progress of the sclerotic changes we see a sheathing of the vessels which ophthalmoscopically appears like a white line accompanying the blood column which may it-

self be reduced to a yellowish blood free thread (Figs. 185, 186). The secondary retinal anoxia manifests itself by a moderate degree of edema, often localized at the posterior pole, whereas the capillaries and veins show signs of transudation and hemorrhages. These features determine the characteristic picture of arteriosclerotic retinopathy consisting of hemorrhages associated with "hard exudates",, indicating deposits secondary to cellular destruction (Figs. 184, 187). The hemorrhages are small, disseminated, superficial or deep, often arranged along the vascular arcades.

The "hard exudates", i.e., yellowish small deposits without accompanying edema, are usually quite stable or change slowly; they occur mainly at the posterior pole (Fig. 188) from where they may extend as a macular star or they may occur along the large vessel (circinate retinopathy). In the more advanced stages degenerative macular lesions develop (macular arteriosclerotic pseudo-hole, senile disciform degeneration of Kuhnt-Junius (Figs. 189, 190) together with more or less diffuse areas of retinal and pigment epithelium atrophy through which the sclerotic vasculature of the choroid becomes visible (Fig. 191). The optic nerve also participates in this process and the disc appears pale, slightly excavated, surrounded by a peripapillary halo of choroidal degeneration and atrophy (peripapillary arteriosclerotic staphyloma) (Fig. 192).

The picture of a vascular pseudopapillitis and of a prethrombotic stage of the central retinal vein may also develop (Fig. 193). The prognosis for visual function is not good, especially because of the accompanying degenerative macular changes and the possibility of vascular complications affecting the large retinal vessels (venous or arterial occlusion) (see pages 121-125).

Fig. 183. Senile ocular fundus. Signs of arteriosclerosis with irregular course and caliber of the arteries, copper wire axial reflex and venous congestion.

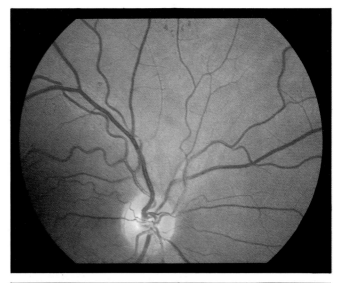

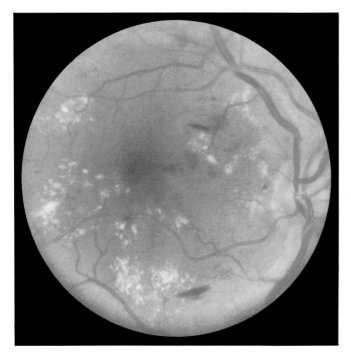

Fig. 184. Mixed retinopathy (arteriosclerotic-diabetic). Gunn and Salus signs of arterio-venous crossing; venous congestione; the arterioles are rectilinear and show a silver wire reflex; retinal hemorrhages and hard exudates.

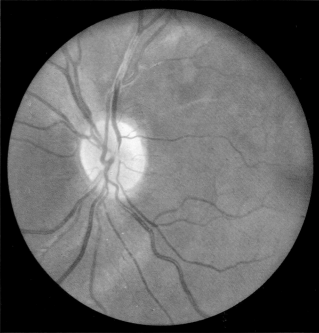

Fig. 185. Arteriosclerotic retinopathy. Conspicuous sclerosis of the entire arterial tree; sheathing of the arterioles and of the upper temporal vein distal from an arterio-venous crossing.

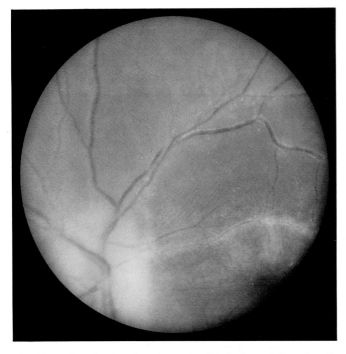

Fig. 186. Arteriosclerotic retinopathy. Marked arteriolar sclerosis with irregular caliber, sheathing and segmental occlusion. Partial optic atrophy, peripapillary edema.

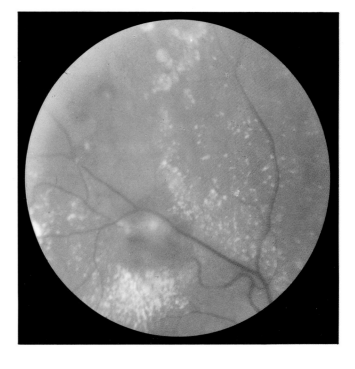

Fig. 187. Arteriosclerotic retinopathy. Hard exudates along the vascular arcades; hemorrhages and transudations accompanying an occluded terminal venule.

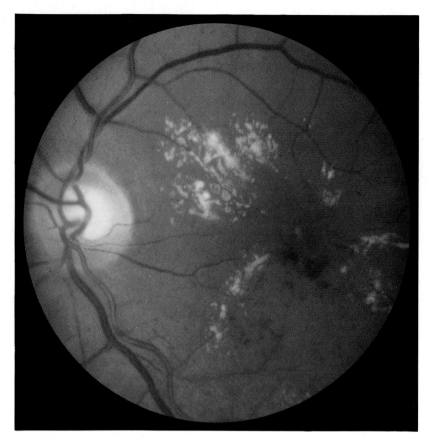

Fig. 188. Diabetic arteriosclerotic retinopathy. Hard exudates disseminated over the posterior pole with marked macular dystrophy and intra-retinal hemorrhages.

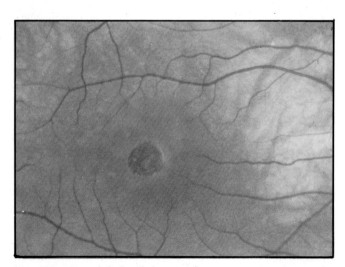

Fig. 189. Pseudohole of the macula.

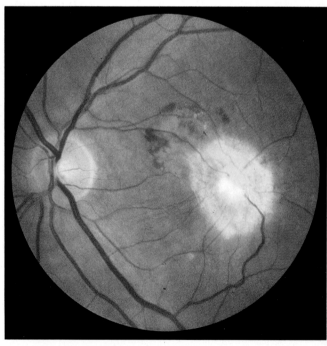

Fig. 190. Age dependent disciform macular degeneration.

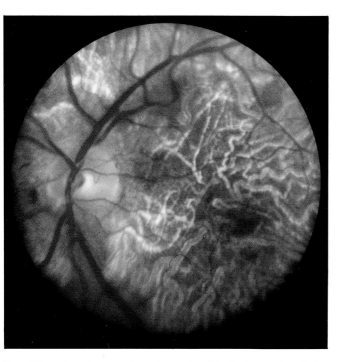

Fig. 191. Arteriosclerotic retinopathy. Marked atrophy of the retina and pigment epithelium; choroidal sclerosis.

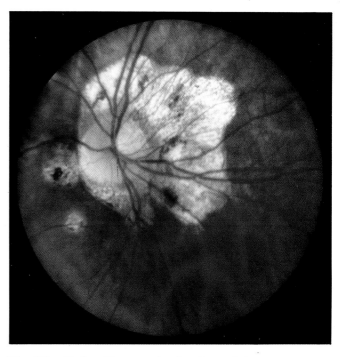

Fig. 192. Peripapillary arteriosclerotic staphyloma.

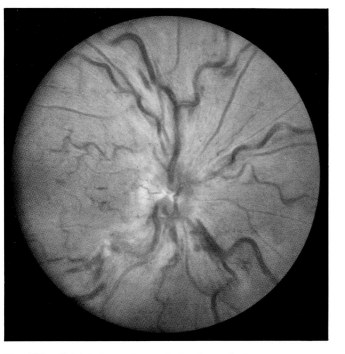

Fig. 193. Initial stage of a central vein occlusion.

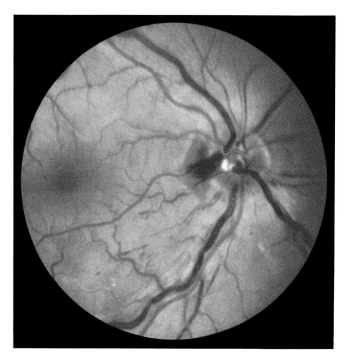

Fig. 194. Arterial hypotension (*aortic arch syndrome*). Disc edema, venous congestion, retinal hemorrhages.

RETINAL CHANGES
IN ARTERIAL HYPOTENSION

These changes are relatively rare and mild and depend upon the hypoxia of the tissues secondary to the arterial deficit involving the head.

The retinopathy begins insidiously and develops slowly. Ophthalmodynamometry is useful to reveal the hypotension in the ophthalmic artery. In the more advanced cases we may see a spontaneous pulsation of the central retinal artery when the patient changes the position of his head. More often we see this condition in occlusion or insufficiency of the internal carotid and in the aortic arch syndrome (pulseless disease, Takayasu disease). Hypotensive retinopathy is characterized by an attenuation of the retinal arterioles, cotton-wool patches, small intraretinal hemorrhages and venous stasis with dilatation or box-car phenomenon in the blood flow, microaneurysms and new-formed blood vessels (Fig. 194).

RETINAL CHANGES
WITH BLOOD DYSCRASIAS

All changes in the composition of the blood, whether of the cells or of the plasma, may give rise to retinal changes. The incidence of such changes will vary with the severity and the nature of the disease.

In the anemias the determining factor is the level of the hemoglobin and retinal hemorrhages can be expected when the hemoglobin is lower than 50% of the normal value, whereas in the leukemias the pathologic element of greatest importance is the progressive increase in the number of leukocytes. In the polycythemias the critical level of erythrocytes in the blood is around $6,000,000/mm^3$.

In all these cases a characteristic ophthalmoscopic picture may develop consisting of hemorrhages, exudates and vascular, especially venous, changes (see Chapter 2).

Polycythemia

The ophthalmoscopic picture is characterized by retinal cyanosis and by the congestion of the entire vascular system. The veins appear extremely dilated, tortuous and slate-grey or violet in color. The arteries are bright red, dilated, and tortuous, while the optic nervehead is edematous and red-purple. Stasis and blood hyperviscosity cause retinal hemorrhages, superficial and deep, as well as occlusion of the central retinal vein or one of its branches.

In secondary polycythemias the retinal lesions are less frequent and less conspicuous.

Anemias

In every type of anemia the ocular fundus is pale and appears washed out. The color intensity of the blood vessels is diminished and there is an attenuation of their caliber. There are flame-shaped and dot-like, pale, fluffy hemorrhages due to the increased permeability of the retinal capillaries; they have a prognostic significance as their number and evolution follow the course of the anemia (Fig. 195). The subretinal hemorrhages are darker in color and originate from localized extravasates in the choriocapillaries. Increased vascular permeability and anoxia secondary to decreased oxygenation of the blood produce focal microinfarcts with the formation of cotton-wool patches, diffuse retinal edema and typical disc edema.

In *pernicious anemia* we may also find changes of the optic nerve (retrobulbar neuritis and optic atrophy) due to the lack of vitamin B_{12}.

In *sickle cell anemia* we find lesions in the retinal periphery which consist of arterial occlusions followed by arteriovenous anastomoses, dilatation and tortuousity of the veins with perivascular sheathing; these changes are the end result of stasis and of the occlusion of small vessels in the retinal periphery, especially on the temporal side. The retinopathy may be proliferative or not. The non-proliferative type is characterized by salmon colored retinal hemorrhages, shiny lipid deposits, hyperplasia and migration of retinal pigment. In the proliferative form we find new-formed blood vessels and fibrovascular proliferation in the area of the posterior arteriovenous anastomoses to infarcted retinal zones producing a proliferative retinopathy (quite similar to the diabetic one or localized as a sea-fan) with subsequent bleeding into the vitreous and the retina followed by a retinal detachment.

Leukemias

The choroidal and retinal involvement in leukemia occur more frequently in the acute than in the chronic types.

Leukemic retinopathy is characterized by retinal edema and a marked venous congestion; the edema involves mainly the posterior pole, but may extend over the entire fundus giving the background a greyish-white, washed out color. The veins are swollen, tortuous and pale with a sheathing due to the leukocytic infiltration of the vessel walls; this infiltration may encompass the entire vessel producing the typical picture of the so-called "white thrombosis". The blood column appears granular. There are retinal hemorrhages of various shape, but characteristic for leukemia are the white-centered hemorrhages (Figs. 196, 197); these are usually found in the macular area and may be bilateral; the white center is due to the leukocytic infiltration whereby the leukocytes tend to agglutinate and separate from the erythrocytes. The latter are pushed toward the periphery of the extra-vasate. In addition to superficial, nonspecific exudates which accompany the retinal edema there are also white, well circumscribed, elevated exudates which appear nodular and constitute true leukemic infiltrates within the retina (Figs. 198, 199 a, b).

In the acute forms the ophthalmoscopic picture is dominated by large hemorrhages (Fig. 200) which stand out in an anemic retina with pale translucent vessels which are nearly empty of blood. The hemorrhages may be within, on, or under the retina. In the most severe cases there is a true apoplexy of the retina.

In all clinical types of leukemia the evolution and variability of the ophthalmoscopic picture are in direct relation to the evolution of the systemic disease and the efficacy of the therapy.

Dysproteinemias

The fundus picture is that of an occlusion of the central retinal vein, whether this is a macroglobulinemia, cryoglobulinemia, or multiple myeloma (Fig. 201 a, b); these diseases produce a true hyperviscosity of the blood. The retinal veins are dilated, tortuous, of irregular caliber, with flame-shaped hemorrhages, more or less extensive striae, "hard" and "soft" exudates with disc edema. These changes are usually bilateral and symmetrical.

Characteristic for this type of blood dyscrasia is the granular and fragmented blood flow in the veins which may be precipitated by pressing on the globe.

The Coagulopathies

Various types of hemorrhages may be observed in these conditions. Their number and extent are in direct relation to the severity of the systemic disease. Retinal involvement is more frequently seen in thrombocytopenia (Fig. 202).

In hemophilia the hemorrhages, often in the vitreous and the retina, follow even minor accidental or surgical trauma.

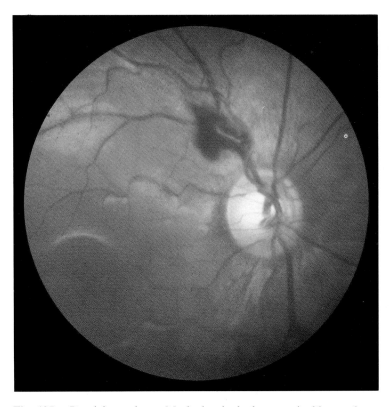

Fig. 195. Pernicious edema. Marked retinal edema, retinal hemorrhage along the upper temporal vein.

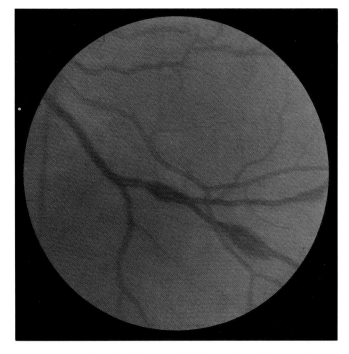

Fig. 196. Leukemia. Characteristic boat-shaped hemorrhages.

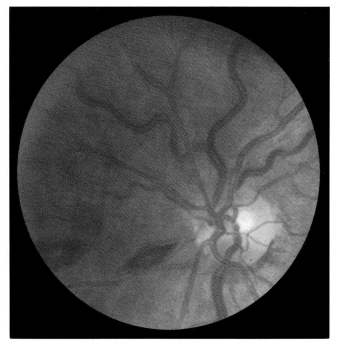

Fig. 197. Leukemia. Marked venous congestion and tortuousity, white centered, sharply outlined, round retinal hemorrhages.

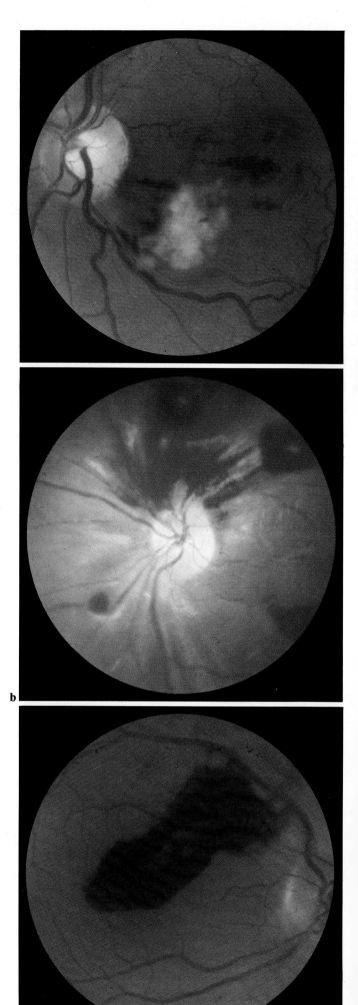

Fig. 198. Leukemic retinopathy. Venous congestion and tortuousity, hemorrhages and cotton-wool patches at the posterior pole.

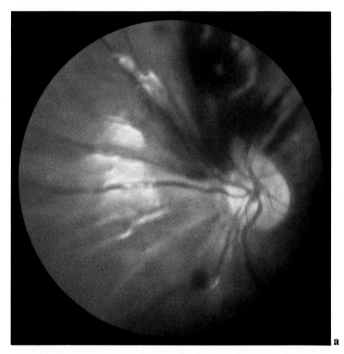

a   b

Fig. 199. **a)** and **b).** Leukemic retinopathy. Diffuse retinal edema at the posterior pole, flame-shaped and round white-centered hemorrhages due to leukemic infiltrates.

Fig. 200. Acute leukemia. Extensive retinal and preretinal hemorrhage in the macular area. In the center is a leukocytic infiltrate.

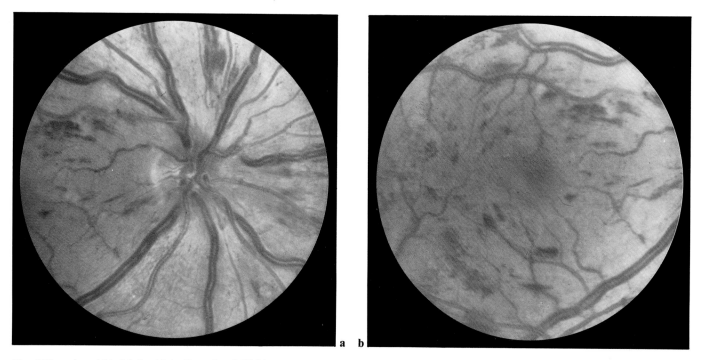

a   b

Fig. 201.   a) and b). Makroglobulinemia of Waldenström. Prodromal stage of a central retinal vein occlusion; edema and hyperemia of the optic nervehead, tortuous and dilated retinal veins, flame-shaped and round retinal hemorrhages at the posterior pole.

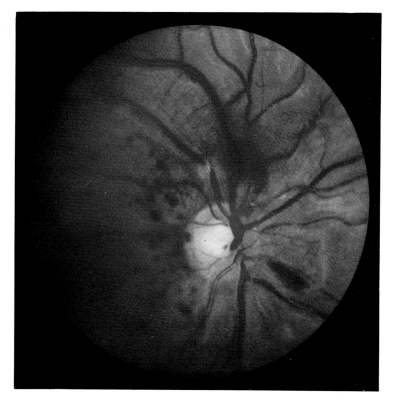

Fig. 202.   Thrombocytopenia. Flame-shaped and dot-like peripapillary retinal hemorrhages.

RETINAL CHANGES
IN COLLAGEN DISEASES

Collagen diseases may give rise to numerous ocular manifestations, especially during the acute phase of the systemic disease; during the last decade the frequency of these conditions has markedly decreased due to the introduction of appropriate and effective treatment with corticosteroids. The ophthalmoscopic changes may be an expression of the retinal vasculitis, may be secondary to the arterial hypertension or to the involvement of the central nervous system. *Toxic retinopathy* is together with the Sjögren syndrome the most frequent ocular manifestation of collagen disease. The retinopathy is observed in a higher percentage among patients with systemic lupus erythematosus, but it may also be seen in all other types. of collagen disease, with the exception of rheumatoid arthritis. This retinopathy is characterized by the development of cotton-wool patches and is the expression of a vasculitis affecting the retinal capillaries with local microinfarcts in the nerve fiber layer of the retina (cytoid bodies). In analogy with other affected tissues in which fibrinoid necrosis develops, the retinal lesions are probably due to the deposition of antigen-antibody complexes in which the antigen consists of free DNA. Ophthalmoscopically there are superficial cotton-wool patches and white deposits, mainly at the posterior pole or in the optic nervehead, which appear suddenly and then disappear after a few weeks leaving barely any or no permanent changes. In addition to these characteristic changes we often see signs of a hypertensive retinopathy and dot—, as well as flame-shaped hemorrhages as a sign of the thrombotic tendency in connective tissue diseases (Figs. 203, 204).

In the more advanced form we may see a retinal vasculitis affecting mainly the arterioles and characterized by multiple, nonembolic occlusions (Fig, 205) causing recurrent episodes of amaurosis fugax; in the acute or hyperacute forms may be also a bilateral occlusion of the central retinal artery or the central retinal vein (see pages 121-125).

The involvement of the optic nerve is mainly seen in panarteritis nodosa and in temporal arteritis producing the typical picture of an anterior ischemic optic neuropathy (vascular pseudopapillitis) (Fig. 206). The bilateral disc edema may also be secondary to an arterial hypertension or may be a disc edema (see Chapter 5) if there is also an involvement of the central nervous system.

Patients with a collagen disease and especially those who are treated for a long time with antimalarial compounds may develop an iatrogenic retinopathy. The *chloroquine retinopathy* is due to the toxic effect of the drug on the retinal pigment epithelium. This layer shows a specific sensitivity to the pharmaceutic agent. Ophthalmoscopically there is a fine granular pigmentation of the macular area which is arranged like a ring around the fovea. This may develop into a redbrown disc in the center, surrounded by an area of depigmentation (Fig. 207 a, b). These bull's- eye changes in the macula are usually bilateral and symmetrical and cause a consideral loss of central vision. Their evolution can be well documented by electrophysiologic tests and with fluorescein angiography. The development of this retinopathy is dose related.

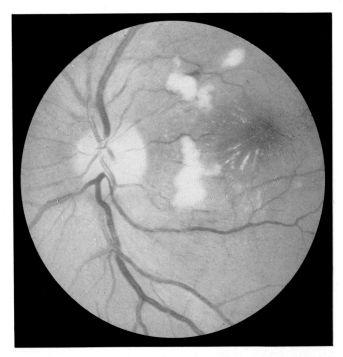

Fig. 203. Systemic lupus erythematosus. Cotton-wool patches at the posterior pole characteristic for the toxic retinopathy occurring in all forms of collagen diseases; signs of a hypertensive retinopaty.

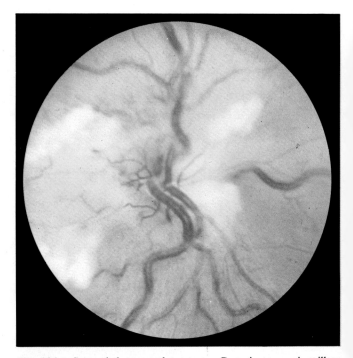

Fig. 204. Systemic lupus erythematosus. Conspicuous peripapillary cotton-wool patches; the disc is hyperemic and the margins are blurred; there are new-formed blood vessels on the disc with intensive retinal edema; congestion and tortuousity of the retinal veins.

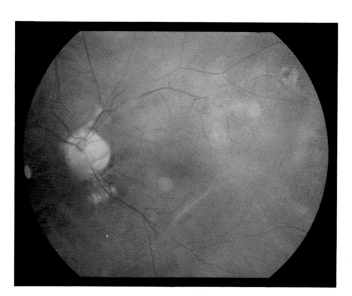

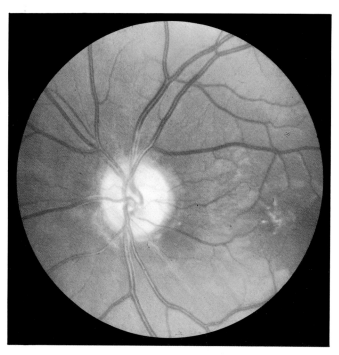

Fig. 205. Panarteritis nodosa. Marked retinal vasculitis with diffuse and segmental arteriolar occlusions; neovascularization with a tenuous proliferative membrane at the posterior pole; partial optic atrophy.

Fig. 206. Temporal arteritis (Horton). Optic atrophy secondary to a vascular pseudopapillitis.

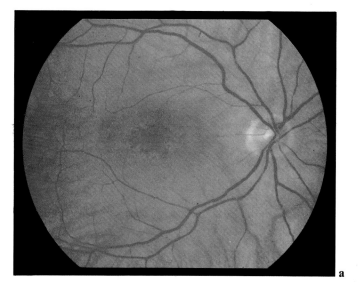

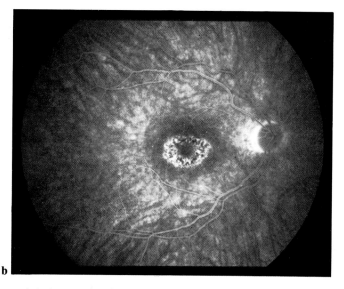

a   b

Fig. 207. Systemic lupus erythematosus. Chloroquine maculopathy: ophthalmoscopic picture (a) and fluorescein angiogram (b).

RETINAL CHANGES IN INBORN METABOLIC ERRORS

These hereditary diseases frequently produce interesting ocular, especially corneal and retinal changes.

We refer here also to the chapter on albinism (Chapter 3) for the alterations of amino acid metabolism.

The anomalies of lipid metabolism may actually be interpreted as hereditary lysosomal diseases; they comprise a group of clinical syndromes classified according to the enzymatic defect into: gangliosidosis (e.g., Tay-Sachs disease), sphingolipidosis (e.g., Niemann-Pick disease), mucopolysaccharidosis (e.g., Hurler and Hunter disease),

cerebrosidosis (e.g., Gaucher disease). The accumulation and overloading of the cells with excessive amounts of fatty substances determine in the various organs the clinical manifestations, e.g., in the gut, nervous tissue and the eyes. All these conditions are transmitted as autosomal recessive factors; the exception is only Fabry's disease which is transmitted as a sex-linked recessive.

The retinal ganglion cells will be infiltrated by the lipid material and this is especially conspicuous in the macula, but absent in the foveola. The infiltrated ganglion cells become white and opaque. This will accentuate the red background color of the foveola giving the area the appearance of the characteristic "cherry red spot" (Fig. 208). Such a macular appearance is most frequently seen in Tay-

Sachs disease, in G.M. 1 gangliosidosis, in Niemann-Pick disease, in metachromatic leukodystrophy and in G.M. gangliosidosis III.

In other lysosomal anomalies (e.g., the mucopolysaccharidoses, Batten-Mayou disease and the juvenile G.M. 2 gangliosidosis III) the changes of the retinal epithelium predominate producing an ophthalmoscopic picture identical to central and/or peripheral retinitis pigmentosa (Fig. 209) frequently accompanied by optic atrophy.

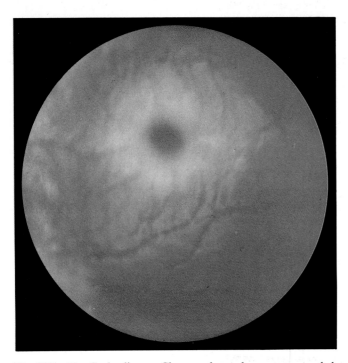

Fig. 208.   Tay-Sachs disease. Cherry red macular spot surrounded by a greyish halo.

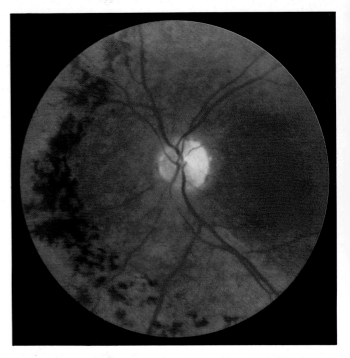

Fig. 209.   Hunter disease. Pericentral semilunar retinitis pigmentosa; partial optic atrophy (*with the kind permission of Prof. C. Santillo*).

RETINOPATHY OF PREMATURITY

This severe condition affects prematurely born children with a birth weight bellow 1,800 g. In the pathogenesis supplemental oxygen plays a dominant role, though this retinopathy may also occur in prematurely born children not exposed to oxygen therapy.

The incidence of this disease has been considerably reduced since it has been established that supplemental oxygen is one of the main etiologic factors.

The supplemental oxygen reduces, through mechanism not yet clearly determined, the endotelial cells in the retinal capillaries which subsequently become occluded.

Retinal circulation remains open via arteriovenous anastomoses. This hypoxemic phase is followed by a proliferation of blood vessels, both in the retina and into the vitreous with secondary connective tissue formation.

The ophthalmoscopic picture varies and depends upon the stage of the disease.

The initial vasoconstriction is followed by a general dilata-tion of the retinal vessels beginning in the periphery; then follows a diffuse new-formation of blood vessels accompanied by hemorrhages. At the same time there is a retianl edema extending from the periphery toward the posterior pole. Progressive neovascularization, hemorrhages and subsequent vitreal retraction produce a retinal detachment which may in the beginning be only peripheral and localized. The subsequent evolution leads to the formation of a white fibrous membrane lying immediately behind the lens (therefore the old name "retrolental fibroplasia").

In this stage the eye is blind. This complete evolution occurs only in about half of the cases of retinopathy of prematurity. The progression may be arrested at any stage of the disease: in these instances the ophthalmoscopic examination will show a more or less extensive fibrosis in the peripheral retina, vascular changes and disturbances of the retinal pigment epithelium.

These incomplete forms of retinopathy are nearly always associated by high myopia which will become manifest at the end of the first year of life (Fig. 210).

CONGENITAL RETINOPATHIES

TUBEROUS SCLEROSIS (BOURNEVILLE'S SYNDROME)

This syndrome of Bourneville is one of the phakomatoses (together with neurofibromatosis, angiomatosis retinae and Sturge-Weber syndrome); it may appear early in life and is characterized by retinal, cerebral and visceral hamartomas, cutaneous angio-fibromas and neurologic deficits, e.g., epilepsy and mental retardation, The retinal hamartomas occur in about 50% of the patients. These lesions are more or less elevated and of varying density.

They are single or multiple and are often round, measuring 1/2 to 4 disc diameters (Fig. 211). Histologically they consist of astrocytes and small blood vessels which may be visible on fluorescein angiography.

The localization of these hamartomas varies: most frequently they are found close to the optic nervehead, rarely in the periphery. When they occur on the disc they may present differential diagnostic difficulties as far as the ordinary drusen are concerned. Vision will be only affected if the hamarthoma lies in the papillomacular bundle but this is rerely the case.

SYSTEMIC NEUROFIBROMATOSIS (VON RECKLINGHAUSEN)

This is also a phakomatosis with neuro-ectodermal involvement. It is transmitted as a dominant mendelian factor and may present itself in numerous organs:

— *cutaneous* form with neurofibromas in or under the skin (Fig. 212). the lesions may vary in size or could be "café au lait" spots;
— *neural and visceral form*, depending on where the neurofribomas develop; the sympatomatology will depend upon the organ involved.

The ophthalmologic manifestation of neurofibromatosis may involve the globe or its adnexa. They may be present at birth. Neurofibromatosis in the *orbit* will cause o slowly progressing exophthalmus; an exophthalmus may also be the product of an optic nerve glioma. *Intraocular neurofibromatosis* may give rise to a congenital secondary glaucoma due to neurofibromatosis of the choroid and the ciliary body combined with anomalies of the chamber angle; neurofibromas may also occur in the conjunctiva, sclera, iris and choroid; in these cases we see greyish nodules, more or less numerous, varying in size from a minute grain of wheat to that of a bean.

The retina is only rarely involved. Ophthalmoscopically we see a nodular elevated mass, mulberry like, yellowish or grey-yellow, of varying size and shape, localized mainly close to the optic nervehead (Fig. 213) and often associated with myelinated nerve fibers.

Five to fifteen percent of the neurofibromas undergo a malignant degeneration.

The prognosis of neurofibromatosis depends primarily upon the location of the lesions; the therapy is only symptomatic.

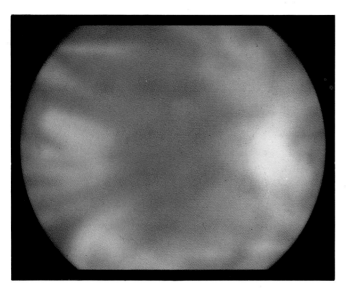

Fig. 210. Final stage of retinopathy of prematurity.

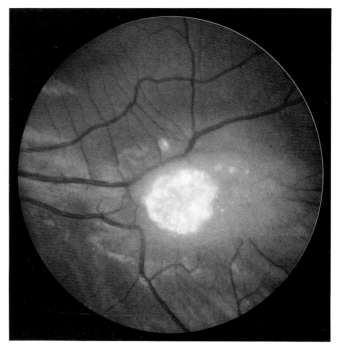

Fig. 211. Tuberous sclerosis (Bourneville). Single retinal hamartoma.

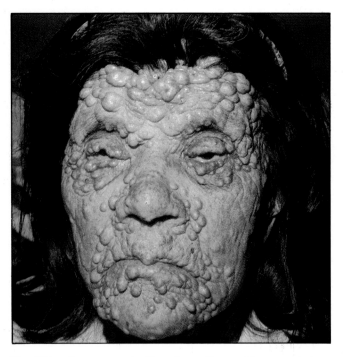

Fig. 212. Cutaneous manifestations of neurofibromatosis (von Recklinghausen). Conspicuous neurofibromas of varying size.

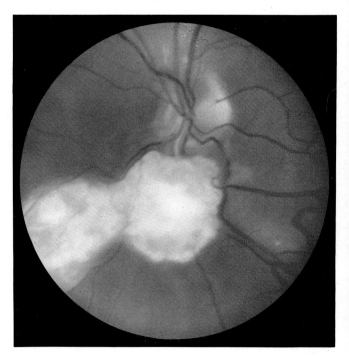

Fig. 213. Retinal astrocytoma in a patient with neurofibromatosis. The hamartoma is unusually large (more than two disc diameters), yellow and biloded.

RETINAL ANGIOMATOSIS

These lesions present a not well defined pathologic entity. They are primarily anomalies of the retinal vasculature, often congenital and frequently hereditary.
The retinal angiomas may be associated with other types of angiomatosis in other organs.
It is important to recognize these retinal vasculopathies though they are rare, because

— of the risk of genetic transmissions in the hereditary types;
— we have to initiate a complete general physical examina-

tion, emphasizing the nuerologic aspects; coexistence of other lesions in other organs is possibile;
— it is possible to treat successfully the initial phases of these progressive or potentially hemorrhagic conditions.

These lesions are usually seen in adolescents or young adults. The first clinical sign is often an involvement of the macula or a vitreous hemorrhage. Frequently the condition is detected by happenstance during a routine eye examination.
We can distinguish several types of retinal angiomas though there are transitional cases which make it difficult to categorize all of them (Table 4).

Table 4. Clinical characteristics of retinal angiomas.

	Con-genital	Heredi-tary	Uni- or bilateral	Sex	Clinical Picture	Fluorescein Angiography	Associated Findings	Treatment
Angiomatosis retinae (von Hippel-Lindau)	+	+ +	Bi	F or M	Tumefaction	Early filling and leakage	Cerebellum, kidney pancreas	Photocoagulation, cryo-treatment, diathermy
Leber-Coats Disease	+		Uni	M	Microangiomas, telangiectasias	Early filling and leakage		Photocoagulation, cryo-treatment, diathermy
Cavernous Hemangioma	+	+ ?	Uni	F	Sessile lesion	Late filling without leakage	Brain, skin (rare)	Photocoagulation, cryo-treatment
Racemose Hemangiomas (cirsoid aneurysm)	+		Uni	F or M	Dilatation of arteries and veins	Arteriovenous anastomoses	Brain, orbit	None

In addition to the ophthalmoscopic evaluation these conditions should also be examined by fluorescein angiography.

On the basis of the ophthalmoscopic picture we may subdivise these retinal angiomas from a clinical point of view into:

— angiomatosis retinae (von Hippel);
— cavernous retinal hemangioma;
— retinal telangiectasia (miliary aneurysm of Leber);
— Coats syndrome (or Leber-Coats disease);
— Racemose hemangioma (cirsoid aneurysm) of the retina.

The hemangiomas of the choroid should be considered as separate entities. These may form part of the encephalo-trigeminal angiomatosis of Sturge and Weber.

Angiomatosis retinae (Von Hippel) (Retinal Angiomas)

A number of vascular anomalies occur in the retina. They may be simple arteriovenous communication, small vascular nodules lying in the retina or on the nervehead which may be regarded as small angiomas or the initial stage of angiomatosis retinae (Figs. 214, 215).

In its typical form the angiomatosis retinae consists of a pair of dilated blood vessels (one arterial and the other one venous) emerging from the optic nervehead. They extend in a tortuous course toward the retinal periphery where they terminate in a more or less voluminous, round tumefaction (the "phakoma") (Figs. 216, 217).

In most of the affected eyes there is only one such lesion. Occasionally these may be multiple and situated in various retinal areas, also in or close to the optic nervehead (Figs. 218, 219).

The tumor may slowly enlarge. During the evolution a few or coalescing retinal exudates may appear; in the far advanced form a retinal detachment may develop which in the final stages may lead to a vitreous hemorrhage or a neovascular glaucoma. The angiomatosis retinae is usually detected in patients between the ages of 10 and 30 years.

The condition may occur in one eye only; in about one-third of the cases it is bilateral, though the second eye may show a minor atypical form of the disease.

It is certainly a hereditary affection. It is transmitted as an autosomal dominant with a variable penetrance, though cases of recessive heredity have also been reported. The condition may be considered as congenital, perhaps a metabolic condition of the capillary endothelium with proliferation of the embryonal endothelial cells. The retinal hemangio-blastoma may be associated with similar lesions in other organs, especially in the cerebellum (von Hippel-Lindau disease) or in parenchymatous organs (kidney, liver).

Xenon or laser photocoagulation is the most satisfactory type of treatment. Cryocoagulation or diathermy my be used in the more advanced and massive cases (Fig. 220).

Cavernous Hemangioma

This constitutes a clinical entity consisting of an accumulation of dark red saccular aneurysms which seem to be isolated from the normal retinal circulation. The caliber of the retinal vessels is normal (Fig. 221).

Fluorescein angiography is useful to confirm the diagnosis: there is no diffusion of the dye across the aneurysms. These fill slowly and sometimes only partly (Fig. 222).

The cavernous hemangioma of the retina is quite rare and may be hereditary as an autosomal dominant. It is more frequently seen in women.

The association with cavernous hemangiomas of the brain and of the skin has been reported.

Treatment consists of photocoagulation, xenon or laser, especially for lesions with hemorrhagic complications.

Cryocoagulation has also been used.

Retinal Telangiectasia (Miliary Aneurysms of Leber)

This is probably a congenital lesion of the retinal vessels. It is usually diagnosed in young individuals.

The vascular lesions appear as vivid red microaneurysms, often limited to one peripheral retinal sector; they may on the other hand involve several areas of the fundus (Figs. 223-226).

They may also occur in the paramacular area. The microaneurysms are associated with ectasia of the arterioles and venules; they may coalesce to form large ampulliform dilatations.

The telangiectasias and the microaneurysms, especially the more pronounced ones, are surrounded by retinal edema and white exudates (Figs. 227, 228).

This exudative process may also develop in a more peripheral area.

These cases may be difficult to distinguish from Coats disease.

The fluorescein angiogram shows the vascular anomalies clearly and reveals also an occasional affection of the capillary network with areas of non-perfusion (Fig. 229).

The angiography also shows alterations in vascular permeability.

In order to localize multiple foci it may be necessary to construct a detailed montage of fundus photographs (Fig. 230).

These telangiectasias occur unilateral, grow slowly, are more frequently seen in male patients and usually involve only the retina.

This is not a hereditary condition.

The pathogenesis is probably an alteration of the retinal vessel wall with disappearance of the endothelial cells and the pericytes and thickening of the basement membrane.

A possibile treatment is photocoagulation or cryo-treatment of the anomalous vessels and of the non-perfused retinal areas (Figs. 231, 232).

Coats Syndrome
(Leber-Coats Disease)

This condition has also been called central exudative retinitis. It is characterized predominantly be the presence of large white-yellow masses, mostly at the posterior pole. They contain birefringent crystals and small hemorrhages (Fig. 233).

Other vascular anomalies are also present, especially in the periphery. These consist of tortuosity, fusiform, spherical, ampulliform, isolated or grouped vascular dilations, more frequently seen at the arterial branch, resembling retinal telangiectasia (Fig. 234).

Here also the retinal angiography will allow a better analysis of the vascular anomalies and will help us recognize the presence of non-perfused retinal areas as well as changes in vascular permeability (Fig. 235).

The predominant picture is that of retinal exudation. The condition progresses more rapidly and more extensively in children than in adults.

We distinguishe:

— the characteristic form in children and in adolescents, with rapidly progressing exudation, followed by massive retinal detachment (the true and actual Coats disease) (Fig. 236);
— the characteristic form in young adults with a tendency for recurrent hemorrhages (these cases have also been called "miliary angiomatosis of Leber");
— minor variations occurring in patients of advanced age, characterized by circumscribed angiectasia with intra- and sub-retinal edema, both in the periphery and the macula.

The type seen in children has a strong tendency for progression and is often complicated by an exudative retinal detachment with secondary glaucoma.

The form seen in young adults may for a long time remain unrecognized and is often revealed by the development of a retino-vitreal hemorrhage.

The form seen in older patients progresses much more slowly and leads to a reduction of central vision because of the macular edema.

It is not always possible to distinguish clearly between Coats disease and retinal telangiectasia.

The first condition characterized by the exudative process may also show vascular lesions typical for telangiectasia. For that reason some authors call this condition "Leber-Coats Disease", recognizing it as a specific entity in which the exudation is secondary to the retinal telangiectasia. Other authors believe that this condition is a clinical, non-specific syndrome, secondary to a number of diseases, congenital or acquired, degenerative or inflammatory.

We also believe that the Leber-Coats angiomatosis is a well-defined clinical entity. Leber-Coats Disease is like telangiectasia a unilateral affection which is nearly exclusively seen in male patients; it is an isolated anomaly, i.e., not associated with pathologic changes in other organs.

It is a hereditary disease.

Xenon or laser photocoagulation can ben applied to telangiectatic lesion with moderate amount of exudates. The non-perfused retinal areas and telangiectasia can be coagulated (Figs. 237, 238).

Cryotreatment or diathermy can also be applied in some cases.

Racemose Hemangioma (Cirsoid Aneurysm)
of the Retina

This lesion consists of fully developed arterio-venous anastomoses.

The ophthalmoscopic picture is characteristic: there is a mass of tortuous, dilated blood vessels extending from the optic nervehead. It is difficult to distinguish the arteries from the veins. Direct arteriovenous anastomoses connect these large vessels. In addition to the typical form there are also formes frustes in which only one segment of the retinal circulation is affected (Figs. 239, 240).

Fluorescein angiography may be useful to demonstrate some of the more subtle arteriovenous anastomoses.

This condition does hardly ever progress.

The anomaly is unilateral and does not show any familial incidence. There is no sex preference.

Frequently associated are similar lesions in other organs, especially the optic nerve, orbit and brain (Wyburn-Mason syndrome).

There is no treatment for the retinal lesions.

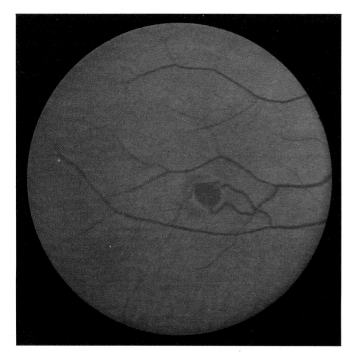

Fig. 214. Angiomatosis retinae (von Hippel). Small round hemangioma with an afferent arterial and an efferent venous vessel.

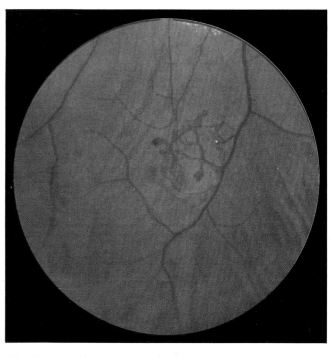

Fig. 215. Capillary retinal hemangioma in a patient with angiomatosis retinae (von Hippel) on the optic nervehead.

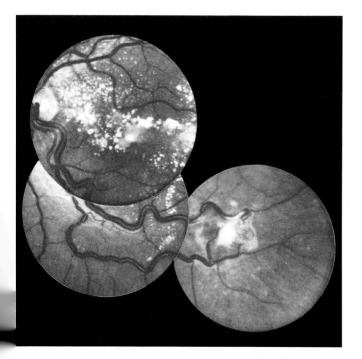

Fig. 216. Angiomatosis retinae (von Hippel). Two dilated vessels, one an artery and the other one a vein, originate from the disc and extend into the lower temporal quadrant terminating in a large round tumefaction: the hamartoma.

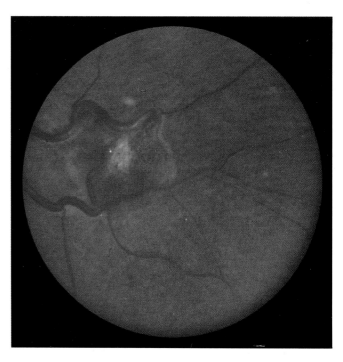

Fig. 217. Detail from fig. 216.

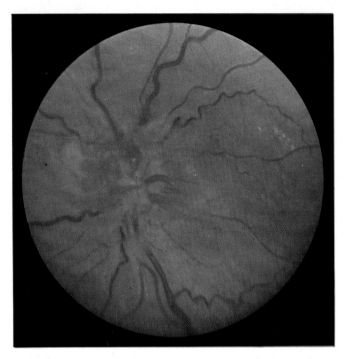

Fig. 218. Angiomatosis retinae (von Hippel) localized on and next to the disc.

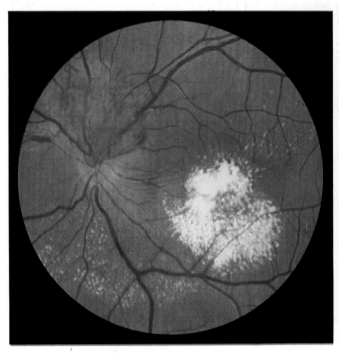

Fig. 219. Angiomatosis retinae (von Hippel) localized on and next to the disc with hard exudates at the posterior pole.

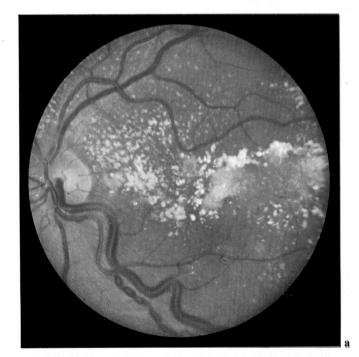

a   b

Fig. 220. Posterior pole in a patient with angiomatosis retinae (von Hippel) (same case as in fig. 216); before (**a**) and after (**b**) photocoagulation treatment. There is marked regression of the hard exudates.

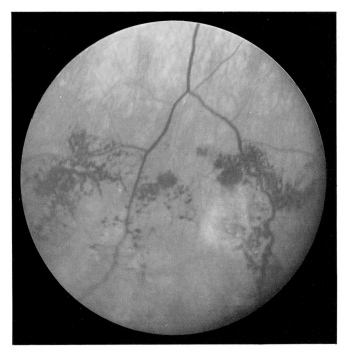

Fig. 221. Cavernous hemangioma of the retina. There are numerous dark red microaneuryms clustered into groups and localized in a single retinal sector.

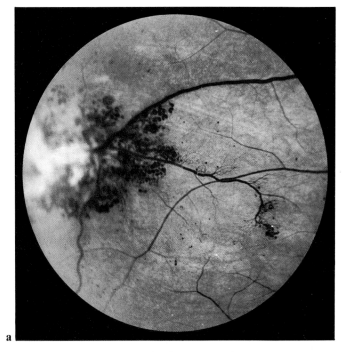

Fig. 222. a)-c). Fluorescein angiograms of a fundus with cavernous hemangioma of the retina; the microaneurysms fill slowly and partially with the dye; this is typical for this form of hemangioma.

a

b   c

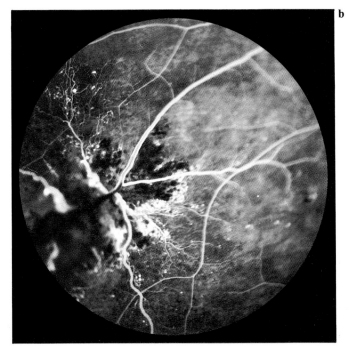

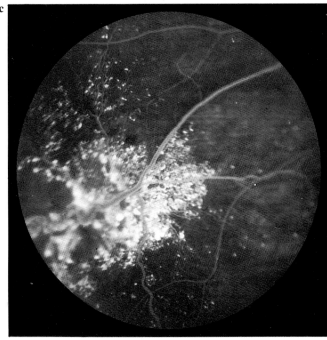

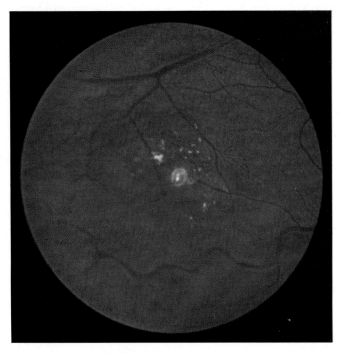

Fig. 223. Leber's miliary aneurysms: in this case the microaneurysms and arterial and venous ectasias occur in only one limited area of the retina. Hard exudates begin to develop.

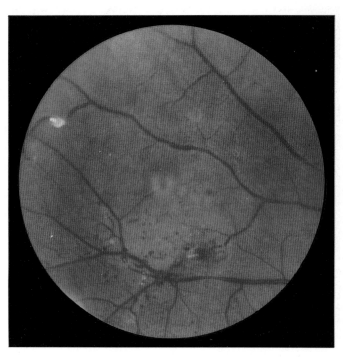

Fig. 224. The telangiectasias occupy a large area, while the capillary circulation in the immediate neighborhood is altered.

Fig. 223-226. Miliary aneurysms of Leber. Various forms of microaneurysms and ampulliform ectasias of the arterioles and venules in a young patient with Leber's disease.

Fig. 225. The arteriolar and venous ectasias are in this case much more conspicuous; in the center of the vascular anomalies is a nonperfused retinal area.

Fig. 226. This case of Leber's telangiectasia shows, similar to the last case, severe alterations of retinal circulation.

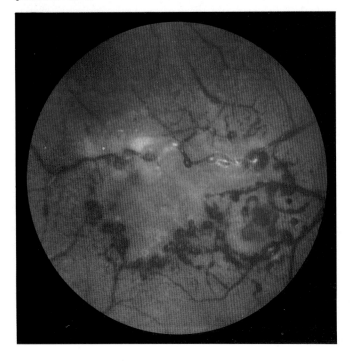

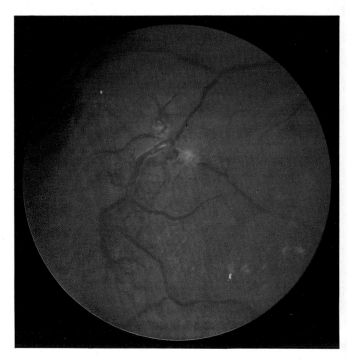

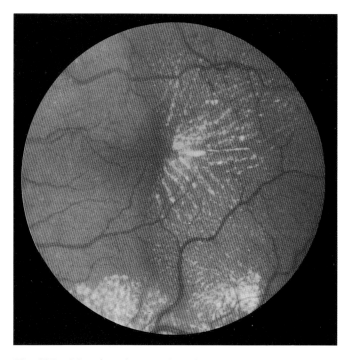

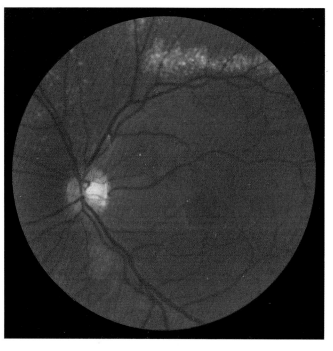

Fig. 227. Macular edema and exudates in a young patient with peripheral retinal telangiectasias.

Fig. 228. Exudates along the upper temporal retinal vessels in a patient with localized telangiectasias, primarily in the periphery of the upper temporal quadrant.

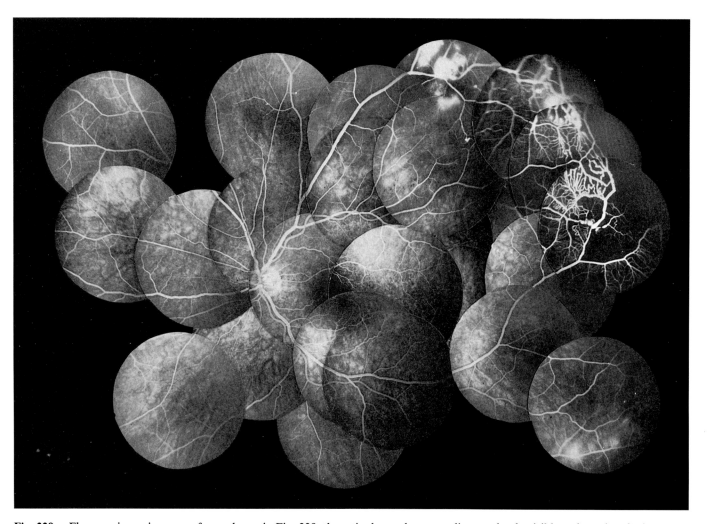

Fig. 229. Fluorescein angiograms of case shown in Fig. 228: the retinal vascular anomalies are clearly visible and consist of microaneurysms, ectasias, reduced capillary network and large areas of non-perfusion.

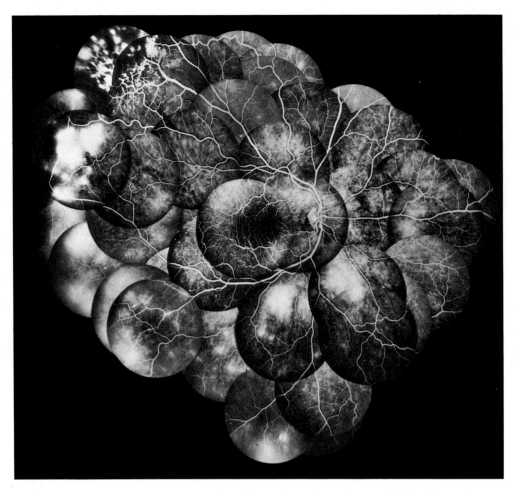

Fig. 230. Peripheral retinal telangiectasia. Fluorescein angiograms put together in a collage in order to show the entire fundus. The telangiectasia involves primarily the upper temporal segment and there is a marked alteration of vascular permeability in various parts of the fundus.

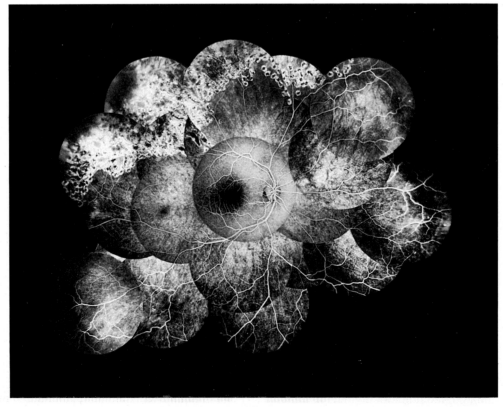

Fig. 231. Fluorescein angiograms of the same case as in Fig. 230 after laser photocoagulation treatment. There is regression of the marked vascular permeability which was present before the treatment.

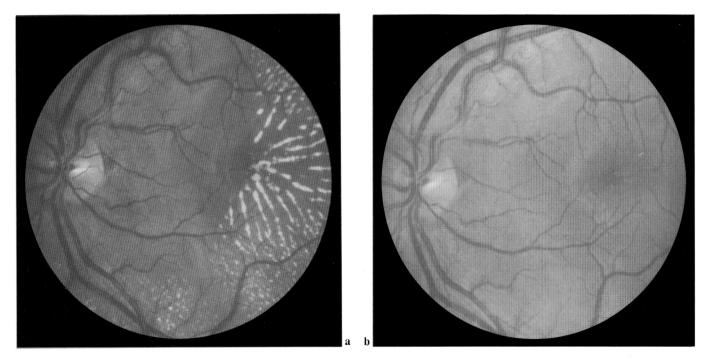

a b

Fig. 232. **a)** and **b).** Peripheral retinal telangiectasia. The posterior pole before **(a)** and after **(b)** laser photocoagulation. There is total regression of the exudates.

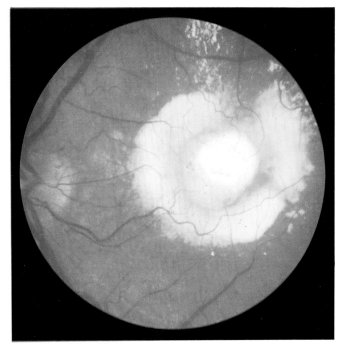

Fig. 233. Large central exudate in a case of Leber-Coats disease in an infant.

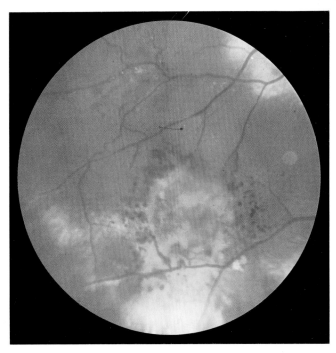

Fig. 234. Leber-Coats disease. Vascular anomalies consisting of aneurysmatic dilatations and telangiectasia, surrounded by a marked exudative process.

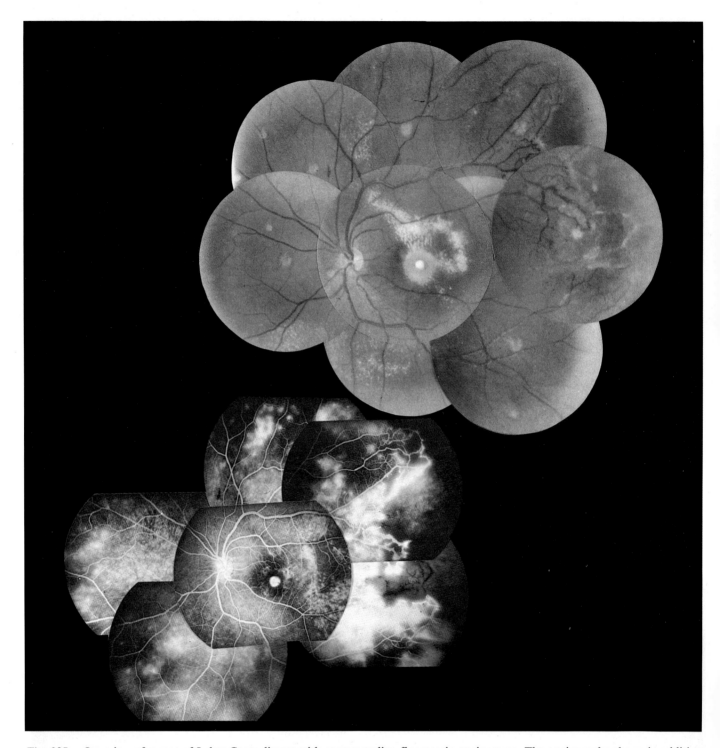

Fig. 235. Overview of a case of Leber-Coats disease with corresponding fluorescein angiograms. The angiography shows in addition to the vascular alterations consisting of ectasia and rarefaction of the capillary network also a marked and diffuse change of vascular permeability.

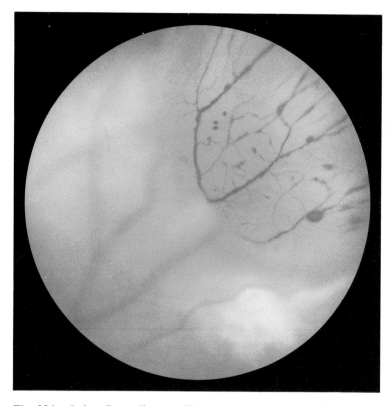

Fig. 236. Leber-Coats disease will frequently cause a secondary retinal detachment as in this case in which the characteristic anomalies of this disease are well visible.

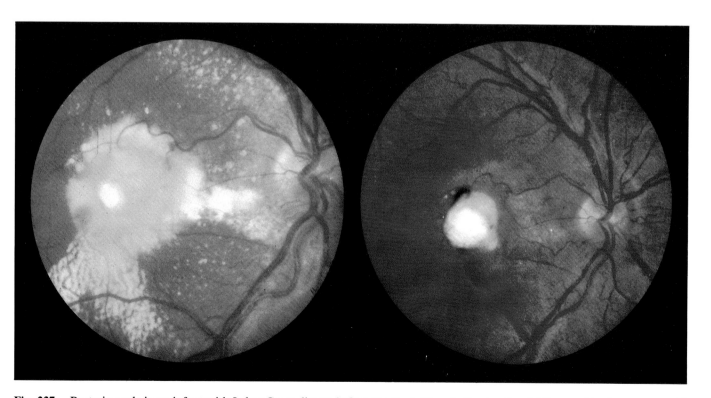

Fig. 237. Posterior pole in an infant with Leber-Coats disease before (on the left) and after (on the right) a combined treatment with cryotherapy and laser photocoagulation. The exudative process has regressed and has given place to a small area of central chorio-retinal atrophy.

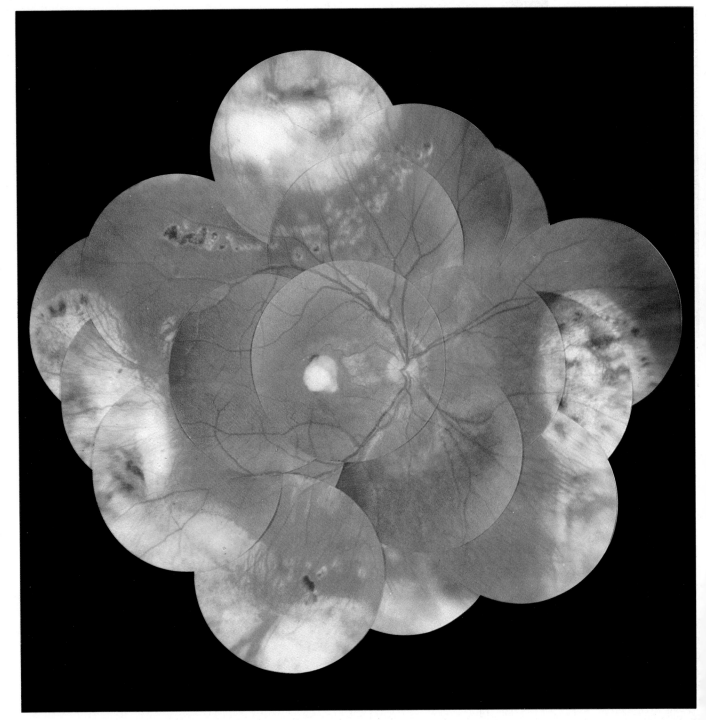

Fig. 238. Overview of the ocular fundus of the case in Fig. 237 obtained by collage of various fundus pictures. The cryotreatment and photocoagulation have produced a regression of the preexisting vascular anomalies.

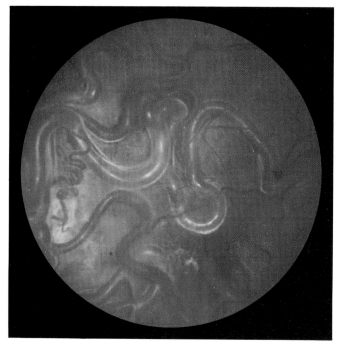 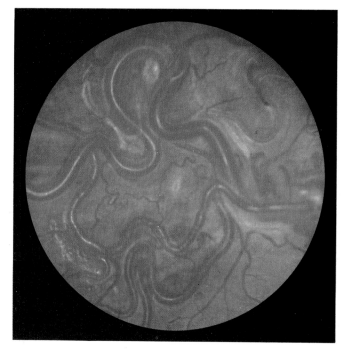

Fig. 239   **Fig. 240**

Fig. 239 and **240.** Typical fundus picture of an eye with racemose hemangioma of the retina. The abnormally dilated retinal vessels originating from the optic nervehead make it difficult to distinguish between an artery and a vein. This distinction can easily be obtained on fluorescein angiography.

DEGENERATIVE MACULOPATHIES

These macular diseases are often hereditary and familial in nature, they may be present at birth or develop during the course of life.

A number of primary macular degenerations have been identified clinically by their ophthalmoscopic appearance, the mode of development, the hereditary nature, the time of appearance and their further course.

Juvenile Retinoschisis

This is a bilateral congenital affection transmitted as a sex linked recessive.

This disease is usually diagnosed in children or young adults. The maculopathy may be associated with a peripheral retinoschisis and with vitreous changes. The ophthalmoscopic picture is characterized by the formation of cystoid deposits in the form of a star; the largest deposits are in the foveola from which they extend in fine stripes (Fig. 241).

This microcystic form changes over the course of years into macrocystic formations resembling honeycombs. A small

central pigmentary atrophy may later develop. The pseudocysts are better appreciated in red-free illumination. The fluorescein angiography is completely negative. In late cases of pigment epithelium atrophy we find the typical ophthalmoscopic picture. Central visual acuity is often more or less decreased. The ERG is usually abnormal. No treatment is available for this central retinoschisis.

Stargardt Disease

This is the most frequent form of juvenile macular degeneration. It can be seen during infancy or adolescence, but some cases have been described in adults in whom the evolution was slow. The condition is usally transmitted as an autosomal recessive. Initially the macular changes observed with the ophthalmoscope are rather minor.

We first see an attenuation or loss of the reflex in the foveola and at the rim of the macula. A wreath of small whitish deposits appear (Fig. 242). Then the macular area looks like granite covered with small fish scales in addition to the small white-yellow round deposits there may be other formations which are larger and resemble a fish: these are the changes seen in fundus flavimaculatus (Fig. 243). There are cases of pure Stargardt disease and others in which the macular changes are associated with a ring of deposits corresponding to fundus flavimaculatus (this may be perimacular or in the periphery) (Fig. 244).

In the course of time the macular pigmentation increases and the pigment accumulates in larger deposits. Other changes occur which give the area a marble-like effect because of the shiny reflexes (Fig. 245). Finally there will develop a more or less extensive area of central atrophy.

Fluorescein angiography is characteristic and quite useful for establishing the diagnosis, especially in the initial stages of the disease. The window effect of the changes in the pigment epithelium gives the lesion a characteristic appearance which has been compared to the eye seen on the feathers of a peacock tail (Fig. 246). The lesions of the flavimaculatus areas are stained with the dye during the early phases and bleach in the late phases. With the evolution of the disease central visual acuity slowly decreases. The electrophysiologic tests do not provide us with information which would be useful for the diagnosis.

The Vitelliform Macular Degeneration (Best Disease)

This is a hereditary bilateral macular dystrophy transmitted as an autosomal dominant. The disease may be manifest already in the newborn or in infants. It is most frequently first observed in young adults because of the relative mild loss in visual function caused by the initial lesions.

The family history is usually quite important for making the diagnosis. The macular changes are bilateral and may present themselves in the following forms:

— an initial stage or a complete disc,
— a stage of evolution,
— an atrophic stage.

The classical ophthalmoscopic picture resembles an egg-yolk on a plate. The disciform lesion may be round or oval, is usually yellow, orange or pink and its center lies in the macular area. The border of the lesion is clear cut and well delineated, sometimes surrounded by a dark red halo (Fig. 247). The size of the lesion may vary from one quarter or one half of a disc diameter to three disc diameters. The lesion is usually single, but may occasionally be multiple and located in various parts of the posterior pole. During the evolutionary stage the material in the vitelliform disc has a tendency to fragment and to accumulate in large clumps or, more frequently, liquify settling at the base of the lesion forming a so-called "pseudohypopyon" (Fig. 248). In rare instances hemorrhages may appear which derive from subretinal neovascularizations.

In the final stage there is macular atrophy which is non-characteristic and therefore difficult to diagnose. The chorioretinal atrophy is well delineated, orange or green in color with pigment deposits in various forms (Fig. 249).

Fluorescein angiography does not contribute any essential information. The disc shaped lesion does not show any fluorescence, but becomes pseudofluorescent in the late stages. During the evolutionary stage of the pseudohypopyon the supernatant is colored with the dye in a rather uneven manner. In the atrophic stage the fluorescein angiogram is similar to that of any other type of chorioretinal atrophy. During the initial stage of the condition visual acuity remains good and contrasts markedly with the clinical appearance of the macular area. In the course of time visual acuity will slowly decrease but will never become extremely poor. The electro-oculogram shows marked changes and is an important indicator. The ERG and the EVP are normal.

The Reticular Dystrophy of the Pigment Epithelium (Sjögren Disease)

This is a rare hereditary condition transmitted as an autosomal recessive. It is usually detected in infancy.

Ophthalmoscopically we see a net-like arrangement of pigment which is more or less geometrical in shape and involves mainly the posterior pole, but may also appear in the periphery.

In some cases the pigment net involves only the posterior pole.

The fluorescein angiogram shows the reticular pigmentation which contrasts with the fluorescence in the loops.

Age Dependent Macular Degenerations

These lesions constitute a frequent pathologic change of the macular area and are a major cause of legal blindness in the aged population. This is a field which is still widely discussed as far as its etiology, pathogenesis, symptomatology and even nomenclature are concerned.

Therefore the colloid degeneration of the macula, the hyaline excrescences (drusen), the disciform macular degeneration, the senile areolar atrophy indicate pathologic changes which are related to each other, but may frequently also be successive stages of one and the same degenerative process.

The colloid degeneration of the macula. More or less numerous deposits of a hyalin substance appear in the cuticular lamella of Bruch's membrane. The deposits are also known under the name of hyalin excrescences, drusen or colloid bodies. In addition to the definite age dependent changes (some of which may occur at a definite pre-senile age) we also know of familial degenerations of this kind which are transmitted as a regular or irregular autosomal dominant.

From a morphological point of view it is difficult to distinguish between the hereditary and the age dependent forms.

The degeneration is often bilateral and symmetrical. Ophthalmoscopically it may appear under a variety of forms and shapes. There may be numerous, small, round, yellow or white structures with sharp outlines, sometimes with a reddish shade and pigmented margins (Figs. 250, 251). They may be dot-like (miliary varicosities) or have the size of a large retinal vessel; several structures may coalesce and form irregular polygonal structures.

These hyalin excrescences may be localized in one sector of the macular area, may involve the entire posterior pole, or may extend to the equator and beyond.

The number and location of these drusen may vary over the course of time. Fluorescein angiography is particularly useful in evaluating the possible evolution toward an exudative type of macular degeneration (disciform degeneration) (Fig. 252 a, b).

These hyalin bodies fluoresce already in the early phase of the angiogram. The fluorescence increases in the later phases without, however, dye leaking into the tissue. The fluorescence then decreases gradually with the decrease in choroidal fluorescence. Visual acuity remains for a long time good. The electrophysiologic tests are generally normal.

Disciform macular degeneration (age dependent exudative macular degeneration). This is a possible and frequent end result of the colloid macular degeneration. When the lesion begins to manifest itself it may herald its evolution by functional disturbance (metamorphopsia) which may precede the ophthalmoscopically recognizable macular lesion. The entity of a colloid degeneration at the posterior pole may represent a pre-disciform stage, the first true phase of such a disease and may manifest itself as a serous detachment of the pigment epithelium accompanied by a subretinal neovascularization stemming from the choroid.

On the other hand, the disciform degeneration may appear suddenly. Ophthalmoscopically it appears as a round or oval, circumscribed lesion with sharp outlines. It is white-grey and may vary in size from one fourth to four disc diameters; it is more or less elevated over the retinal surface (from 0.5 to 2-3 diopters) (Fig. 253). The seat is the macular or paramacular area. The initial lesions constitute a detachment of the pigment epithelium which may remain unchanged for a long time and even regress. More often it has a tendency to evolve, losing its sharp outlines by diffusion of the serous detachment into the subretinal space and into the retina itself. We therefore see in addition to the original lesions hard exudates often arranged to a wreath.

The serous detachment of the pigment epithelium is frequently complicated by hemmorrhages causing a serous hemorrhagic detachment of the pigment epithelium which produces the typical degenerative age dependent lesion of the macula. In this phase the subretinal neovascularization becomes evident leading to the hemorrhagic component (Figs. 254, 255).

In some cases, however, this last stage of development is not due to the appearance of a neovascular membrane, but to a rupture of the pigment epithelium and of Bruch's membrane which by traction also involves the inner most layers of the choriocapillaries.

In the course of time these serous and hemorrhagic fluids diffuse into the inner layers of the retina, elevating the retinal surface and giving the lesion a pseudotumor-like appearance. The margins often become indistinct and frayed

due to exudation inside the retina. The fluid has a tendency to gravitate downward toward the deeper layers. Sooner or later the lesion will develop fibrovascular proliferations which modify the picture. This will produce the cicatricial aspect which presents itself as a disciform, oval or geographic, yellowish lesion with rather sharp borders (Fig. 256), sometimes associated with large pigment deposits arranged in various forms.

Fluorescein angiography is useful in order to define the detachment of the pigment epithelium, but it is essential to prove the presence of a neovascular membrane (Figs. 257 a, b).

The age dependent macular degeneration is usually bilateral though different stages may be present in the two eyes. The central visual acuity is generally reduced, moderately in cases of circumscribed serous paramacular detachment, severely when the serous detachment is complicated by hemorrhages.

The electrophysiologic tests are abnormal.

Medical treatment is not successful. Laser photocoagulation is useful to treat the subretinal neovascularization provided that the stage of the disease and the seat of the lesion allow such a treatment.

Atrophic age dependent macular degeneration. This is another aspect of the age dependent macular degenerations. It could be regarded as a progressive stage of the colloid degeneration, but it may also occur independently from the latter. Ophthalmoscopically it consists of indistinct patches of hyper- and hypopigmentation with irregular outlines associated with drusen (Fig. 258); in the areas of pronounced atrophy the underlying choroidal vasculature can be seen (Fig. 259).

If the atrophy is round and has sharp outlines we also speak of an age dependent areolar atrophy of the macula. The fluorescein angiogram in this type of lesion is characterized by alterations of the pigment epithelium with hyperfluorescence due to the window effect, and with hypofluorescence due to the masking effect of the accumulated pigment.

Visual acuity is usually markedly decreased.

Age dependent pseudocystic macular degeneration. This type of age dependent primary degeneration is usually bilateral though it may occasionally appear in one eye only. It presents itself in three successive stages: the first stage is difficult to detect ophthalmoscopically. The foveal area may show a slight marble-like appearance or may resemble honeycombs. This stage is known as the "microcystoid phase".

The next stage is the "macrocystoid phase". Ophthalmoscopically we see a central, foveolar, round defect which is dark red and surrounded by a greyish halo (Fig. 260). With the slit lamp we see that the anterior wall is intact and consists of coalescing small pseudocysts which formed during the initial stage.

In the final stage the clinical picture is that of a "macular hole"; this is a round macular dehiscence with a dark red excavation, often with small whitish deposits which constitute cellular debris (Fig. 261). The margins appear elevated and underminded.

Fluorescein angiography does not contribute significantly

to the diagnosis. In advanced cases there may be fluorescence in the depth of the hole due to the changes in the pigment epithelium. The loss of visual function is in direct relationship to the evolution of the microcystoid degeneration. Vision will be considerably reduced in cases of a macular hole. It would be unusual for the hole to cause a retinal detachment. Photocoagulation is therefore only indicated in exceptional cases.

Maculopathy with Angioid Streaks

Middle-aged patients with angioid streaks frequently show an involvement of the macula (see Chapter 8, Angioid streaks, page 253). The macular changes may be regarded as a final stage of the damage produced by the angioid streaks in the macular area. The macular lesions may manifest themselves as

— atrophic macular degeneration,
— exudative macular degeneration,
— atrophic and hypertrophic degeneration.

The atrophic macular degeneration is the rarest form and resembles ophthalmoscopically the areolar atrophy of the macula.

The exudative macular degeneration shows, analogous to the disciform age dependent degeneration, a first stage of sero-hemorrhagic exudation (Fig. 262) with the frequent development of a subretinal neovascular membrane coming from the choroid. This lesion then is transformed into the atrophic-hypertrophic type which is ophthalmoscopically characterized by coalescing areas of hyperpigmentation and atrophy.

The loss of visual acuity is connected with the phase of the disease and the site of the lesion. The closer the angioid streaks lie to the macula, the more severe will be the macular damage. Fluorescein angiography may be of considerable help.

No effective medical treatment is known. Reasonably good results may be obtained from photocoagulation in those cases in which a subretinal neovascular membrane has developed.

Myopic Maculopathy

The macular lesions occurring in eyes with degenerative myopia (see Chapter 4) may be divided into three ophthalmoscopic pictures:

— the atrophic form;
— the hemorrhagic form;
— the serous-hemorrhagic form.

The atrophic form consists of the usual myopic degeneration; ophthalmoscopically we see more or less extensive whitish areas of chorioretinal atrophy; these are round or geographic in outline sometimes transversed by atrophic lines corresponding to breaks in Bruch's membrane (lacquer cracks) (Fig. 263).

The hemorrhagic type is characterized by a dark red area probably representing a small subretinal hemorrhage. It is not surrounded by any retinal elevation; the cause of this hemorrhage is often a rupture of Bruch's membrane with subsequent involvement of the underlying choriocapillaries (Fig. 264).

The serous-hemorrhagic type appears ophthalmoscopically as a small spot or a grey nodule, one quarter to one half of a disc diameter in size, surrounded by a greenish halo or by a dark red hemorrhagic border (Fig. 265) which in some cases may expand so that it covers the posterior pole. Other small hemorrhages may be observed somewhat away from the macular lesion. The central nodule corresponds to a serous detachment of the pigment epithelium, whereas the hemorrhagic halo is often an indication that a subretinal vascular membrane is present.

A fluorescein angiographic examination is absolutely necessary to prove the presence of such a neovascular membrane (Fig. 265 b). An extension of the membrane will be accompanied by new hemorrhages. In the final stages the fibrovascular scar is partially covered or surrounded by more or less extensive pigment deposits. This picture is known under the name of "Fuchs spot" (Fig. 266). The atrophy of the pigment epithelium and of the choriocapillaries gives the final stage of this condition the aspect of a coloboma. This is quite a characteristic development in this condition.

The loss of visual acuity is also connected with the site and extension of the lesion.

In some cases photocoagulating the neovascular membrane may be of some benefit.

The Syndrome of Retraction at the Vitreo-Retinal Interface (Irvine-Gass Syndrome)

This syndrome may be acquired, usually after a surgical procedure, or may be idiopathic. The idiopathic form usually occurs in patients of advanced age and probably represents a type of vitreal degeneration. The other type is secondary to inflammatory processes, retinal vasculopathy or surgical procedures. The ophthalmoscopic picture is characterized by a tortuousity of the retinal vessels, principally of the perimacular vessels. This is directly due to the vitreal traction. The vessels of the papillomacular bundle are dragged toward the temporal side (Fig. 267). Fluorescein angiography shows a leakage of the dye through the affected retinal vessels. In rare cases there may be a cystoid macular edema.

Visual function is decreased to a varying degree due to the vitreous retraction itself.

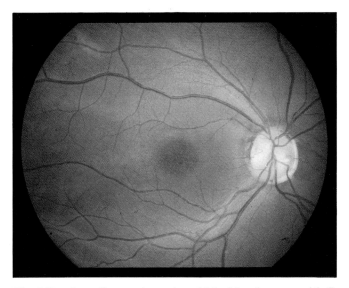

Fig. 241. Juvenile macular retinoschisis. Macular cysts with fine radial striae extending from the center and giving the lesion a starlike appearance.

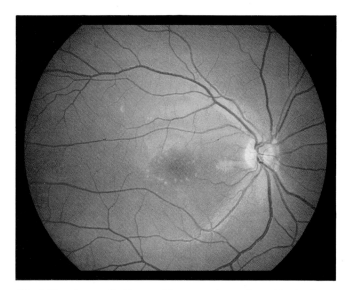

Fig. 242. Stargardt disease. The normal macular reflex is obscured by small, round, white-yellow lesions surrounding the macula.

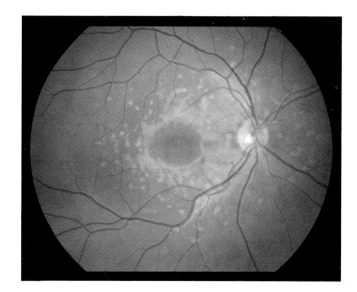

Fig. 243. Stargardt disease with a ring of flavimaculatus lesions. The macular dystrophy is surrounded by a wide wreath of white-yellow lesions.

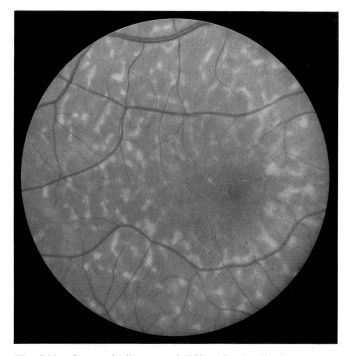

Fig. 244. Stargardt disease and diffuse fundus flavimaculatus. The macular dystrophy is associated with diffuse fish-shaped flavimaculatus lesions.

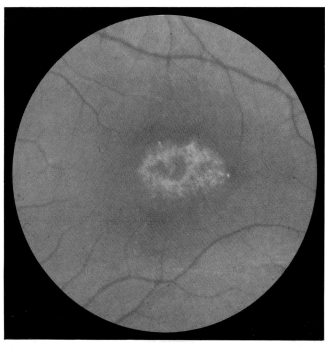

Fig. 245. Stargardt disease. Detail from the posterior pole with marble-like appearance of the macular area surrounded by a wreath of subtle white lesions.

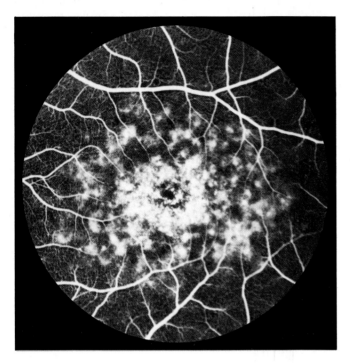

Fig. 246. Fluorescein angiogram of the macula in a case of Stargardt disease.

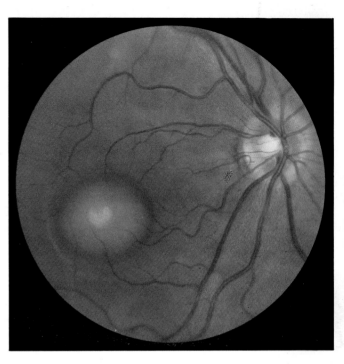

Fig. 247. Best disease (vitelliform macular degeneration). In the macula is a round, yellow-orange lesion surrounded by a darker halo.

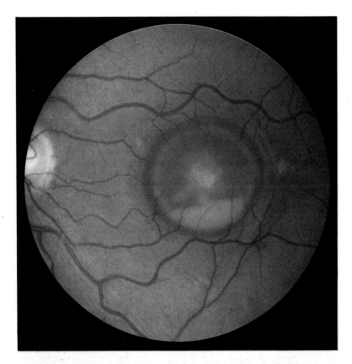

Fig. 248. Best disease (vitelliform macular degeneration). The vitelliform lesion shows a ''pseudohypopyon'' produced by sedimentation of the material contained in the cyst.

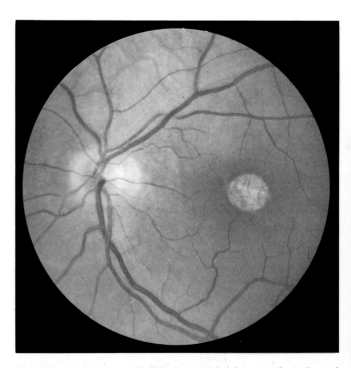

Fig. 249. Best disease (vitelliform macular degeneration). Round central atrophic scar developing during the late stage of the disease.

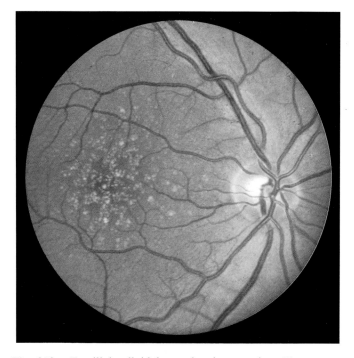

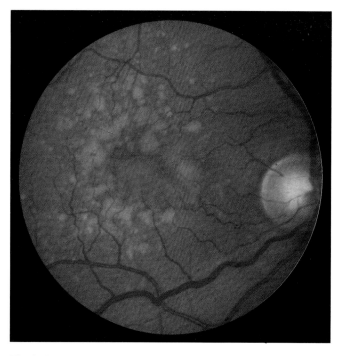

Fig. 250. Familial colloidal macular degeneration. Numerous small white lesions scattered over the posterior pole.

Fig. 251. Age dependent colloidal macular degeneration. White-yellow lesions (drusen) of various size located at the posterior pole.

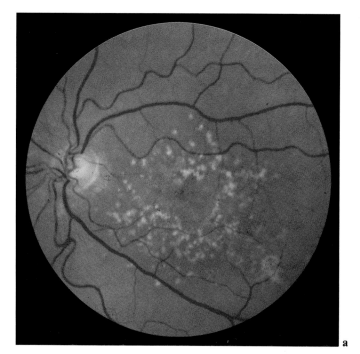

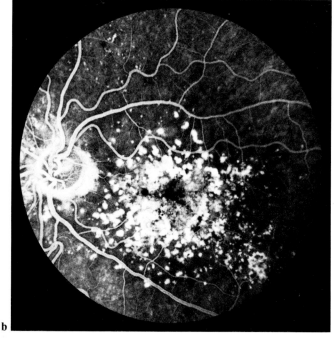

a b

Fig. 252. Age dependent colloidal macular degeneration.
a) The ophthalmoscopic examination shows small white lesions (drusen) disseminated over the posterior pole. **b)** The fluorescein angiogram is characterized by a marked fluorescence of these verrucosities which does not change in the late phases of the angiogram.

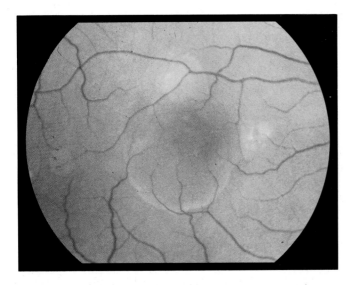

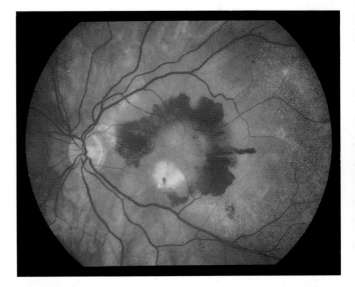

Fig. 253.

Fig. 254.

Fig. 253. Age dependent exudative macular degeneration. Large oval lesion, elevating the retina and involving the macular area representing a serous detachment of the pigment epithelium.

Fig. 254. Age dependent exudative macular degeneration. Central serous detachment surrounded by a massive halo of hemorrhages, produced by a probable break in pigmented retinal epithelium.

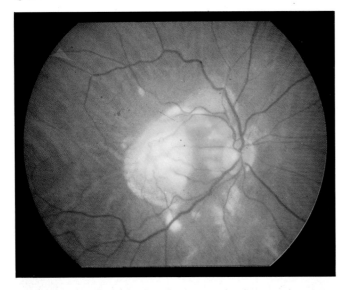

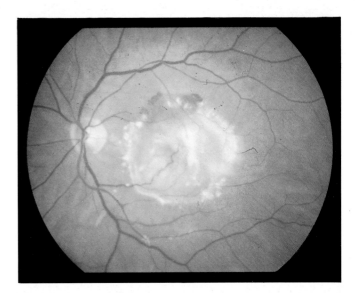

Fig. 256. Age dependent macular degeneration. Cicatricial stage of an advanced disciform degeneration.

Fig. 255. Age dependent exudative macular degeneration. Marked disciform elevation with hemorrhage in the upper part and small hard exudates arranged like a wreath around the disciform detachment.

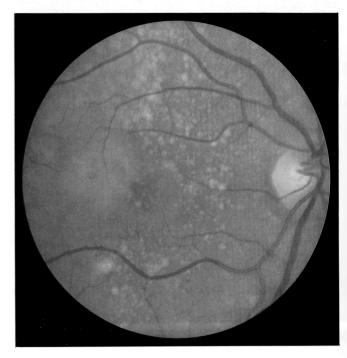

Fig. 257. **a)** and **b).** Age dependent exudative macular degeneration.
a) Fundus photo.

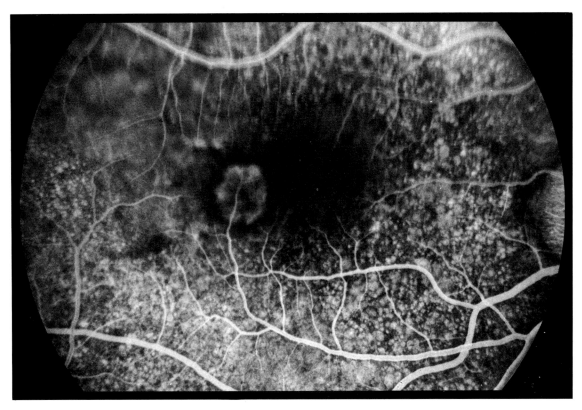

Fig. 257. Age dependent exudative macular degenaration.
b) Fluorescein angiogram: a neovascular membrane is present in the context of a diffuse colloidal degeneration.

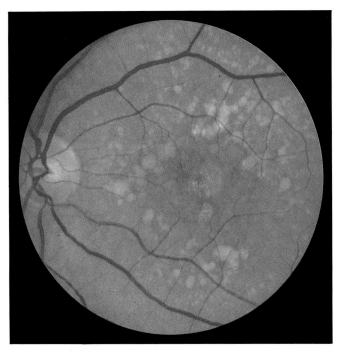

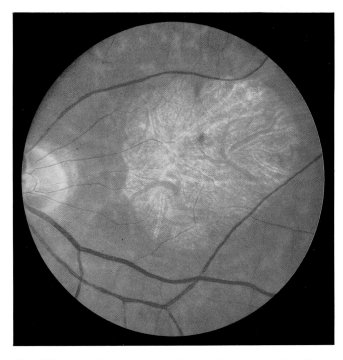

Fig. 258. Age dependent atrophic macular degeneration. Small round area of retinal atrophy surrounded by a halo of hyperpigmentation within the framework of a colloidal degeneration.

Fig. 259. Age dependent atrophic macular degeneration. Large round central area of retinal atrophy.

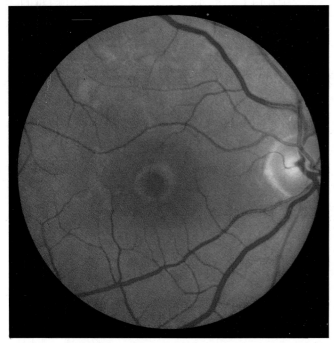

Fig. 260. Age dependent pseudocystoid macular degeneration. There is a central dark red cyst-like structure in the fovea. It is surrounded by a grey-yellow margin.

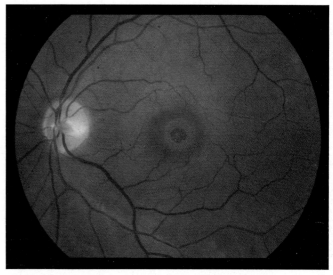

Fig. 261. Age dependent pseudocystoid macular degeneration with the formation of a macular hole. Central punched out dehiscence, on the dark red bottom of which is white cellular debris.

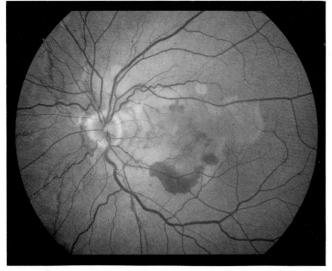

Fig. 262. Macular degeneration with angioid streaks. The typical lesions of angioid streaks are associated with severe changes at the posterior pole constituting an exudative hemorrhagic process.

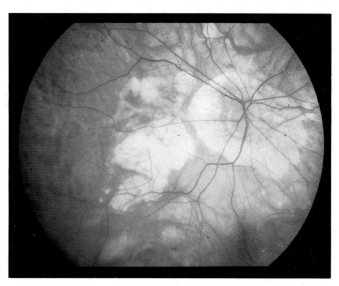

Fig. 263. Atrophic myopic maculopathy. Large white areas of chorioretinal atrophy involving also the posterior pole.

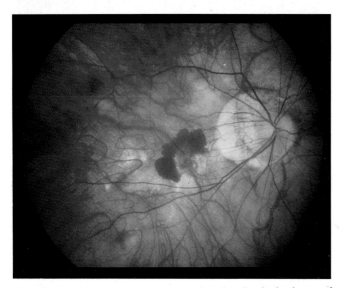

Fig. 264. Hemorrhagic myopic maculopathy. On the background of chorioretinal atrophy lies a hemorrhage resembling red lacquer.

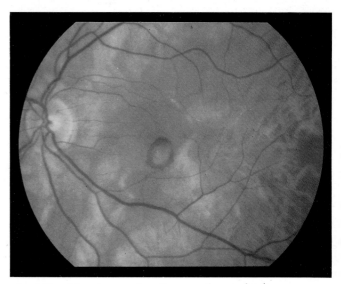

Fig. 265. Myopic maculopathy, sero-hemorrhagic.
a) Fundus photo: an oval grey paramacular lesion is surrounded by a hemorrhagic halo.

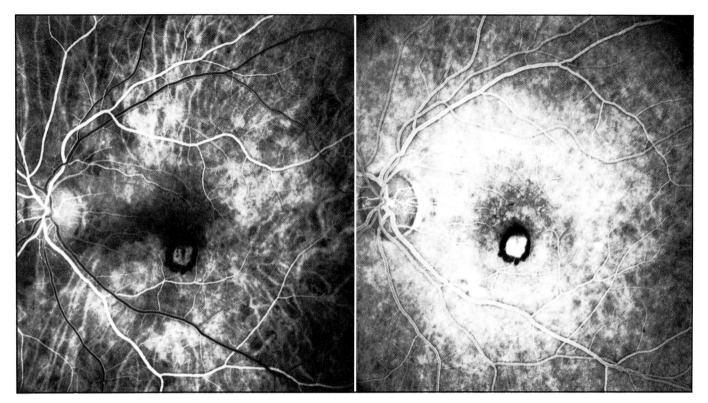

Fig. 265. Myopic maculopathy, sero-hemorrhagic.
b) Fluorescein angiogram (early and late phases): a subretinal neovascular membrane can be seen.

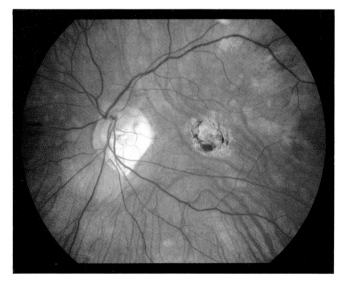

Fig. 266. Cicatricial myopic maculopathy. Central pigmented lesion, the end stage of a serous hemorrhagic process, the so-called "Fuchs spot".

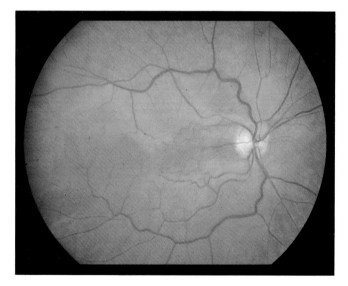

Fig. 267. Retraction of the vitreo-retinal interface. Tortuosity of the retinal vessels between the macula and the optic nervehead due to vitreous traction and directed toward the macula.

TAPETORETINAL DEGENERATIONS

A number of chorioretinal degenerative conditions are grouped under this heading. They are usually hereditary, progressive and of varying appearance. They may occur in various members of the same family or even in the same patient.

They are grouped under one heading because they have several elements in common: the hereditary nature, the defects in light sense and in color vision, loss of visual field and a pathologic electroretinogram.

The basic pathology is an abiotrophic process which primarily leads to a degeneration of the photoreceptors, but may involve the pigment epithelium (tapetum nigrum) and the choriocapillaries.

Symptoms and electroretinographic changes accompany the

early ophthalmoscopic signs. Characteristic is the night blindness reflected in a change of the dark adaptation curve. There may be an absence of the cone or of the rod component leading to a monophasic curve in which the normal break is missing.

The changes in color vision affect mainly the blue-yellow axis and may lead to a dichromatic vision. The defects in the visual field correspond to the topographic location of the degenerative process. There may be a ring scotoma with progressive extension and breakthrough toward the periphery so that finally only a tunnel field around the central vision remains. This occurs in the peripheral forms of tapeto retinal degeneration. Central scotoma with early reduction of visual acuity occurs in those degenerations which are located at the posterior pole.

The ERG has a diagnostic importance: in the peripheral types of tapetoretinal degeneration the ERG is completely extinguished, even in the early stages of the disease. In other forms of degeneration the ERG is subnormal.

Table 5.   Classification of tapetoretinal degenerations.

Peripheral forms	with little pigment without pigment confined to one fundus quadrant occurring in one eye only progressive retinitis albipunctata fundus albipunctatus fundus flavimaculatus
Diffuse form	Leber's congenital amaurosis
Central or hereditary macular forms	infantile form of Best juvenile form of Stargardt form appearing during puberty pre-senile form of Behr senile form of Sorsby

The classification of these dystrophies (Table 5) is primarily on a topographic basis and distinguishes a peripheral (retinitis pigmentosa, with little or without pigment, confined to a quadrant, unilateral, progressive retinitis albipunctata, fundus albipunctatus, fundus flavimaculatus), a diffuse form (congenital retinal dystrophy of Leber), and a central or macular form (classified according to the age when the disease first manifests itself: infantile form of Best, juvenile form of Stargardt, a type that appears with puberty, the pre-senile form of Behr, and the senile form of Sorsby). The central forms of tapetoretinal degenerations merit a special chapter because they present a clinical picture which is distinctly different from the other two types. In these patients we have day blindness, photophobia, central scotoma, normal ERG, dischromatic vision according to the green-red axis (see pages 163-165).

In the **peripheral pigmentary form** (retinitis pigmentosa) the characteristic findings are the bone corpuscle-like, branching pigment deposits which occur in groups or solitary, first in the equatorial area and finally progressing and coalescing toward the posterior pole which itself remains free (Figs. 268 a, b; 269; 270). The retinal vessels are attenuated and seem to be sheathed by pigment; the arterioles are thread-like. Here and there non-pigmented areas remain in which

the choroidal vessels become visible. The optic nervehead is pale, grey-yellow and atrophic. The histopathologic examination reveals absence of the photoreceptors, proliferation of glial elements and of the pigment epithelium, the melanin of which migrates into the retinal tissue and accumulates around blood vessels (Fig. 271). The condition is usually hereditary and in the majority of cases follows an autosomal recessive pattern. The patients complain about night blindness and progressive constriction of the visual field until finally only a small central tubular field remains or the patient becomes totally blind. The ERG is extinguished.

In addition to this classical form we have atypical forms: *little pigmentation* (Figs. 272, 273), *without pigment* (Fig. 274), *affecting only one quadrant or only one eye*. The characteristic features of these atypical forms are usually indicated by the name of the disease. The *progressive retinitis albipunctata* is clinically very similar to retinitis pigmentosa. Ophthalmoscopically it is characterized by white or yellowish, round or oval deposits involving the entire retina. They are of uniform size and may be accompanied by the typical pigmentary changes; the *fundus albipunctatus* shows a less wide extension of the degenerative process, always sparing the fovea. The condition is stationary and has a good prognosis (Fig. 275). The *fundus flavimaculatus* is a retinal dystrophy characterized by yellowish spots at the posterior pole. They vary in size and may in the center have a pigmented area (Fig. 276); this is associated with a macular lesion leading to loss of visual acuity with a normal or subnormal ERG. The prognosis is rather good because the condition develops slowly; it affects mainly young patients; fluorescein angiography may show the lesions as of the initial stages because of the early hyperfluorescence of these degenerative spots.

Leber amaurosis (neuro-epithelial dysgenesis). This is a diffuse tapetoretinal dystrophy. It is congenital and the affected children are blind as of the first months of life due to the atrophy of the photoreceptor cells. The degeneration begins in the periphery and shows ophthalmoscopically white spots and pigment dots which increase in size and number. The general aspect is that of a "pepper and salt" fundus. The optic nervehead is pale, the vessels attenuated and the ERG extinguished. There is complete afferent pupillary areflexia, pendular nystagmus and sometimes the digito-ocular sign of Franceschetti.

Medical treatment is inadequate and ineffective for all types of tapetoretinal degenerations, except for the dystrophy associated with hypobetalipoproteinemia and acanthocytosis (Bassen-Kornzweig) in which vitamin A orally is indicated.

We have to keep in mind that the tapetoretinal degeneration is frequently only one aspect of a widespread systemic involvement: the fundus condition may be associated with degenerative lesions in the central nervous system or the pituitary, as for instance in the Laurence-Moon-Bardet-Biedel syndrome (retinitis pigmentosa, obesity, polydactyly, hypogenitalism and mental retardation) and with the Cockayne syndrome (retinitis pigmentosa, deafness and progeria).

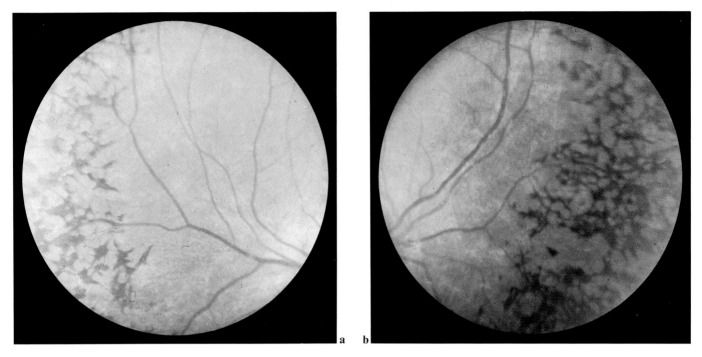

Fig. 268. **a)** and **b).** Tapetoretinal degeneration (true retinitis pigmentosa). Typical black pigment accumulations resembling bone corpuscles.

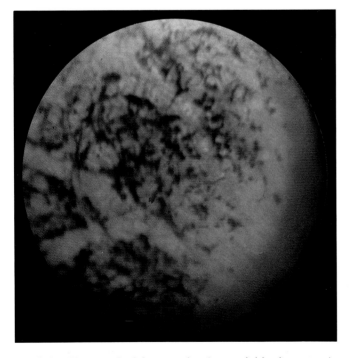

Fig. 269. Tapetoretinal degeneration (true retinitis pigmentosa). Characteristic pigmentation in the retinal periphery.

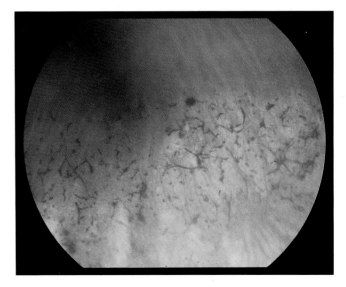

Fig. 270. Tapetoretinal degeneration (true retinitis pigmentosa). Pigment accumulations at the equator resembling bone corpuscles.

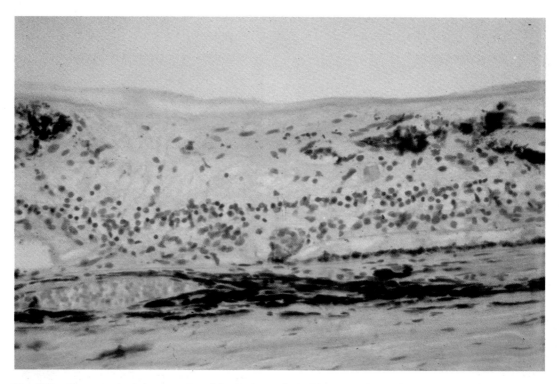

Fig. 271. Tapetoretinal degeneration (histologic section). Pigment migration is evident: the coarse pigment deposits lie in the internal retinal layers and the retinal cyto-architectonic is profoundly changed.

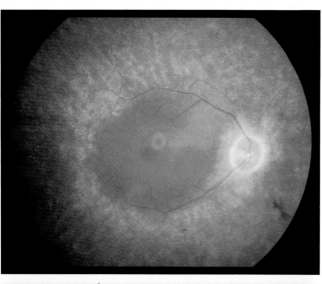

Fig. 272. Tapetoretinal degeneration (retinitis pigmentosa with little pigment). Partial optic atrophy and conspicuous attenuation of the retinal vessels. Only the posterior pole seems not yet affected whereas the rest of the fundus is sprinkled with small, dystrophic yellow spots and with a few characteristic pigment deposits.

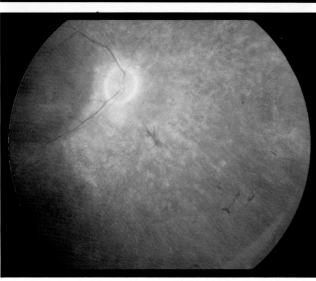

Fig. 273. Tapetoretinal degeneration (same ad Fig. 272). In the lower nasal segment are a few bone corpuscle-like pigment deposits.

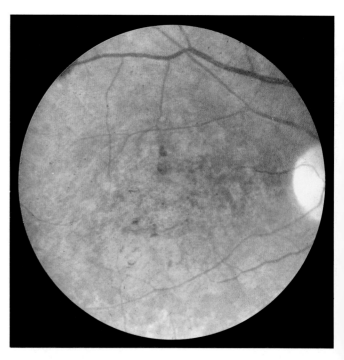

Fig. 274. Retinitis pigmentosa sine pigmento. Detail of the fundus picture showing the posterior pole in high magnification.

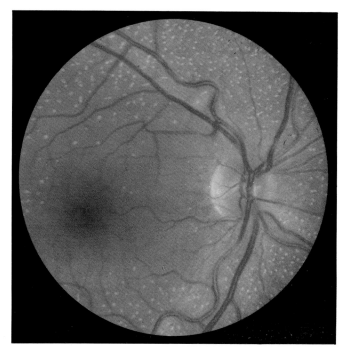

Fig. 275. Fundus albipunctatus. The whole retina is sprinkled with yellow shiny dots which spare the fovea.

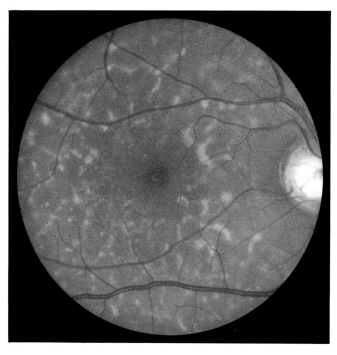

Fig. 276. Fundus flavimaculatus. Characteristic white-yellow fishlike changes seen over the entire fundus and associated with degenerative macular lesions.

PERIPHERAL RETINAL DEGENERATIONS WHICH MAY OR MAY NOT CAUSE A RETINAL BREAK

The degenerations of the peripheral fundus consist of a series of lesions affecting the retina, the choroid, and the vitreous, nearly always due to a two-fold series of factors which are mixed to a varying degree: one series is constitutional and hereditary, the other one is degenerative (of vascular origin) as could be proven by fluorescein angiographic and recent histopathologic studies. These factors are often associated with high myopia, have a direct relation to age and are situated anterior or barely posterior to the equator.

These changes are only rarely directly responsible for retinal breaks with subsequent retinal detachment; and indeed in order for such a severe complication to develop it is in-dispensable that similar changes occur in the vitreous gel with the subsequent formation of pathologic vitreo-retinal adhesions causing traction. The first distinction, therefore, can be made between rhegmatogenous and nonrhegmatogenous types: in the rhegmatogenous changes there is always a participation of the vitreous with destruction of its physical and chemical integrity and liquifaction of the gel (Table 6).

The **non-rhegmatogenous lesions** involve mainly the external retinal layers. The most frequent clinical types are: *paving stone degeneration* and *pigmentary degeneration*.

Table 6. Classification of non-rhegmatogenous and rhegmatogenous peripheral retinal degeneration.

Non-rhegmatogenous	
Paving stone degeneration	degeneration of the external retinal layers
Pigmentary degeneration	
Rhegmatogenous	
Peripheral cystoid degeneration	intraretinal degeneration
Lattice degeneration (oval plaques of well delineated retinal thinning)	
Snail track degeneration (degeneration with white glistening dots)	
White with and without pressure	vitreo-retinal degenerations
Pigment clumps	
Paravascular adhesions	

Both occur often in highly myopic eyes and have a tendency to progress with age; they are in direct relation to a deficit of vascular flow. They have a favorable prognosis as they only under unusual circumstances produce a retinal break; prophylactic treatment is therefore not necessary.

Pavingstone degeneration occurs mainly in the inferior temporal sector and is on ophthalmoscopic examination characterized by white-yellow spots which are oval and sharply outlined; the chroidal vessels are often seen in the center of the lesion. These areas are surrounded by a pigmentary ring (Figs. 277 a, b). Histopathologically they present atrophic lesions in the pigment epithelium, the external retinal layers and the choriocapillaries; the vitreous is not affected (Fig. 278).

The **pigmentary degeneration** is usually at the equator and may involve one or several quadrants. We therefore distinguish degenerations affecting one, or several segments, or the entire circumference. Ophthalmoscopically we see areas of chorio-retinal atrophy and zones of depigmentation alternating with zones of pigment dispersion (Figs. 279-281).

The **rhegmatogenous** degenerative lesions are the main causes for the idiopathic retinal detachment. As mentioned above, we are dealing here with a double mechanism: on one hand there is a progressive thinning of the retina until this organ perforates; on the other hand there is vitreous traction on the margin of the lesion. We distinguish various types differing in clinical picture and course. The main types are the following:

Peripheral cystoid (or microcystoid) **degeneration** hardly ever leads to a retinal hole: the lesion is intraretinal and the most advanced end result is senile retinoschisis. It is present to a varying degree in nearly all adult eyes and is situated just posterior to the ora serrata. Ophthalmoscopically the pre-equatorial retina appears as a greysh band subdivided into round holes separated by thin septa. Histologically we see large cystoid spaces which encompass the entire thickness of the sensory retina (Fig. 282). The prognosis is generally good. Only 10% of these eyes will develop a retinal break.

Lattice degeneration is according to some authors present in 20 to 65% of all eyes undergoing treatment for retinal detachment. This degeneration does indeed evolve frequently into a retinal hole or tear. The lesions usually involve one segment of the fundus and appear ophthalmoscopically as a thin red retina with oval well-delineated plaques which appear lighter than the adjacent retina. They show linear, white-greyish lines and an irregular pigment dissemination inside the lesion (Figs. 283-288). Above this area of retinal degeneration the vitreous is liquified and there are often vitreo-retinal adhesions along the margins of the oval plaque. The degeneration is most often seen in the upper temporal quadrant between the equator and the ora serrata. Histologically there is retinal atrophy mainly limited to the inner limiting membrane and the nerve fiber layer, hyalinization of the retinal blood vessels with intraretinal proliferation of perivascular glia (white lines); there are associated choroidal (thickening of Bruch's membrane and vascular

sclerosis) and vitreal (liquifaction of the central and condensation of the peripheral vitreous) alterations. Fluorescein angiography confirms the vascular etiology: the lesion is arranged around a vein, the arterial blood flow is diminished or absent, whereas the surrounding vessels appear normal.

Snail track degeneration is often found in connection with myopia. The lesions are usually bilateral and symmetrical, most frequently situated in the upper temporal quadrant, at or in front of the equator. Clinically they may present themselves in three forms with different prognoses: a *diffuse form*, a *focal* one and one *associated with other degenerative* lesions, usually lattice degeneration (the two last types have a higher propensity to form retinal breaks). Ophthalmoscopically these lesions appear as milky zones in which numerous scintillating, white-yellow, reflecting elements are deposited. The lesions are parallel to the equator and there are vitreous adhesions around them (Figs. 289-291). Histologically the lesions involve mainly the retinal neural elements thereby liberating neutral fat causing a secondary proliferation of glial cells which phagocytize the lipid molecules. Fluorescein angiography shows a vascular deficit or ischemia.

White with and **without** pressure is a form of rhegmatogenous retinal degeneration. The white color is only visible when the sclera is indented. The lesion usually affects the temporal fundus between the equator and the ora. It is usually bilateral. It may appear as an isolated degenerative phenomenon or may be associated with other rhegmatogenous lesions. Ophthalmoscopically we see ischemic, pale, festooned areas alternating with retinal zones that appear darker. The fundus in general has a stippled appearance (Figs. 292, 293). Histopathologically there is retinal atrophy with the formation of intraretinal argentaffin fibers ("spiderlike bodies") localized mainly in the inner retinal layers accompanied by a proliferation of collagen fibers and vitreo-retinal adhesions around the lesion. In 10% of these eyes the vitreo-retinal retraction will lead to a flap tear.

Coarse pigmentation is a degeneration that increases with age and is most often found in emmetropic eyes. It is most frequently seen in the upper temporal segment of the fundus; there is no tendency for bilaterality or symmetry. It appears in two clinical forms: isolated or associated with other retinal degenerations, e.g., paravascular adhesions. Some authors have felt that these two conditions are closely related. A prophylactic treatment is necessary because 26% of these eyes will develop a retinal break. Ophthalmoscopically wee see pigmented, well-delineated lesions usually behind the equator and surrounding the retinal blood vessels giving the appearance of a retinal elevation. If the lesion is associated with paravascular adhesions we see localized vitreo-retinal connections (Figs. 294, 295).

Finally the **paravascular adhesions** belong to the primary vitreous changes; they lie between the equator and the ora serrata, usually over retinal vessels, mostly at bifurcations or crossings. Ophthalmoscopically they are practically invisible. With slit lamp examination and indentation we see small whitish structures which are dense, elevated, conical with the base on the retina and the peak toward the vitreous

They constitute initially traction strands which may cause a retinal break (Fig. 296).

The symptomatology of peripheral retinal degenerations is associated with the various alterations responsible for these lesions. Phosphenes are pathognomonic for retinal ischemia, whether it is functional or organic; floaters may be present in vitreal disorganization as well as in a posterior vitreous detachment; scotomas are indicative for retinal changes and correspond to the projection of areas where the retina is detached.

As far as treatment is concerned we believe that the non-rhegmatogenous retinal degenerations do not need any prophylaxis; on the other hand, rhegmatogenous changes may need to be treated. If a cystoid degeneration progresses to a retinoschisis prophylactic treatment will be obligatory when the lesion extends up to three disc diameters from the macular area or when holes develop both in the internal and the external wall of the schisis. Photocoagulation, cryotherapy or diathermy is indicated in all other types of rhegmatogenous degenerations and for retinal tears produced by vitreous adhesions. Argon laser photocoagulation will not make these lesions disappear but will limit them and isolate them from the adjacent normal retina produc-ing a ring of scars which spot welds the two layers of the schisis together thereby arresting the retinal splitting and the development of a true retinal detachment.

Cryotreatment or diathermy destroys the lesion which will be incorporated in a scar following the necrosis produced by the physical energy (Fig. 297). The end result is similar in the two modes of treatment.

Diathermy is now regarded as obsolete (mainly because it produces necrosis of the superficial sclera). The choice between laser photocoagulation and cryotreatment can be made on the basis of various factors.

Cryotherapy is indicated for children in whom the treatment has to be performed under general anesthesia; it is also indicated when the refractive media are opaque, when the degenerative lesions lie in the far periphery or are too diffuse in their extension. Laser treatment, on the other hand, is indicated for more posterior lesions and for those lesions which are focal and localized (Figs. 287, 288, 291, 296).

These treatments with physical modalities may be supplemented by mechanical surgical treatments (exoplant, encircling band) if the vitreo-retinal traction is so strong that a counterpressure from the outside is necessary to balance the forces of traction.

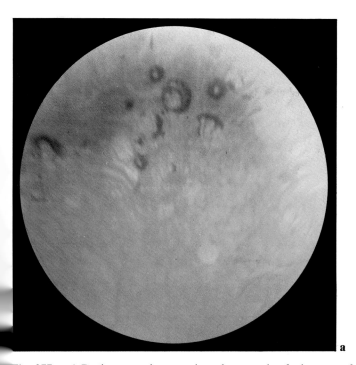 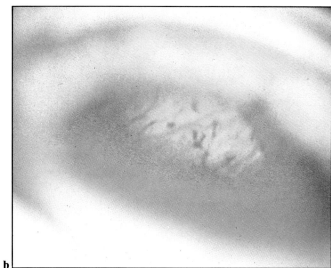

a b

Fig. 277. a) Pavingstone degeneration: degenerative foci, some of which are delineated by pigment dispersion. At the depth of these lesions choroidal vessels are visible.
b) Pavingstone degeneration (slit lamp picture of the peripheral retina). Inside of the white lesions, which are well delineated by a fine pigment dispersion, the choroidal vessels can be seen.

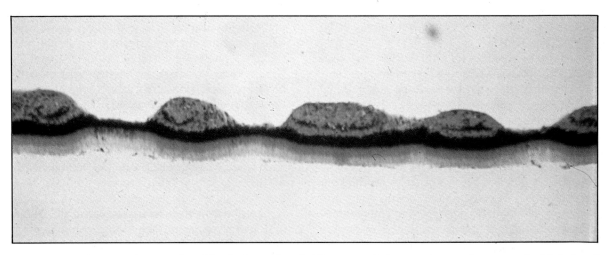

Fig. 278. Pavingstone degeneration (histologic specimen). The areas of degeneration are interspersed with isolated parts of the retina that are only partially changed in their cyto-architectonic, especially as far as the internal layers are concerned.

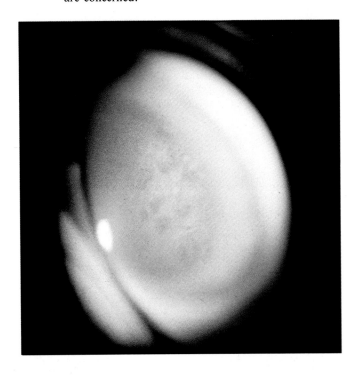

Fig. 279. Pigmentary degeneration (slit lamp picture of the peripheral retina). Tigroid fundus with areas of pigment dispersion in the periphery in the form of a non-rhegmatogenous degeneration.

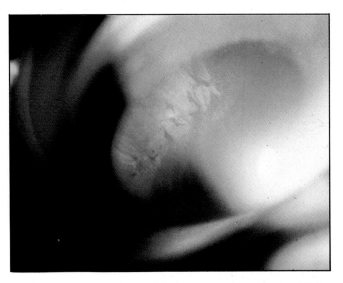
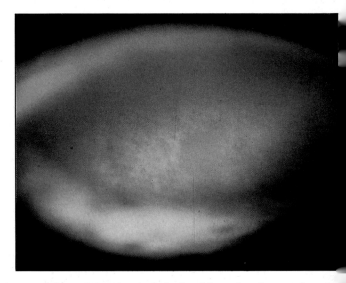

Figs. 280 and 281. Equatorial pigmentary degeneration (slit lamp picture of the peripheral retina). Isolated irregular pigment deposits are seen.

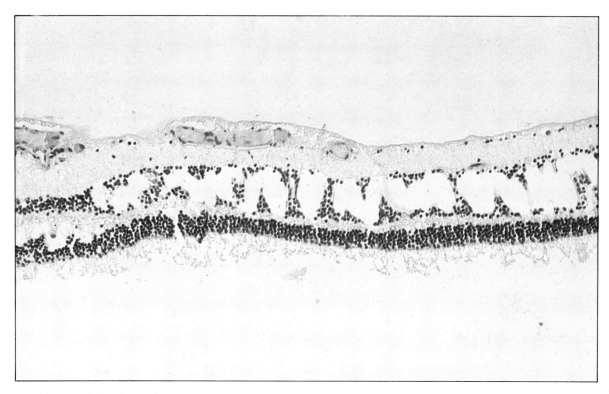

Fig. 282. Peripheral cystoid degeneration with a possible evolution toward retinoschisis (histologic section).

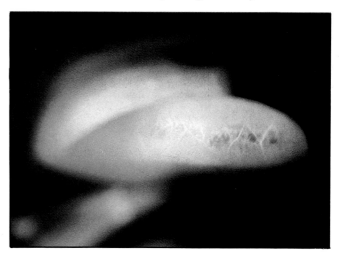

Fig. 283. Lattice degeneration (retinal thinning in the form of a well outlined oval plaque) (slit lamp picture of the peripheral retina). Segmental focal lesion with wide white stripes — occluded vessels —, and coarse pigment deposits).

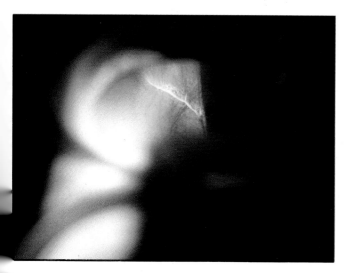

Fig. 284. Lattice degeneration (slit lamp picture of the peripheral retina).

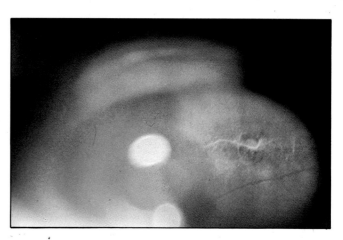

Fig. 285. Lattice degeneration (slit lamp picture of the peripheral retina). The occluded vessels and a few small holes are visible in the area of the degeneration.

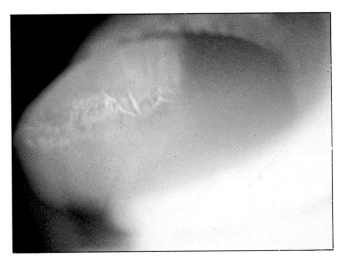

Fig. 286. Lattice degeneration (slit lamp picture of the peripheral retina).

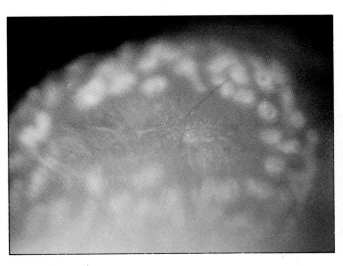

Fig. 287. Lattice degeneration soon after photocoagulation treatment (slit lamp picture of the peripheral retina).

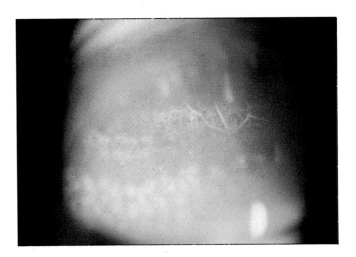

Fig. 288. Lattice degeneration (slit lamp picture of the peripheral retina). Scars, partly already pigmented, after photocoagulation treatment.

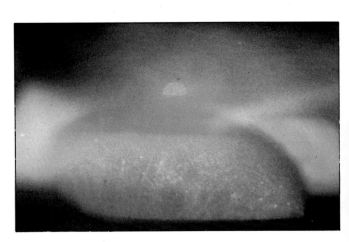

Fig. 289. Snail track degeneration showing the white shiny deposits (slit lamp picture of the peripheral retina). These deposits are partly coalescing to larger foci.

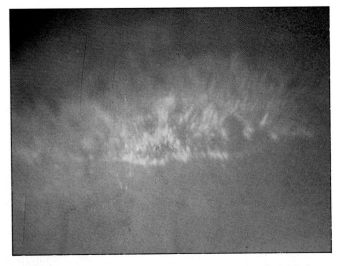

Fig. 290. Snail track degeneration with coalescing foci (slit lamp picture of the peripheral retina). There are some small holes, often only lamellar, within the lesion.

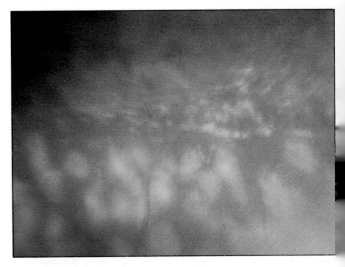

Fig. 291. Snail track degeneration (slit lamp picture of the peripheral retina). The same case as in Fig. 290 in higher magnification soon after photocoagulation treatment.

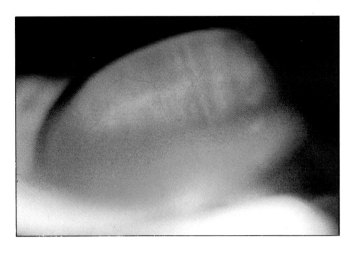

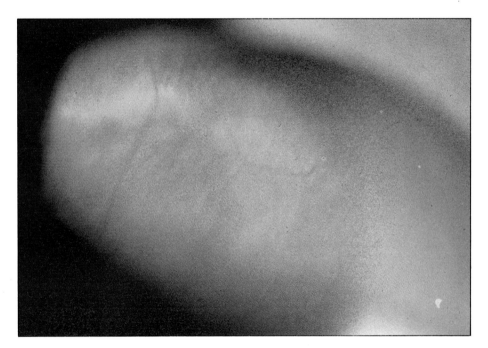

Fig. 292. White without pressure (slit lamp picture of the peripheral retina). The undulating (festooned) posterior margin separates the pale degenerative zone from the healthy, intensively colored zone. It is frequently the site of vitreo-retinal adhesions.

Fig. 293. White without pressure (slit lamp picture of the peripheral retina). Detail of Fig. 292 in higher magnification.

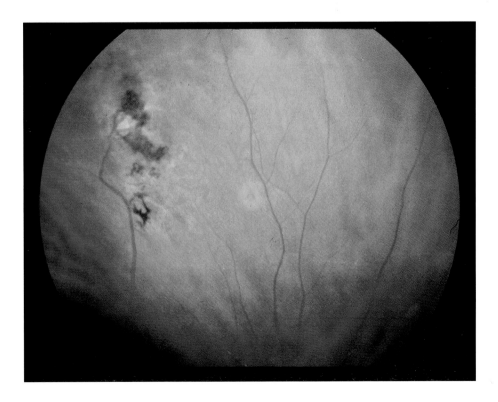

Fig, 294. Coarse pigment deposits and associated paravascular adhesions. These adhesions develop in an area of retinal thinning. Large pigment deposits are seen confirming the frequent association of the two types of degeneration.

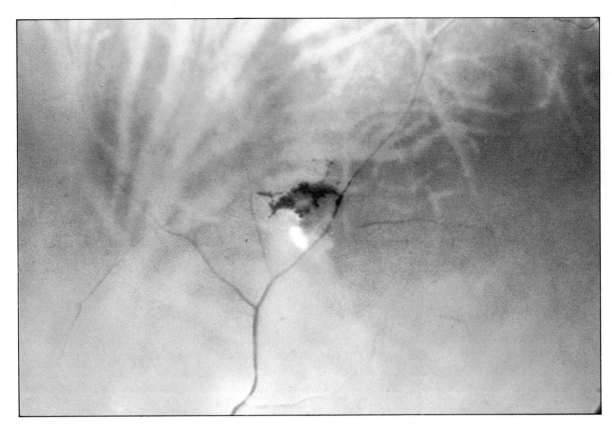

Fig. 295.   Macroscopic specimen of a fresh retina in a sectioned globe: coarse pigment deposit surrounding a retinal vessel on which there is vitreo-retinal traction (paravascular adhesions).

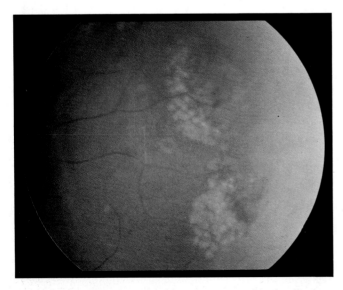

Fig. 296.   Paravascular adhesions: two areas of such adhesions are ringed by argon laser coagulations.

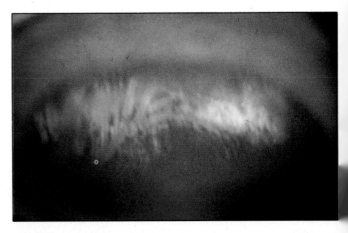

Fig. 297.   Area of peripheral retinal atrophy treated with cryo-applications; the end result is an adherent chorio-retinitis (slit lamp picture of the retinal periphery).

RETINAL HOLES AND TEARS

Retinal breaks constitute a discontinuity of the sensory retina due to degenerative (usually called rhegmatogenous), vascular, inflammatory or traumatic lesions which are associated with vitreous changes. They are usually located in the mid or extreme periphery, rarely at the posterior pole or in the macula. On the basis of their morphologic characteristics they can be divided into: holes, flap tears and retinal disinsertion.

Retinal holes are formed by a progressive thinning and focal destruction of retinal tissue which in the majority of cases is caused by vascular lesions. There is usually no vitreous traction. There is a dissolution of retinal continuity without the development of a flap. Sometimes the operculum is visible, completely detached from the retina floating freely in the vitreous (Figs. 298, 299). The holes appear with the ophthalmoscope and with the slit lamp dark red varying in size from the diameter of a large retinal vessel to one half to two thirds of a disc diameter. They are usually round or oval with sharp margins; the adjacent retina may be edematous or show radial folds and signs of elevation (Figs. 299-302).

We distinguish *primary* and *secondary holes*: the primary holes are round or oval, punched out, usually peripheral and not accompanied by retinal or vitreal lesions or degenerations. They are generally asymptomatic. They are found in 15% of persons over the age of 30. Secondary holes derive from preexisting rhegmatogenous degenerative areas and are associated with organic and functional changes in the vitreous, e.g., retinal holes in myopic or aphakic eyes. Macular holes can also be regarded as secondary holes as they represent, according to some authors, the end stage of a cystoid macular degeneration (Figs. 303-308).

Retinal tears, on the other hand, have obvious pathologic vitreoretinal adhesions at the flap which exert traction detaching the surrounding retina.
The tears often show a horseshoe shape and their size varies. The flap is somewhat triangular, mobile and floats in the vitreous (Figs. 309-311). The base of the flap points toward the ora serrata and its margins are often rolled up. The dark red choroid is visible at the bottom of the tear; the latter is sometimes traversed by intact retinal vessels (Figs. 312, 313). The so-called "acute retinal tears" are absolutely unpredictable and develop in retinal areas which appear clinically normal. In this case, the lesion is the result of two pathogenic mechanisms: an acute vascular occlusion in a retinal area causing a necrotic infarct, and a traction factor exerted from the vitreous (Figs. 314 a, b; 315).

Retinal disinsertion may be secondary to trauma or an intraocular inflammation (pars planitis). The disinserted retinal flap appears white, is often elevated and with margins showing the typical teeth and bays of the ora serrata; in the flap we sometimes see the signs of the precipitating condition. In cases of trauma we may find hemmorrhages, fibrin, localized clouding of the vitreous cortex; in cases of inflammation we may see white intraretinal exudates (cotton-wool patches) and an inflammatory condensation of the vitreous which has been called "snow banks". The disinsertion is most often seen in young individuals, even in children (with pars planitis), but may manifest itself in all age groups following a severe trauma.

Giant tears or *dialyses* are always localized in the extreme periphery; they involve more than a quadrant of the retina and are usually found in the lower temporal fundus. They are sometimes bilateral. The condition affects often young emmetropic or highly myopic individuals. It is due, at least in part, to congenital malformations. The dialysis appears as a wide cleft with the major axis parallel to the ora. It becomes more evident on indentation (Fig. 316).

The patients may have no symptoms at all, as for instance in case of peripheral retinal holes; on the other hand, more commonly, they experience phosphenes and floaters.
Loss in central visual acuity occurs in cases of macular holes and in eyes with a vitreous hemorrhage usually due to a torn vessel lying in the depth of the retinal break. A retinal hole will only rarely enlarge or cause a retinal detachment, especially when the vitreous is normal; a horseshoe tear, on the other hand, will because of the concomitant vitreo-retinal traction produce a detachment in a considerable number of cases.
Predisposing conditions for a retinal detachment are diffuse retinal degenerative changes (whether acquired or hereditary), alterations of the vitreous gel, aphakia, myopia, a positive family history as far as the detachment or vitreo-retinal pathology is concerned. Argon laser coagulation is presently the treatment of choice for retinal holes or tears if the retina is still attached. With this treatment we isolate the affected areas from the surrounding healthy retina producing a marked and obvious reactive pigmentary dissemination (photocoagulation barrier) which spot welds the two neural layers together preventing an extension of the pathologic process (Figs 302; 305 a, b; 314 b).
Transconjunctival cryotreatment is an alternative approach. It provokes a reactive edema in the treated zone and a complete adhesion (adhesive chorioretinitis) with destruction of the sensory retina.

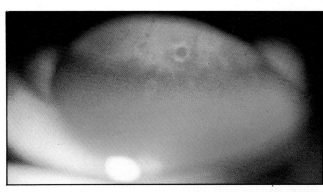

Fig. 298. Equatorial retinal hole with a halo of perifocal edema. The operculum is visible in the vitreous (slit lamp picture of the retinal periphery).

Fig. 299. Retinal hole. Detail of Fig. 298 in higher magnification.

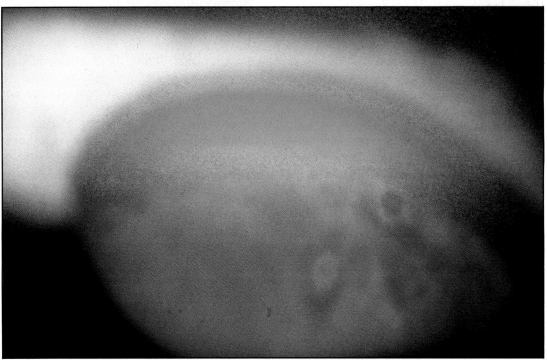

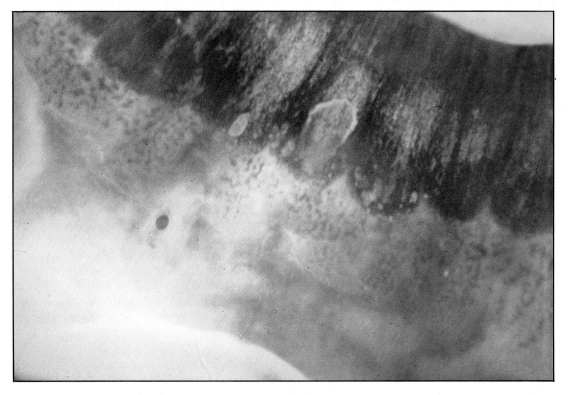

Fig. 300. Macroscopic specimen of a fresh retina in a sectioned globe: localized retinal hole just posterior to the ora serrata in an area of peripheral cystoid degeneration.

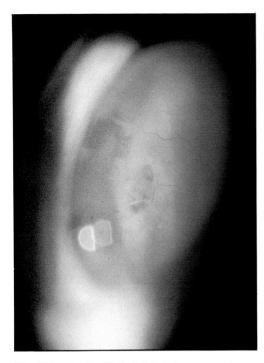

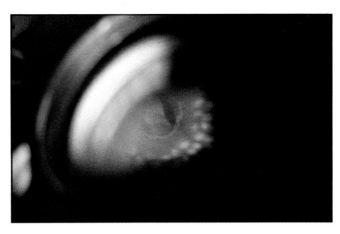

Fig. 302. Retinal hole recently treated with a ring of photocoagulation (slit lamp picture of the peripheral retina). The margins of the hole are still elevated.

Fig. 301. Retinal hole behind the equator in an area of retinal thinning (slit lamp picture of the peripheral retina). Within this area are other rhegmatogenous elements of lattice degeneration: occluded vessels (white striae) and pigment accumulation.

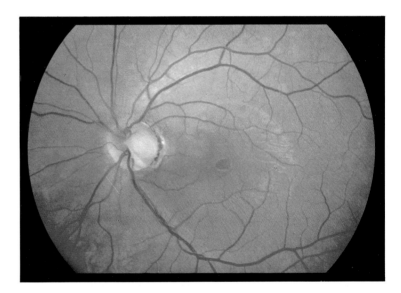

Fig. 303. Macular hole. Moderate retinal edema around the lesion. There is an optic nerve coloboma in one sector.

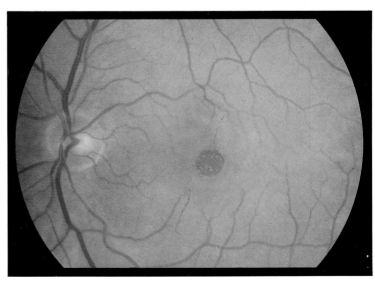

Fig. 304. Macular hole.

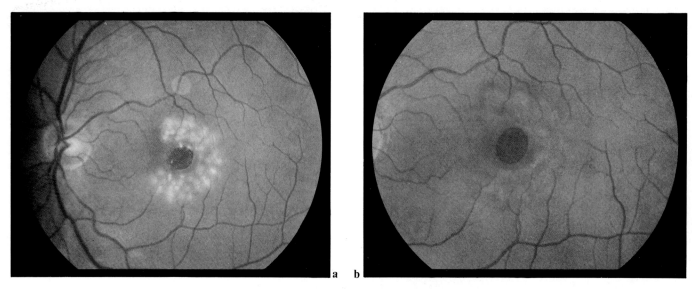

Fig. 305. Macular hole (same case as in Fig. 304) soon after treatment by a horseshoe shaped barrier of argon laser treatment (**a**); after some time the photocoagulated area shows evidence of pigment and scar formation (**b**).

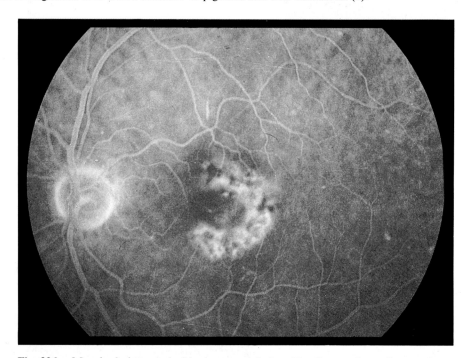

Fig. 306. Macular hole treated with photocoagulation. The fluorescein angiogram shows the window effect (same case as in Figs. 304 and 305).

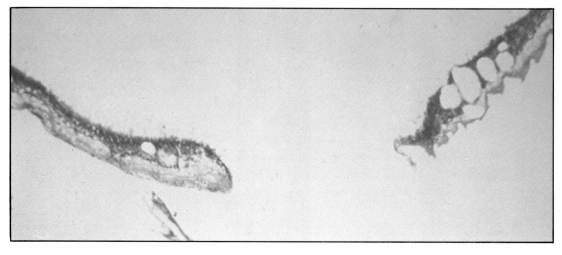

Fig. 307. Histologic section of the retina. Retinal hole; on both sides of the hole are micro- and macrocystoid degenerations of the retina.

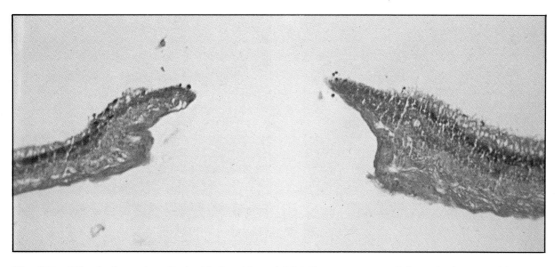

Fig. 308. Histologic section. Retinal hole with an initial disarrangement of the retinal cyto-architecture on both sides of the hole.

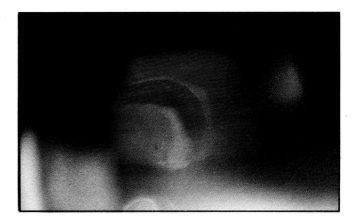

Fig. 309. Flap tear with adherent retina (slit lamp picture of the peripheral retina).

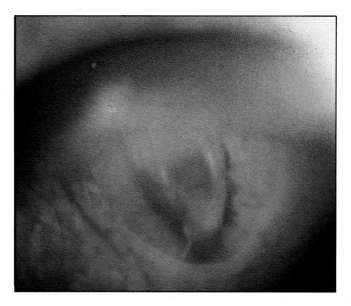

Fig. 310. Flap tear of the retina, recently treated with argon laser (slit lamp picture of the peripheral retina). There is a pigmented spot on the flap, probably part of a preexisting rhegmatogenous degeneration.

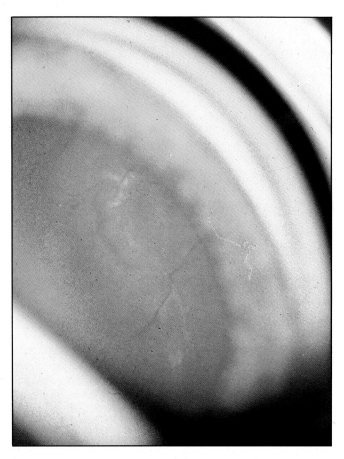

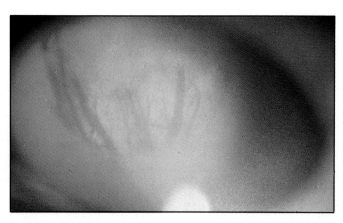

Fig. 312. Everted flap tear on the detached retina (biomicroscopic picture of the peripheral retina in high magnification). Choroidal vessels can be seen in the depth of the tear.

Fig. 311. Flap tear on the detached retina (biomicroscopic picture of the peripheral retina).

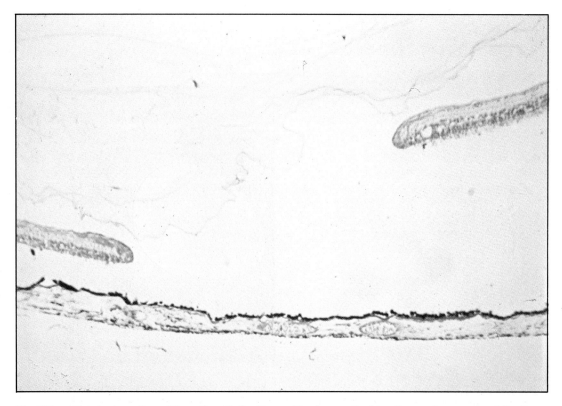

Fig. 313. Histologic section of the retina. Retinal tear with vitreo-retinal traction on the margin of the flap.

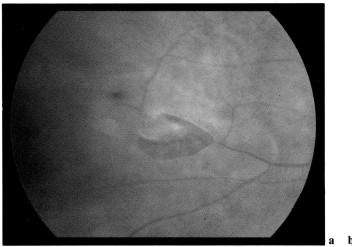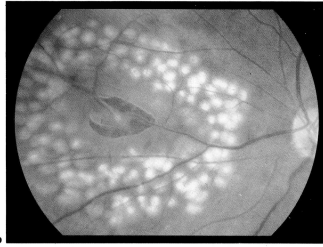

a b

Fig. 314. **a)** Large, recent flap tear of the nasal retina due to vascular changes with rupture of a large vessel. Edema of the adjacent retina; two small retina hemorrhages.
b) Argon laser treatment of the retinal tear.

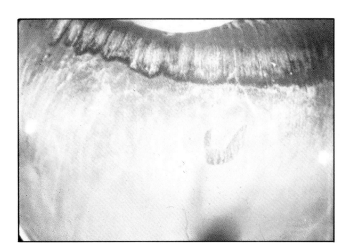

Fig. 315. Fresh macroscopic specimen of a dissected globe. Recent retinal flap tear just posterior of the ora.

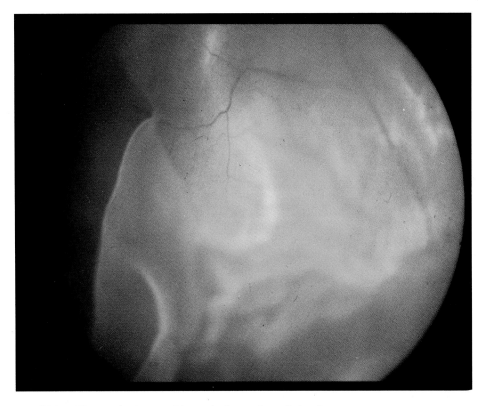

Fig. 316. Giant retinal tear with marked eversion of the flap.

RETINOSCHISIS

In retinoschisis the *sensory epithelium is divided into two layers*. This may be the consequence of trophic lesion caused by a choroidal or chorioretinal inflammation, but in the majority of cases it is the consequence of degenerative processes, which may be hereditary in type and occur in young patients, or may be acquired and appear in adults. The most frequent localizations are the two areas where the retina is thinnest and least vascularized, i.e., the periphery and the macula. Retinoschisis affecting older patients is usually located in the periphery and represents the terminal stage of a cystoid degeneration; in these cases central vision is not affected.

The juvenile retinoschisis is usually bilateral. It is the sequel of hereditary vitreo-retinal degenerations. The transmission may be autosomal dominant (Wagner disease), autosomal recessive (Goldmann-Favre disease) or sex linked. The diagnosis is based not only on the clinical examination but also on the ERG which is extinguished in Goldmann-Favre disease and subnormal in the other two conditions (see page 163). Ophthalmoscopically retinoschisis appears like a translucent veil which corresponds to the internal limiting membrane. It is white, transversed by retinal vessels and does not move with the eye. It is elevated over the retinal surface (Figs. 317, 318). It usually lies in the lower temporal quadrant. We frequently find oval or round dehiscences of the internal lamella. Through similar dehiscences of the external lamella the choroid becomes visible. There may be an associated lattice (or reticular) degeneration with vitreal changes; in these cases the pathologic adhesions and tractions may lead to a retinal hole and subsequent retinal detachment. The retinal vessels show in congenital retinoschisis anomalies and in the senile degenerative form neovascularizations. Fluorescein angiography will reveal whether the vessel walls are permeable to fluorescein or not.

The histopathologic specimen shows that retinoschisis begins with the formation of true cavities in the retinal tissue; these are due to atrophy of neural elements; these lacunae are initially limited to the outer plexiform layer, but as they progress will extend to the entire sensory retina. These cavities have a tendency to coalesce. The schisis will appear when the septa disappear thereby forming large cavities dividing the retina into two layers (Figs. 319, 321). There may be discontinuities, both of the internal lamella (pseudohole) as well as of the external lamella.

Initially the patients do not experience any symptoms and the diagnosis of a retinoschisis is often made incidentally during a routine examination of the ocular fundus; only later will the disease be associated with a constriction of the visual field when the retinal changes extend posterior to the equator. Decreased central vision with central scotoma will develop when the macula is involved.

Argon laser photocoagulation can be used as a prophylactic treatment in order to ring the split retina; surgical intervention will be necessary when there is a frank retinal detachment.

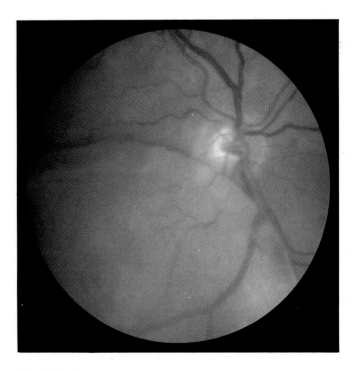

Fig. 317. Peripheral retinoschisis.

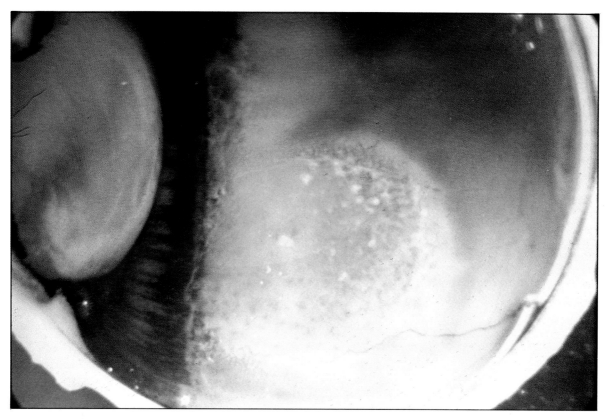

Fig. 318. Retinoschisis (macroscopic specimen of a dissected globe).

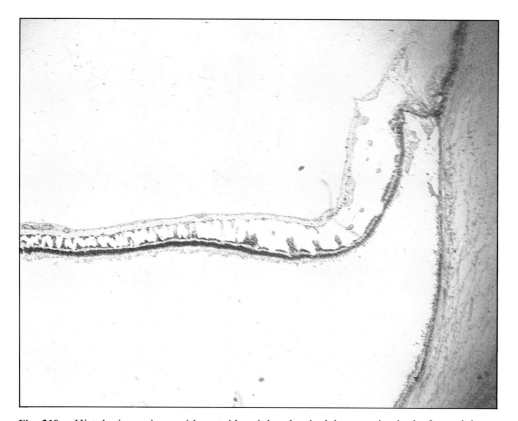

Fig. 319. Histologic specimen with cystoid peripheral retinal degeneration in the far periphery, progressing toward a retinoschisis.

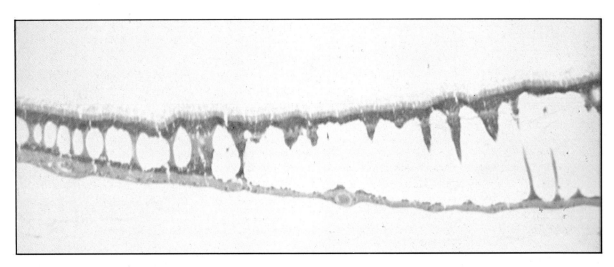

Fig. 320. Histologic specimen of retinoschisis. The peripheral cystoid degeneration on the left goes over into a true retinoschisis on the right.

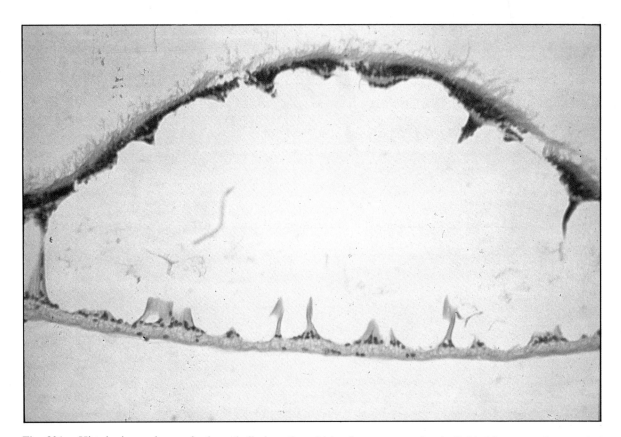

Fig. 321. Histologic specimen of a large bulla in retinoschisis; the sensory retina is divided into two characteristic lamellae.

RETINAL DETACHMENT

In order to understand the pathogenesis of a retinal detachment we have to refer to the embryology of the human eye: the optic cup has two layers: the external layer which develops later into the pigment epithelium, the inner layer which is produced by the in-folding of the optic vesicle gives rise to the sensory retina. There remains a virtual space between the two layers, i.e., between the outer members of the photoreceptors and the villi of the pigment epithelial cells. A subtle connection between the two layers is effected by a mucopolysaccharide matrix which is produced by the pigment epithelium and which also acts like an ion pump. This pump removes fluid from the subretinal space. The juxtaposition of these two layers is also guaranteed by the integrity of the vitreous which has a supporting and tamponading effect. Lack of one of these factors will produce a condition predisposing to a detachment, if not directly causing this event. Density of pigmentation favors a stronger adhesion and for this reason retinal detachment is less frequently seen in the black races.

The normal relation between pigment epithelium and sensory retina is lost in cases of primary or idiopathic detachment which constitutes the most frequent type of this condition. The virtual space becomes a real one as liquid accumulates. The fluid may be derived from either the vitreous or from the choroid. From a pathogenetic point of view we distinguish a primary or idiopathic (rhegmatogenous) retinal detachment from a secondary (exudative, traction, solid) detachment.

Primary or **rhegmatogenous** or **idiopathic retinal detachments** are always due to a tear or hole in the retina, subsequent to retinal degenerations. The vitreal fluid seeps through the break thereby extending the detachment.

The degenerative lesions are characterized by a variety of alterations of the retina, of the choroid and of the vitreous. These lesions may be hereditary or acquired and are predominantly vascular in nature (see Non-rhegmatogenous and rhegmatogenous peripheral retinal degenerations, pages 177-184). These lesions lie usually in the periphery and involve mainly the upper temporal quadrant. The retinal break and therefore the detachment can only occur when there is a parallel change of the vitreous gel with liquifaction and the formation of pathologic vitreo-retinal adhesions and tractions.

The most frequent rhegmatogenous retinal degeneration is the *lattice degeneration* of the retina which according to various authors is seen in 20 to 65% of the eyes treated for a detachment. The hereditary factors explain the tendency for bilaterality: we find in the contralateral eye frequently (20% of the cases) degenerative areas, often symmetrical to the zones in which the break (or the breaks) are found in the eye with the detachment. Other predisposing factors, in addition to advanced age, are high myopia and aphakia. In myopia we find in addition to degenerative lesions a higher percentage of vitreous liquifaction and therefore less vitreo-retinal adhesions (the posterior vitreous detachment is, according to various statistics, 20 to 35 times more frequent in the myopic eye than in the emmetropic eye). In the aphakic eye we find following an intracapsular extraction an anterior dislocation of the vitreous (endophthalmodonesis) with the possibility of traction on pathologic vitreoretinal adhesions, especially in older individuals in whom in addition to poor local circulatory conditions the vitreous is already liquified and collapsed.

The **exudative detachment** is characterized by an accumulation of fluid within the retina or choroid; this may be secondary to an inflammatory disease of the choroid, a detachment of the pigment epithelium, a central serous retinopathy, or secondary to tumors, either malignant (e.g., melanoma or retinoblastoma) or benign (e.g., angiomatosis retinae or choroidal hemangioma).

The subretinal fluid may shift and has a tendency to accumulate in the lower segments when the patient is in an erect position. Its location may change with the position of the head. Fluorescein angiography may identify the origin of the exudate: a more or less rapid diffusion of the dye across the barrier of the pigment epithelium may be observed. The integrity of the pigment epithelium is fundamental because it will not allow the passage of fluid from the choroid into the subretinal space. The same applies to the walls of the retinal vessels which constitute the blood retina barrier. If damaged there will be leakage of the dye into the retinal tissue.

The **traction retinal detachment** is due to fibrous bands in the vitreous developed from secondary organizations of inflammatory exudates or hemorrhages. Retinal neovascularization may also produce connective tissue or vascular strands between the retina and the vitreous. As the retina is not elastic their contraction will lead to a detachment. Traction bands may be formed in numerous systemic diseases, e.g., diabetes and sickle cell anemia, as well as in ocular conditions, e.g. pars planitis, retinopathy of prematurity, intraocular parasitic infestations, perforating injuries and contusions, cataract extraction with loss of vitreous and some forms of chronic and progressive severe uveitis. Retinal traction detachment is frequently associated with diabetic proliferative retinopathy: in these cases a preretinal or vitreous hemorrhage may be followed by the formation of vascular and connective tissue membranes which cause a traction detachment of the retina (see page 128).

The **solid retinal detachment** is usually due to a pathologic process outside the retina (primarily choroidal neoplasms); in these cases all the retinal layers (neuro-epithelium plus sensory retina) may be elevated. In advanced cases the formation of an exudative fluid will often allow the correct diagnosis. In these cases echographic examination will clearly show a solid mass beneath the subretinal fluid.

The clinical diagnosis of a retinal detachment can be made on the basis of the ophthalmoscopic picture, whether this is an idiopathic or a secondary detachment. The ophthalmoscopic picture varies, however, depending on the type of the detachment the direct illumination through the pupil may allow us to suspect a retinal detachment: the detached part of the retina appears in a different color (lighter) compared to the red color of the normal adjacent fundus. Careful direct and especially indirect binocular ophthalmoscopic examination permit us to distinguish the exact nature of the detachment, its location and extension. In cases of *idiopathic retinal detachment*, the detached part (retinal bulla) appears white-grey and moves with the motions of the eye; the vascular network of the retina is well visible and follows the undulations of the elevated sensory retina. These characteristics are the same in various bullous detachments, if they are extensive and involve more than one segment (Figs. 322-324). Once the presence of a detachment has been ascertained it is most important to find the holes and/or tears and to localize them (Fig. 325). The examination should be repeated after a few days of bed rest which may flatten the bullous detachment and thereby make retinal breaks visible which originally had been hidden in the bullae or retinal folds. Subretinal fluid will accumulate in the lower parts following gravity, even if the retinal break is in an upper quadrant; it extends in preferential directions which depend in addition to the position of the break on chorio-retinal adhesions, mainly at the ora and the optic nervehead. The most frequent finding is a large bulla in the inferior quadrants. The intraocular pressure is always low. Echographic examination will corroborate the diagnosis. In the ERG the b-wave will be subnormal or absent.

The ophthalmoscopic appearance of an *exudative detachment* is similar to the above description but varies in two fundamental aspects: there is no retinal hole or tear and there is less subretinal fluid accumulated.
The area of an exudative retinal detachment appears moist and shiny. It is transversed by subtle retinal folds which are a little elevated. Its color is more intense similar to that of the normal retina. Within the area of detachment there may be some degenerative deposits, as well as cotton-wool patches and fibrin, also perivascular sheathing and, depending on the etiology, other manifestations of vascular permeability (small hemorrhages) (Fig. 326). The overlying vitreous shows signs of inflammation, subtle pigment dissemination and some floating exudates. On fluorescein angiography we find in exudative detachments always leakage and accumulation of the dye.

In *traction detachment* the peak of the elevated retina corresponds to the insertion of the vitreous strand. This mechanism does not produce a bullous retinal detachment, but concave surfaces which are often oriented and directed in an irregular fashion in relation to the traction (Fig. 327). Ophthalmoscopic and biomicroscopic examination will determine the direction of the vitreous strand, its extension, as well as the vitreous opacification secondary to inflammatory reactions, characterized by a condensation in the vitreous and on the retina, together with pigment and fibrin in the vitreous gel.

The ophthalmoscopic appearance of a *solid retinal detachment* differs from the two above described types by the deeper color of the detached retina, at least when dealing with a choroidal melanoma, by the rigidity of the elevation and its volume (Figs. 328, 329). In these cases we find neither rhegmatogenous degenerations, nor breaks and holes. The retinal vascular tree maintains its characteristic features because the retina is still adherent to the underlying tissues. If the tumor mass is voluminous the ophthalmoscopic examination may be difficult and may resemble a choroidal detachment; the history and other clinical parameters will point toward the correct diagnosis. Occasionally we find on the surface of a solid retinal detachment small hemorrhages and coarse pigment. This large intraocular mass often allows a visualization of the extreme retinal periphery and of the ora serrata by a mechanism which is similar to an indentation.
The patients frequently experience prodromal symptoms, e.g., phosphenes and floaters, the first indicating a change

in retinal function and the second a beginning disorganization of the vitreous. A scotoma with sharp outlines corresponding to the detached area (but in the opposite direction) will appear. If the detachment is peripheral and extends gradually to the macula, the patient will experience metamorphopsia (distorted vision of objects) and decreased central acuity.

The therapy of a retinal detachment is exclusively surgical. There is, however, the possibility of a prophylactic treatment in order to avoid progress of rhegmatogenous lesions. Argon laser photocoagulation is sufficient for focal degenerative lesions or for punched out holes with no major changes in the vitreous. It is, however, prudent to add an encircling buckle to the photocoagulation or cryotreatment if the degenerative foci and holes are multiple and extensive and if there are also marked vitreous changes. A pars plana vitrectomy is indicated in cases of massive post-traumatic vitreous opacities with vitreo-retinal traction secondary especially to a perforating injury with an intraocular foreign body. Such an approach will probably prevent the major complication, i.e., massive vitreo-retinal proliferation (MVP) which will cause blindness in the majority of affected eyes.
The surgical treatment of a detachment aims in the first place to close by a scar the retinal break. This is done with physical energy (cryo-application or diathermy) which produces a dense chorio-retinal scar in the affected area (Fig. 330). Draining the subretinal fluid can be performed before or after the closure of the break depending upon the nature of the case. We then try to reapproach the pigment epithelium to the outer retinal layers by applying external pressure using a silicone exoplant (Fig. 331) and/or a circumferential scleral buckle. The buckle should always be behind the retinal break and serves to reduce the volume of the globe. In addition it produces a new ora serrata lying posterior to the anatomical one (Figs. 332, 333). The prognosis of such an operation is quite favorable: anatomical cure can be obtained in about 80% of the cases though this does not always guarantee a physiologic cure. The latter depends to a great extend upon the involvement of the macular area, on other clinical aspetcs and on the duration of the detachment.

The possible intra- and post-operative complications should not be under-estimated: among the first we should mention the serous or sero-hemorrhagic choroidal detachment produced by pressure or traction on the vorticose veins, ocular hypotony secondary to draining of the subretinal fluid, as well as secondary congestion due to excessive cryotherapy.

Organization of the vitreous with vitreo-retinal traction may develop during the post-operative course. There may also be a massive preretinal retraction, macular pucking, cystoid macular edema, changes in the macular pigment epithelium and finally secondary glaucoma due to blockage of the vorticose veins.

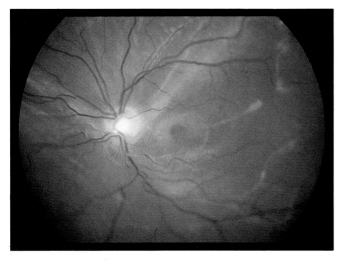

Fig. 322. Idiopathic (rhegmatogenous) retinal detachment. Coarse vitreo-retinal traction lines converge toward the posterior pole producing a retinal detachment.

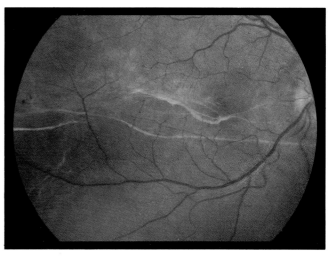

Fig. 323. Idiopathic (rhegmatogenous) retinal detachment. Massive vitreal organization in the form of straight bands which traverse the entire posterior pole in an attempt to demarcate the detachment. The upper line has already produced vitreo-retinal tractions.

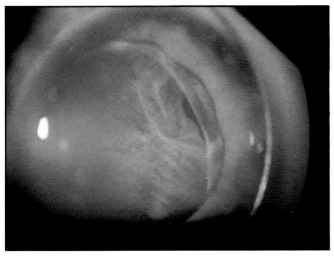

Fig. 324. Old total retinal detachment with giant tear in the upper nasal segment in an aphakic globe. With dilated pupil massive remnants of lens capsule and fibers are seen extending between 11 and 5 o'clock.

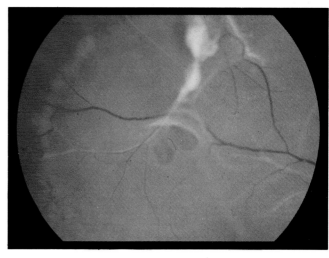

Fig. 325. Idiopatic (rhegmatogenous) retinal detachment. Vitreous traction band tethering two retinal holes beneath the upper temporal arcade. The retinal detachment also distorts the retinal vessels.

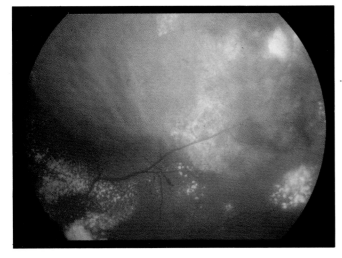

Fig. 326. Exudative retinal detachment in the upper temporal fundus. Numerous hard exudates in the detached retina and surrounding areas.

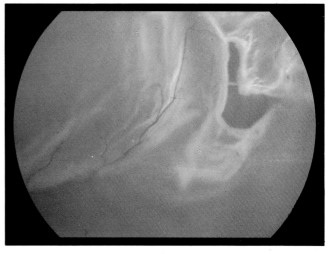

Fig. 327. Traction retinal detachment. The flap tear is well visible on the taut retina showing vitreo-retinal traction signs.

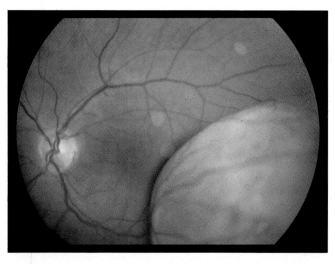

Fig. 328. Solid retinal detachment in the lower temporal segment partly covering the posterior pole.

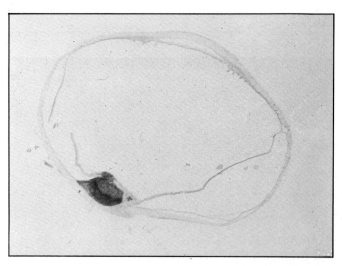

Fig. 329. Solid retinal detachment. Histologic specimen of a bissected globe: a mushroom shaped pigmented juxtapapillary choroidal tumor can be seen at the posterior pole causing a retinal elevation.

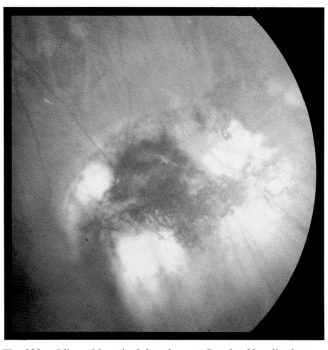

Fig. 330. Idiopathic retinal detachment. Result of localized cryotherapy: atrophic areas of chorioretinal adhesion.

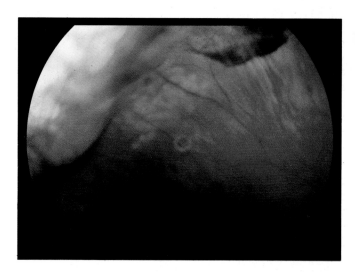

Fig. 331. Result of a retinal detachment operation. Localized indentation by an exoplant with adhesive chorioretinitis. The results of a recent photocoagulation treatment can be seen at the posterior margin of the indentation. The coagulation rings a retinal hole posterior to the indented area.

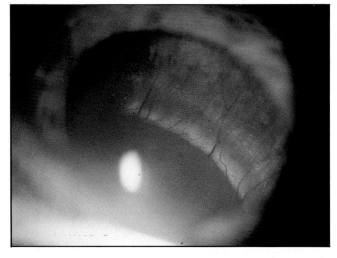

Fig. 332. Result of a retinal detachment operation (biomicroscopic picture of the peripheral retina): detail of the circular indentation produced by the buckle.

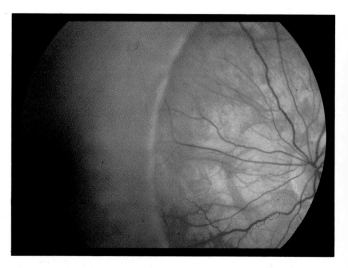

Fig. 333. Result of a retinal detachment operation. In front lies the buckle which is here out of focus, In the depth the adherent retina with myopic chorioretinal atrophies.

RETINAL FOLDS

We distinguish congenital and acquired retinal folds.

The **congenital folds** are associated with other developmental anomalies of the visual apparatus (see Chapter 3); in microphthalmic eyes these folds are visible as a kind of septum running from the posterior pole toward the lens (frontal septum of Heine); in cases of persistence of the hyaloid artery the folds present themselves as falciform elevations which course radially from the optic nervehead toward the retinal periphery (see Figs. 109, 334).

The **acquired form** is seen more frequently and represents a sequel of vitreo-retinal traction, traumatic lesions and deformations which the globe undergoes secondary to intraocular or orbital neoplasms. The traction folds represent wrinkles of the sensory retina. Ophthalmoscopically they appear as white striae with flat and poorly outlined terminations. Sometimes they are surrounded by a reactive edema; initially they are mobile, but they tend to become fixed in the course of their development. Morphologically we distinguish star-like and linear folds (Figs. 335, 336). The first type is of varying size (from quite small to more than a disc diameter) and is usually located between the posterior pole and the equator, frequently in the inferior quadrant. The linear folds represent, on the other hand, a rectilinear course along a meridian or parallel to the retinal equator.

Traction folds are due to changes in the vitreous structure which occur secondary to the organization of a vitreous or epiretinal hemorrhage or an inflammatory exudate; these have a tendency to contract (a typical example is that of a proliferative diabetic retinopathy); traction folds may also occur in connection whith rhegmatogenous peripheral retinal degenerations and as a sequel to old retinal detachments (see page 194 and following) (Figs. 335-338).

The folds running parallel to the equator originate from a condensation of the peripheral vitreous with retraction of the vitreous at the site of major vitreo-retinal adhesion, i.e., at the equator and at the ora.

In case of massive vitreal retraction (MVP) the folds are radial extending from the posterior pole to the equator; they are usually associated with extensive high retinal detachments.

Retinal folds indicate a poor prognosis and are frequently the reason for surgical failures in retinal detachment operations, at least when it is not possible to dissolve them surgically (vitrectomy, Yag laser, etc.); recurrent detachments are due to the formation of new retinal breaks, the reopening of treated breaks or to the recurrence of traction forces. Irregular star-like folds may also be seen in consequence to a pronounced hypotony of the globe or may be due to the incarceration of retina between choroid and sclera after an accidental or surgical trauma. Folds which develop when the globe undergoes marked deformation and is indented by an intraocular or orbital neoplasm are usually mobile and pliable. In these cases the course of the folds reflects the location of the tumor. They appear in parallel lines with varying extension. They are sometimes so conspicuous that the surface of the retina resembles the lobes and fissures of brain.

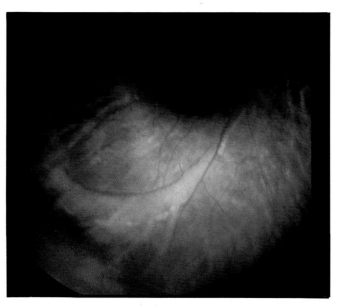

Fig. 334. Congenital retinal fold. Large elliptical fold extending from the posterior pole in an arcuate shape toward the mid periphery; the surrounding retina appears pale and the retinal vessels deviate from their course because of the thickness of the fold.

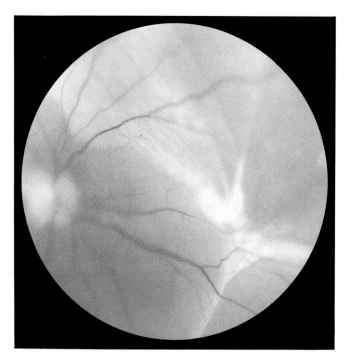

Fig. 335.   Large retinal fold estending in a star-shaped fashion. Beginning traction detachment of the retina, deviation of the retinal vessels due to the fold.

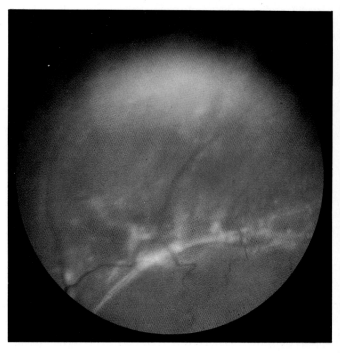

Fig. 336.   Retinal fold with radial thickening, parallel to the course of the vascular arcade; the traction causes conspicuous changes in the course of the vessels. Exudative foci are disseminated on both sides of the fold (the white area in the upper temporal part of the picture is a technical artifact).

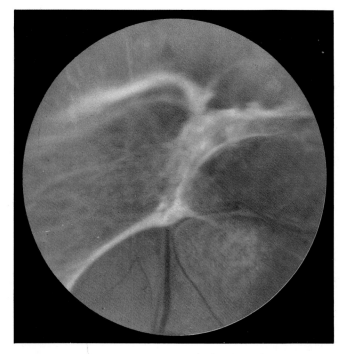

Fig. 337.   Retinal folds. Large, arcuate fibrous and connective tissue proliferation producing marked traction and a retinal detachment in the temporal segment.

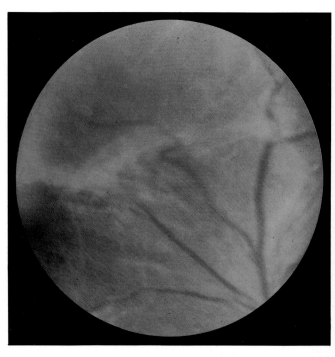

Fig. 338.   Retinal folds. Detail in high magnification. The traction effect is well visible on the elevated retinal surface and along the vascular trunks.

RETINAL VASCULITIS

Inflammatory changes in the vessel walls give rise to retinal vasculitis which is clinically not always distinguishable from the occlusive retinal vasculopathies which are non-inflammatory (essential hypertension, diabetes, hemoglobinopathies and hyperviscosity of the blood). On fluorescein angiography we see a characteristic leakage of the dye from the affected vessels into the retinal tissue.

The inflammatory process may affect either the arteries or the veins; they may be peri-or endo-vasculitis; most frequently seen is the retinal periphlebitis. Characteristic for any vasculitis are sheating and cellular infiltration of the vessel wall not altering the blood flow (see Chapter 2).

In *periphlebitis* the veins are surrounded on both sides by a white line which runs parallel to the vessel sheathing it segmentally or diffusely. In the segmental form the vessel appears granular or like the branching of a fungus (similar to a twig covered with frost), whereas in the diffuse form there is usually a certain degree of perivascular edema. In some cases the sheathing may involve the entire circumference of the vessel and the vein appears like a white chord without being necessorily completely occluded (Figs. 339, 340).

With the progress of the vasculitis there will be changes in the caliber of the vessel with attenuation and partial occlusion.

In the majority of cases the periphlebitis begins in the periphery and extends toward the posterior pole, though there are also cases in which the sequence is reversed. The natural history of the condition varies a great deal and the inflammation may remain stationary for a long time. The complications are related to venous occlusions which cause bleeding into the retina and into the vitreous, neovascularization and subsequent proliferative retinopathy.
In retinal vasculitis an arterial involvement frequently accompanies the venous disease.

Periarteritis is ophthalmoscopically similar to periphlebitis (segmental or diffuse sheathing, segmental attenuation of the caliber of the vessel). Signs of an *arteritis obliterans* with edema and localized retinal infarcts (cotton-wool patches) are seen here more frequently. There may also be retinal ischemia and neovascularization (Figs. 341, 342).

In the further course of a retinal vasculitis there will inevitably be involvement of the optic nerve with disc edema and secondary optic atrophy; the posterior pole may show a cystoid macular edema. Characteristic are the paravascular pigmentary changes which follow a vasculitis and which may resemble the bone corpuscle like pigmentation of a tapeto-retinal degeneration (Fig. 389).

Retinal vasculitis may be primary as in Eales disease, or secondary to a uveo-retinitis or a systemic disease (Table 7).

Table 7. Retinal vasculitis.

Primary or idiopathic vasculitis	Eales disease
Vasculitis secondary to a uveo-retinitis	Pars planitis Sarcoidosis Tuberculosis Syphilis Toxoplasmosis Behçet disease Bilateral acute retinal necrosis
Vasculitis secondary to a systemic disease	Systemic lupus erythematosus Polyarteritis nodosa Wegener's granulomatosis Multiple sclerosis Behçet disease

The signs of a vasculitis seen in the course of an acute retinitis are generally reversible when the primary retinal inflammation resolves.

In *pars planitis* or *basal uveo-retinitis* the signs of a vasculitis are characteristic and represent the most important retinal signs of this condition, together with changes in the vitreous. The examination of the fundus periphery shows fine white vitreous opacities that are round and dense (similar to a snowball or an ant egg) which project their shadow onto the retinal surface; in addition there are large and dense vitreous exudates resembling snow banks (Fig. 343 a) or a membrane, obviously manifestations of retinal vasculitis with preretinal exudates. The venules show segmental periphlebitis (Fig. 343 b) and, more rarely, an occlusive vasculitis. In most instances the vasculitis remains confined to the periphery with a tendency to remain stationary. In some cases the process may extend toward the posterior pole and also involve the arterioles. Among the retinal complications of such a pars planitis are in addition to paravascular pigmentary changes a cystoid macular edema and a peripapillary edema (Fig. 344).
The characteristics of other uveo-retinitis types are discussed in Chapter 7.

Retinal periphlebitis is an important and interesting sign of *multiple sclerosis*. Its incidence is only somewhat lower than that of a retrobulbar optic neuritis. The condition is nearly always asymptomatic and hardly ever progresses so that it is often unrecognized. The process involves mainly the veins as they emerge from the disc. There is usually sheathing of the vessel wall. The peripheral periphlebitis appears often as a paravenous nodular type and may be associated with a peripheral uveitis. A relation between periphlebitis and uveitis cannot always be established, but a uveitis is certainly much less frequent in multiple sclerosis than a vasculitis. All types of systemic vasculitis may involve the retinal vessels. In collagen diseases (pag. 146) we find mainly an involvement of the arterioles with occlusion of the vessel and fibrinoid necrosis of the vessel wall.

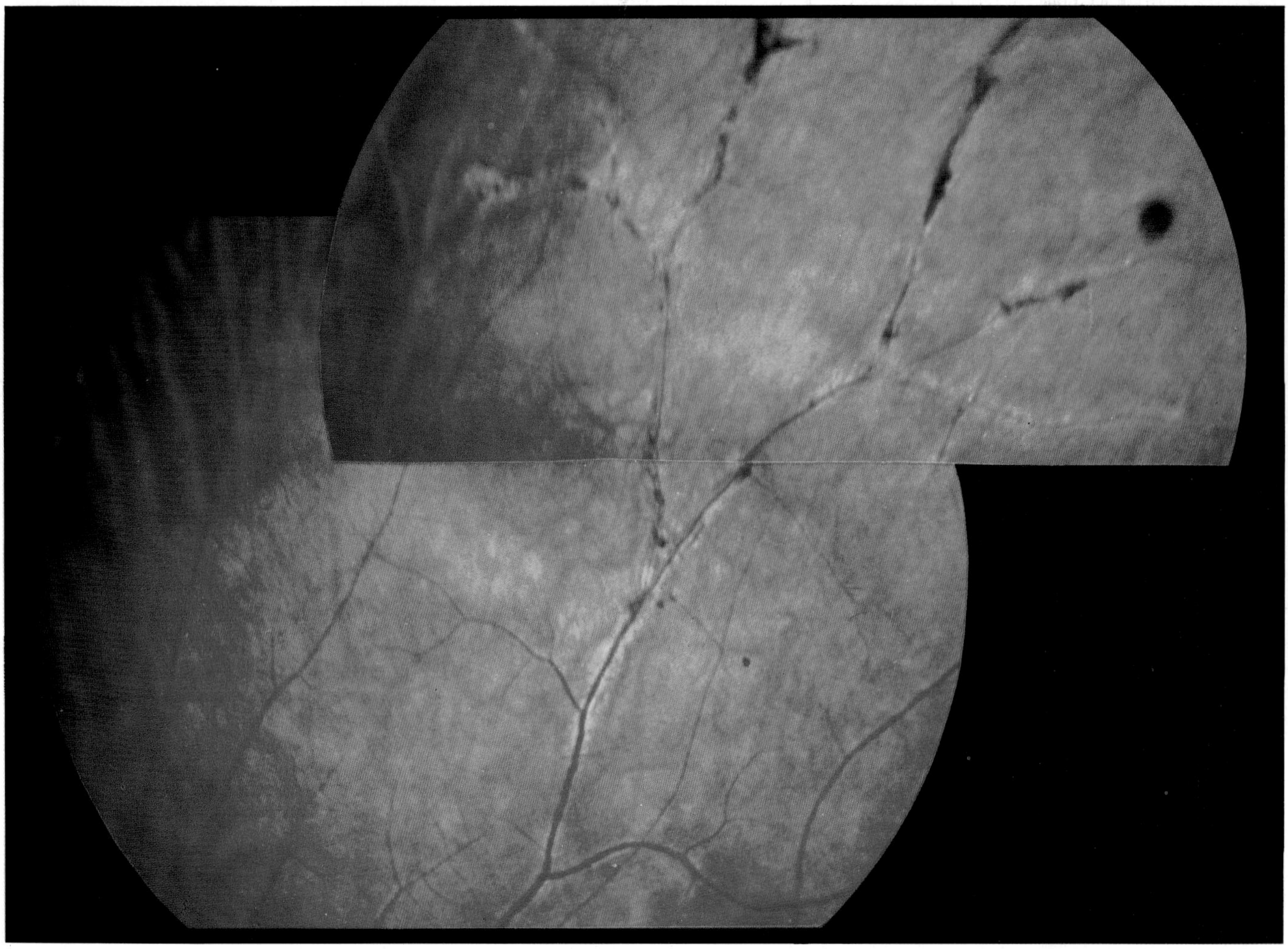

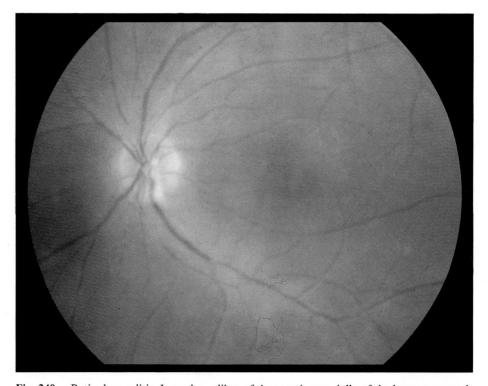

Fig. 339.   Retinal periphlebitis. Perivasal sheathing and segmental irregularities of the caliber; paravascular pigmentation.

Fig. 340.   Retinal vasculitis. Irregular caliber of the vessels especially of the lower temporal vein; perivascular edema; post-edematous macular degeneration (uveo-retinitis).

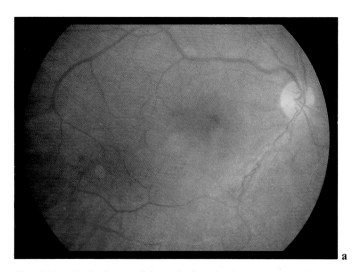 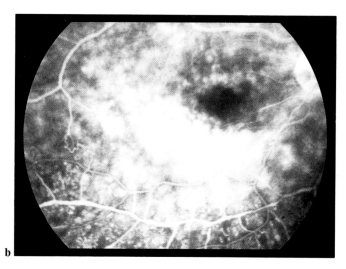

Fig. 341. Retinal vasculitis occluding the lower temporal arcade and conspicuous neovascularization (systemic lupus erythematosus).
a) Fundus photo.
b) Fluorescein angiogram: areas of non-perfusion and obvious vascular leakage, cystoid macular edema, neovascularization.

Fig. 342. End stage of retinal vasculitis with the vessels reduced to white threads, diffuse ischemic retinal degeneration (Behçet disease).

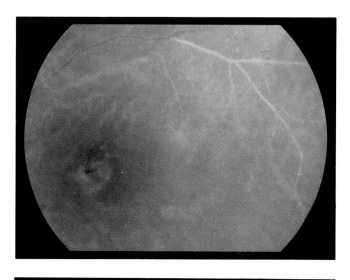

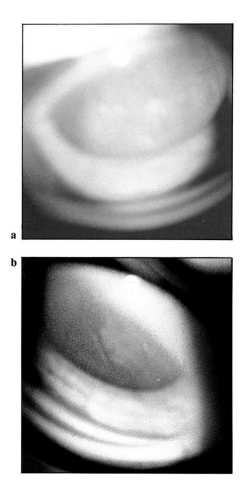

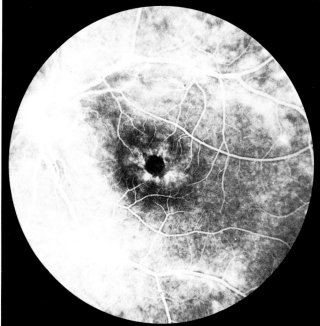

Fig. 343. Pars planitis (slit lamp examination).
a) Preretinal exudates at the vitreous base.
b) Peripheral periphlebitis.

Fig. 344. Pars planitis (fluorescein angiogram). Cystoid macular edema; segmental leakage of the dye along the upper and lower temporal veins.

EALES DISEASE

Eales disease (recurrent retino-vitreal hemorrhages in young men) is an idiopathic retinal perivasculitis characterized by peripheral periphlebitis, neovascularizations and recurrent vitreo-retinal hemorrhages. It affects mainly young men between the ages of 20 and 30 and is bilateral in 90% of the cases. In women often only one eye is involved. The etiology is unknown. A presently most acceptable hypothesis assumes that there is a pecular familiar vascular lability complicated by toxic, allergic and vaso-motor factors.

Fluorescein angiography and histologic examinations confirm the presence of a vasculitis, primarily involving the veins. There may be obliteration of the lumen with proliferation of the endothelial cells. In the final stage the entire vascular tree is transformed into fibrous tissue.

The patients initially notice small scotomas, transient obscurations and floaters caused by the peripheral retinal hemorrhages. Finally there will be a decrease in central acuity when the posterior pole and the vitreous are involved. The onset of the disease may be sudden with a severe visual loss due to massive vitreous hemorrhage.

Ophthalmoscopically we see initially a retinal periphlebitis involving mainly the peripheral venous branches in one or several segments of the fundus. The sheathing appears like fine white lines which delineate the two sides of the blood column. The extension of the sheath may vary. The venules appear rigid, more rectilinear, and are surrounded by white, dot-like exudates and small hemorrhages located in the superficial retinal layers. Later the hemorrhages become more extensive and involve the entire nerve fiber layer. Characteristic are in this stage the anastomoses which connect two adjacent vessels. The arterioles may also be involved in the inflammatory process (Figs. 345 a, b)

As the vasculitis progresses there will be an attenuation of the peripheral retinal veins which appear like white fibrotic lines, eventually surrounded by pigment; the periphlebitis may then extend to the larger vessels and finally toward the optic nervehead (Figs. 346, 347). The initial peripheral exudative and hemorrhagic lesions may disappear and may be substituted by connective tissue which strangles the small vessels; there may be decreased caliber and varicosities in the adjacent venules. The retinal hemorrhages increase in intensity and frequency, both at the equator and at the posterior pole. The vitreous becomes opaque due to the repeated bleedings.

The progressive occlusion of peripheral vessels will produce ischemic retinal areas with subsequent neovascularization, characterized by subtle tortuous blood vessels which form convolutes and may advance toward the vitreous contributing to the formation of a proliferative retinopathy. The hemorrhages become more numerous and massive, lie beneath the hyaloid membrane and extend into the vitreous making it often impossible to examine the fundus. The blee-

ding comes mostly from ruptured, new-formed blood vessels. The hemorrhages may recur and their absorption is slow and uncertain. The proliferative retinopathy consists of glial elements and perivascular connective tissue with organized vitreous hemorrhages (Figs. 348, 349) (see pag. 128).

In addition to the usual peripheral form there is also a central form of Eales disease involving predominantly the large vessels. Here we find sheathing of the veins at their entrance into the optic nervehead, hyperemia of the disc and macular edema.

The prognosis is not good because of the tendency for recurrences and the propensity of the disease to progress. Nevertheless, there are cases with little progression and spontaneous resolution after a certain period of activity. In these cases the visual prognosis is obviously better. In peripheral forms laser photocoagulation may retard, but does not arrest, the progression of the disease. The coagulation should destroy the ischemic areas which are responsible for neovascularization and from which the final vitreo-retinal complications originate (massive vitreous hemorrhage, traction detachment of the retina and neovascular glaucoma). In the central form of the disease repeated administrations of high dosage corticosteroids have been advised.

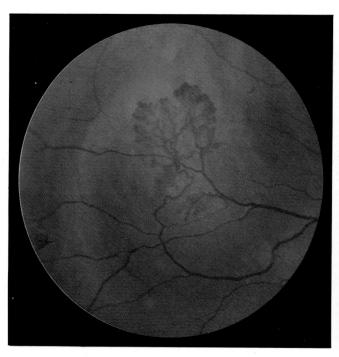

Fig. 345. Eales disease. Peripheral epiretinal neovascularization. **a)** Fundus photo.

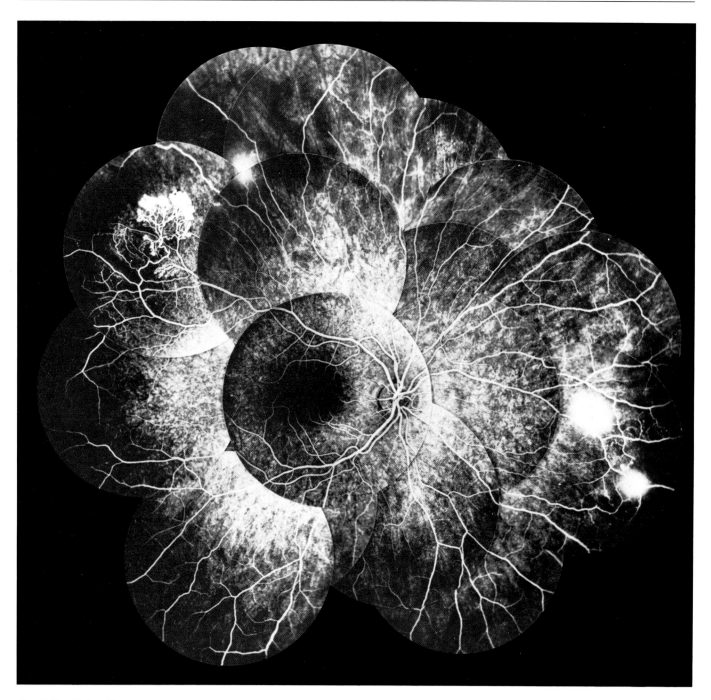

Fig. 345. Eales disease.
b) Collage of luorescein angiograms. Peripheral epiretinal neovascularization in the upper temporal segment, retinal neovascularization and areas of hyperfluorescence in the periphery indicating active periphlebitis.

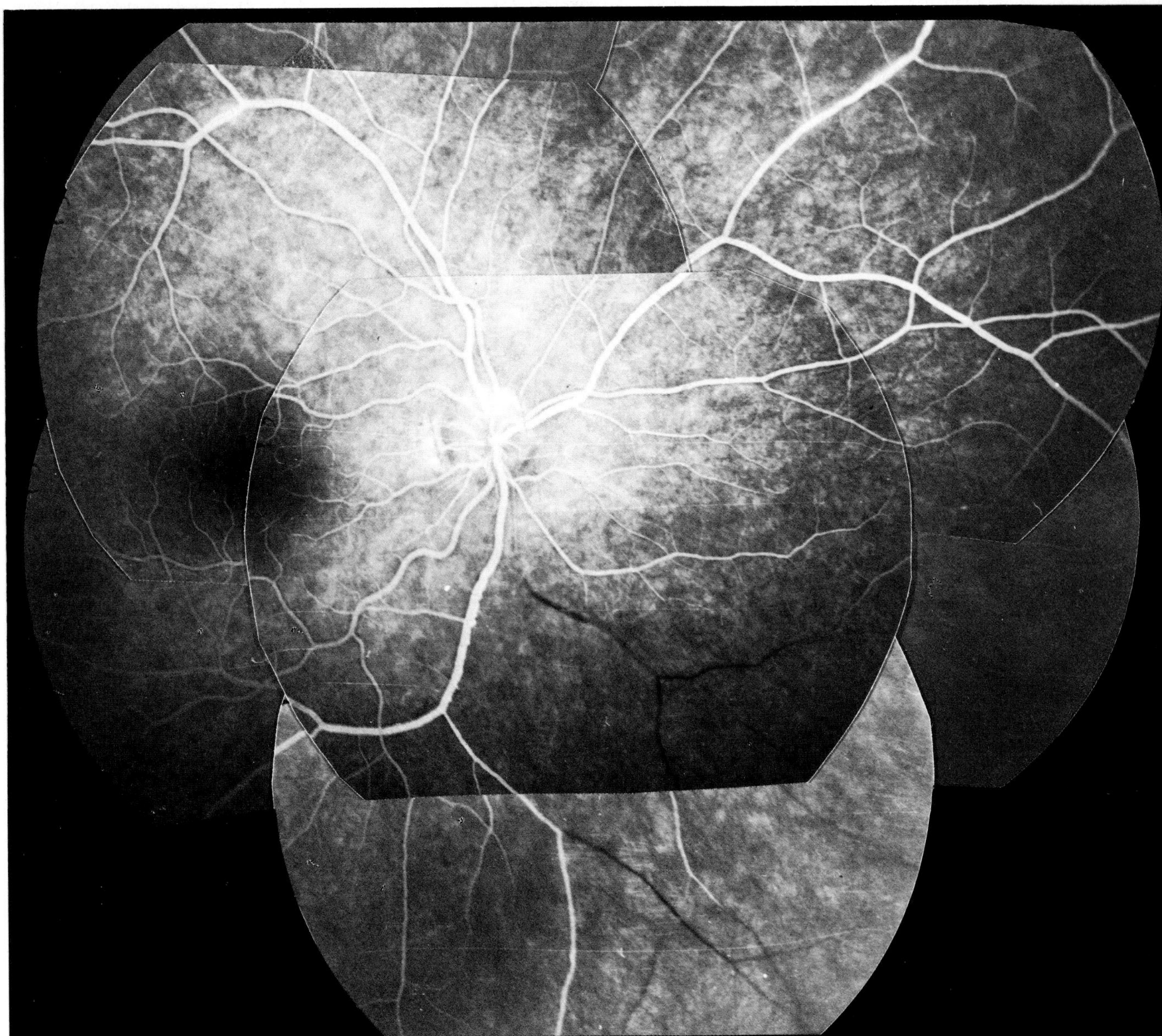

Fig. 346. Eales disease (fluorescein angiograms). Complete occlusion of the lower nasal vein and of a branch of the lower temporal vein; areas of segmental hyperfluorescence in mid periphery along other vascular trunks indicating a phlebitis.

Fig. 347. Eales disease. Progression of the periphlebitis toward the optic nervehead; paravascular pigmentation.
a) Fundus photo.
b) Fluorescein angiogram: active periphlebitis, more pronounced in mid periphery, where there are areas of pigment epithelium atrophy associated with pigment accumulations along the vessels.

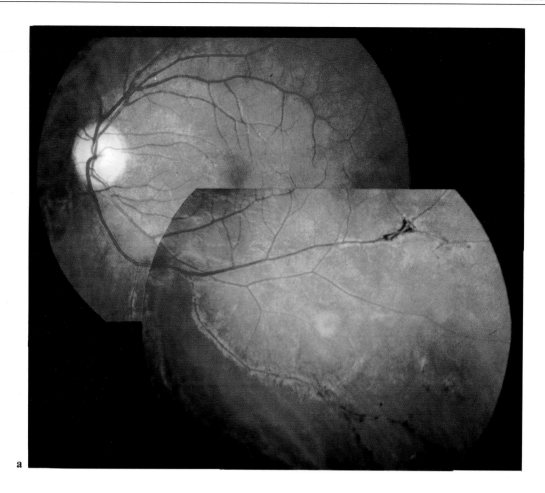

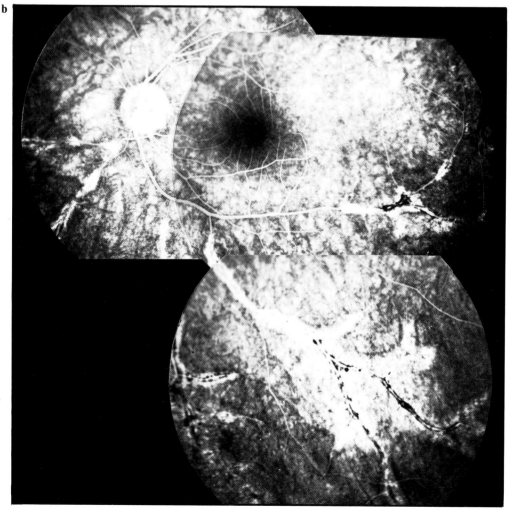

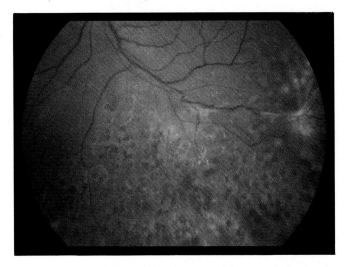

Fig. 348. Eales disease. Periphlebitis and neovascularization in mid periphery, with hemorrhages and proliferative retinopathy; result of laser treatment.

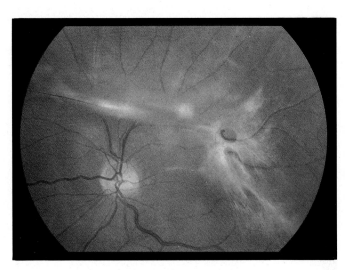

Fig. 349. Eales disease. Proliferating vitreo-retinal membrane at the posterior pole with distortion and neovascularization; perivascular sheathing and irregular caliber as an indication of periphlebitis.

ACUTE POSTERIOR MULTIFOCAL PLACOID PIGMENT EPITHELIOPATHY (BENIGN DIFFUSE EXTERNAL EXUDATIVE RETINITIS)

The benign diffuse external exudative retinitis was described by Scuderi in 1948 and corresponds from a clinical and ophthalmoscopic point of view to the acute posterior multifocal placoid pigment epitheliopathy of Gass (1968).

The disease affects primarily young patients between the age of 15 and 25; there is a slight predominance of male patients.

The condition is usually unilateral, but may be present in both eyes simultaneously or the second eye may be involved after an interval of several months. The initial symptom is frequently a metamorphopsia (macropsia, micropsia), but generally the patient notices loss of central vision with an absolute or relative central scotoma which can be plotted on a visual field and constitutes the most important sympton.

The ophthalmoscopic picture varies with the stage of the disease. In the acute stage we see at the posterior pole, primarily in and around the macula, spots of various dimensions, which are round or oval, often with blurred outlines, sometimes coalescing, exudative in nature and white-yellow in color. These lesions are later surrounded or sprinkled with fine pigment disseminations (Figs. 350, 351 a, 352). The lesions are never elevated but seem to be confined to the external retinal layers. There is no subepithelial serous exudation. There are no changes in the retinal vasculature, nor are there signs of choroidal involvement (vitreous opacities, etc.). We find in the literature also cases of epitheliopathy complicated by and associated with a uveal reaction, papillitis, subretinal or peripapillary hemorrhages, retinoschisis, retinal detachment or Eales disease.

In the healing phase (usually after two to three weeks) the spots clear progressively. This process starts in the center and extends toward the periphery until the exudates disappear. Finally there remains only a subtle pigment dissemination forming brown or black designs and small areas where the choriocapillaris becomes visible. Characteristic and in some aspects pathognomonic is the fluorescein angiogram. During the acute phase the normal choroidal flush is missing in the area of the lesions, while during the late and extremely late phases there will be a progressive and irregular staining of these areas. Once the lesions have healed we see hyperfluorescence in the area of depigmentations and dark areas of various forms, size and location corresponding to the zones of hyperpigmentation (Figs. 351, 353).

The ERG remains normal in all stages of the disease, but there are changes of the electrooculogram which usually becomes normal after clinical healing has occured. In a good number of patients there is a dyschromatopsia in the blue-yellow axis.

In general the disease resolves, especially the pure form of the condition and there is good functional prognosis as the visual acuity recovers after a few weeks or months. Only rarely will there be a marked and permanent visual defect depending upon the site of the lesion, the extension of the pathologic process and above all on the degree of damage to the sensory retina. Recurrences are often seen and they may occur one month or several years after the first attack has healed.

There are three different theories concerning the etiology of the condition: tuberculosis, allergy or a viral infection. Indeed, the epitheliopathy frequently occurs concurrently with a simple viral infection (upper respiratory infection, common cold, influenza, etc.). On the basis of experimental investigations, some authors have put forward a vascular and an autoimmune hypothesis as far as the pathogenesis is concerned.

Treatment with corticosteroids, antiphlogistics and immune suppressive medications probably permits a quicker healing with a more benign course and a low tendency for recurrences.

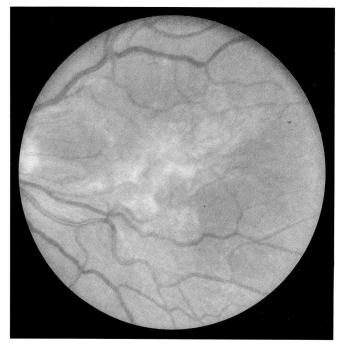

Fig. 350. Acute posterior multifocal placoid pigment epitheliopathy; exudative, yellow areas with blurred outlines at the posterior pole.

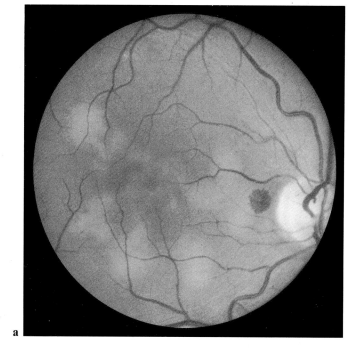

Fig. 351. a-c) Acute posterior multifocal placoid pigment epitheliopathy.
a) Numerous yellow spots at the posterior pole; juxtapapillary hemorrhage.
b-c) Fluorescein angiography. In the early phase **(b)** numerous diffuse areas of hypofluorescence at the posterior pole. In a late phase **(c)** these areas become hyperfluorescent.

a

b c

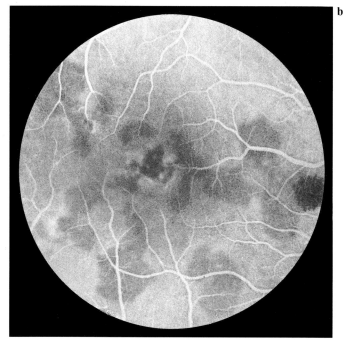

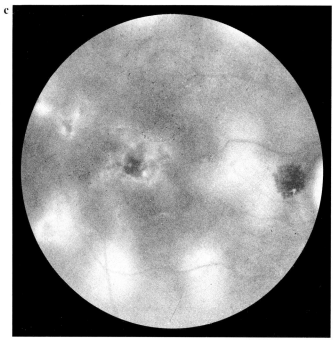

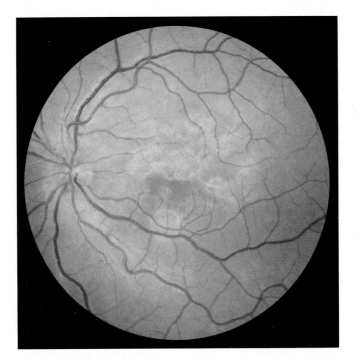

Fig. 352. Acute posterior multifocal placoid epitheliopathy. Numerous yellow round deposits surrounded by a pigment halo are seen in the macular area.

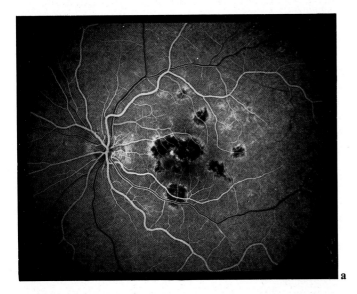 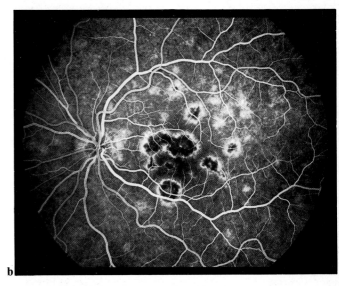

a   b

Fug. 353. a) and **b)** Acute posterior multifocal placoid pigment epitheliopathy. Fluorescein angiography (same case as in Fig. 352).
a) Arterio-venous phase: Areas of hypofluorescence in the macula.
b) Venous phase: these areas appear partially hyperfluorescent.

CENTRAL SEROUS RETINOPATHY

This condition is characterized by an accumulation of serous fluid between the pigment epithelium and the sensory retina.

Its occurs predominantly in the macular area and affects mainly young male patients. The etiology is unknown and therefore it is often called idiopathic. There are usually no changes in general health, nor is there any evidence of familial occurrence. The affected patients are often in a state of severe anxiety with a profound concern about their disease.

The basic pathogenetic process is an anatomical or functional break in the blood-retina barrier.

The symptoms are typical for any macular lesion: a relative central scotoma, metamorphopsia, hypersensitivity to photo stress exposure and dyschromatopsia.

The diagnosis of the condition is in most cases easy, but the examination of the fundus should always be performed with the pupil widely dilated.

Ophthalmoscopically (Figs. 354-356) we see a retinal, well delineated elevation, round or oval, usually in the macular area but often decentered as far as the foveola is concerned.

The retinal elevation appears darker than the adjacent normal retina and is demarcated by a bright halo which can be better appreciated in red-free illumination. The foveolar reflex is absent.

The size of the lesion varies from one disc diameter to three disc diameters and more. Fluorescein angiography is of fundamental importance to corroborate the clinical diagnosis and to study the evolution of the condition.

On fluorescein angiography we see initially a dot-like area of hyperfluorescence (compared to a "smoke stack") which increases progressively in extension and intensity during the successive phases of the angiogram. It persists even in the late phases (Figs. 357-359).

The fluorescein angiogram allows us to determine precisely:

— the number of hyperfluorescent spots: single or multiple;
— their morphology: dot-like, round, convoluted, comet-like or like a smokestack;
— its site: foveolar, foveal, parafoveal or perifoveal;
— the stage of evolution: initial, acute, cicatricial, recurrent.

The prognosis of the condition is in its typical form favorable even without any treatment though it may take some time to regress.

The duration of the epithelial detachment may last several weeks and up to six months. Recurrences can be expected in 30 to 50% of the cases.

A recurrence may affect the same eye or the contralateral eye. In about 30% of the patients the condition is bilateral; the contralateral eye may show the acute or the regressive stage of the condition.

During the remission we see small yellow shiny dots (Figs. 355, 356), whereas the central retinal elevation regresses and its borders disappear (Fig. 360). This is accompanied by subtle areas of pigmentation and depigmentation in the pigment epithelium (Fig. 361).

The fluorescein angiogram also changes. There is hyperfluorescence which appears earlier than in an active phase, but no leakage, nor increase in dye intensity during the later phases: the "smoke stack" phenomenon is therefore transformed into a typical "window effect" by localized changes in the pigment epithelium (Fig. 362).

There is at present no medical treatment known for this condition. Only laser photocoagulation has shown a certian efficacy, especially in shortening the duration of the disease. The precise indications for phototreatment are still unknown.

DIFFUSE RETINAL EPITHELIOPATHY

In addition to the typical form of the idiopathic central serous retinopathy which is defined as a serous retinal detachment with a subretinal area of diffusion, usually solitary with mild changes in the pigment epithelium, there is also an atypical form characterized by extensive changes in the pigment epithelium which is referred to as "diffuse retinal epitheliopathy". These changes become conspicuous on fluorescein angiography. (Figs. 363, 364) and may be areas of depigmentation (Fig. 365), single or multiple, individual or coalescing, or direct tears and rips directed toward the deeper layers (Fig. 366). This last aspect is somewhat similar to the end results of a chronic subretinal exudation which because of gravitational forces will accumulate in the lower part of this space (Fig, 367).

Within the extent of these more or less wide alterations of the pigment epithelium it is possibile to see one or two leakage points similar to a central serous retinopathy.

Diffuse retinal epitheliopathy is also an idiopathic disease, but can be considered as a definite clinical entity which differs from central serous retinopathy by the following characteristics:

— the loss of central vision is more pronounced and the prognosis is less favorable;
— affects older patients;
— frequently both eyes are affected;
— the retinal elevation is not clearly demarcated and there are one or several foci of subretinal diffusion of the dye within the framework of a marked alteration of the pigment epithelium, often in the macula, but more frequently peripapillary or paramacular;
— chronic course of the disease.

The actual cause of this condition is also unknown. Laser photocoagulation seems to be useful when the leakage points apparently reduce central vision.

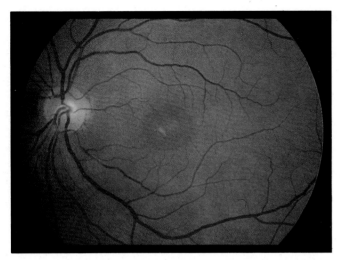

Fig. 354.   Central serous retinopathy. Ophthalmoscopically we see a central bulla, a typical sign of an elevation of the macular sensory epithelium.

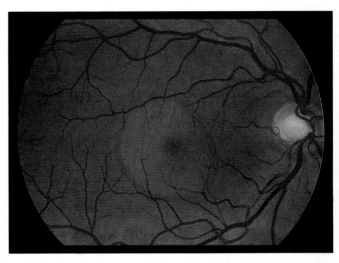

Fig. 355.   Central serous retinopathy. Phase of beginning remission; there are small yellow dots in the area of the retinal elevation.

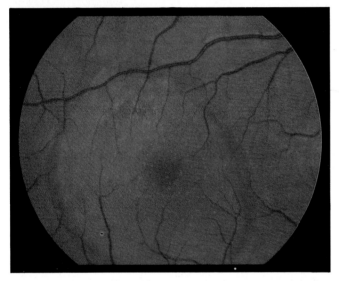

Fig. 356.   Same case as fig. 335 in higher magnification. Especially conspicuous are the dot-like yellow precipitates in the area of the retinal elevation.

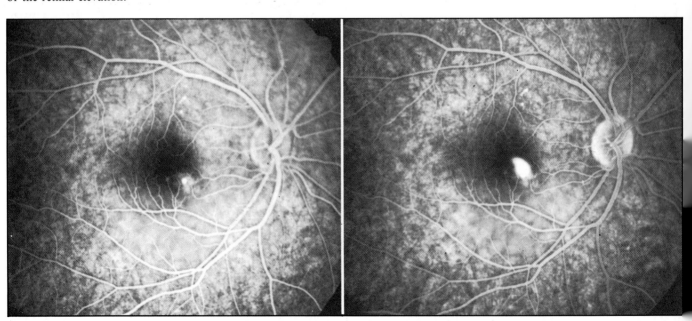

Fig. 357.   Central serous retinopathy. Typical fluorescein angiograms with a single focus of dye diffusion shown in two phases of angiography: the first one is in early phase, the second one at a late phase.

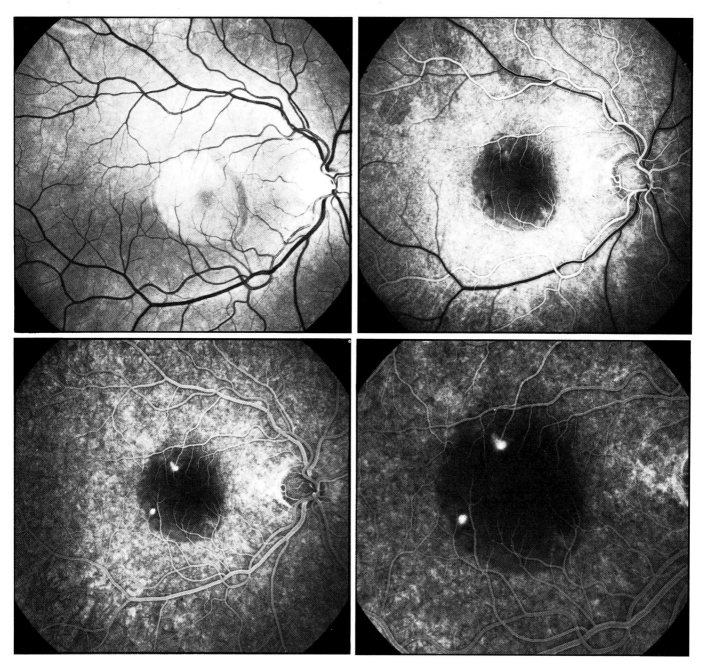

Fig. 358. Central serous retinopathy. Typical angiographic picture. In red free light the demarcation line between the elevated retina and the surrounding tissue is well marked; in the initial phase of angiography we see two small dots of dye diffusion which become more extensive and intensive during the later phases of the angiogram.

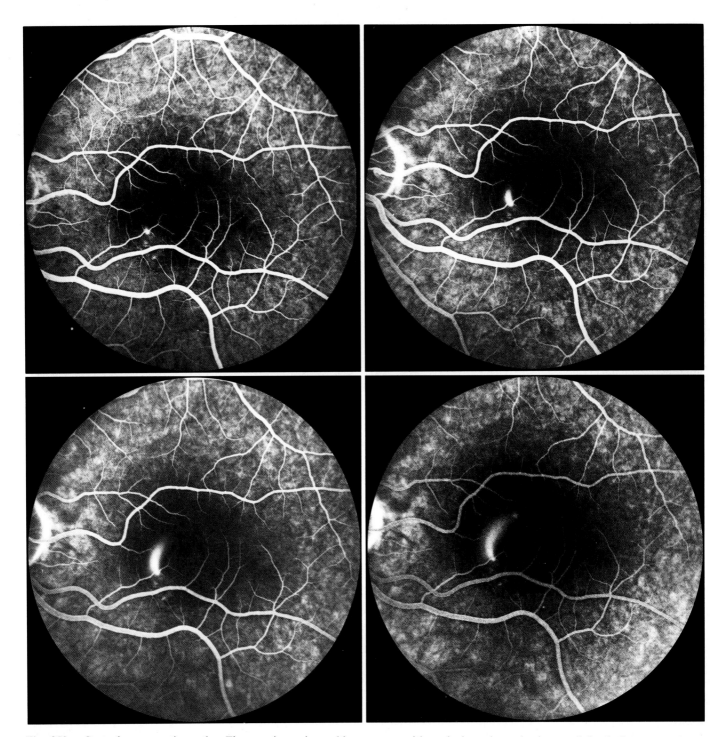

Fig. 359. Central serous retinopathy. Fluorescein angiographic sequence with typical smokestack picture of dye leakage.

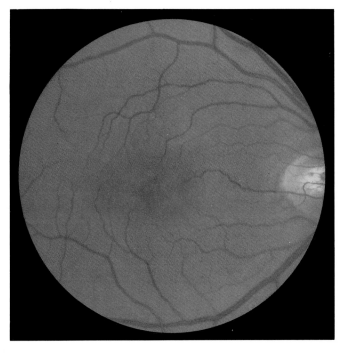

Fig. 360. Old central serous retinopathy. The central serous elevation has flattened out; there is subtle alteration of the retinal pigment epithelium.

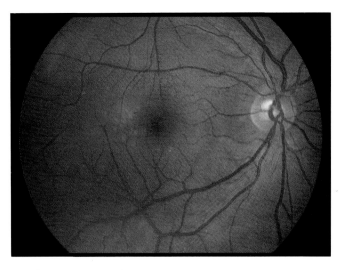

Fig. 361. Old central serous retinopathy. There is fine pigmentation in the involved macular area preceding a retinal elevation.

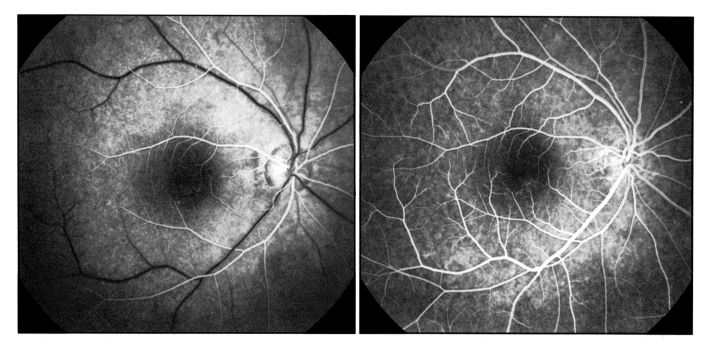

Fig. 362. Central serous retinopathy. Fluorescein angiography in the cicatricial stage. There is a subtle hyperfluorescence due to the transmission of abnormal retroretinal fluorescence (a window effect), it remains constant and does not increase during the late phases.

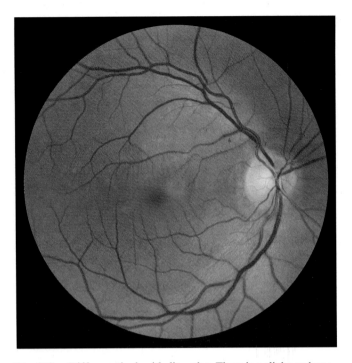

Fig. 363. Diffuse retinal epitheliopathy. There is a slight and uneven retinal elevation without sharp borders.

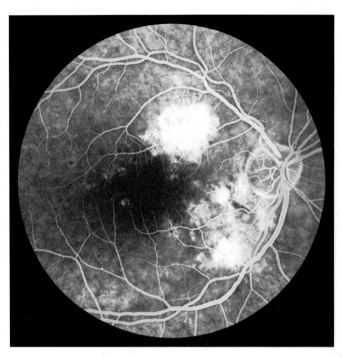

Fig. 364. Fluorescein angiogram of Fig. 363.
There are multiple foci of dye diffusion with a serous retinal detachment and alterations of the pigment epithelium.

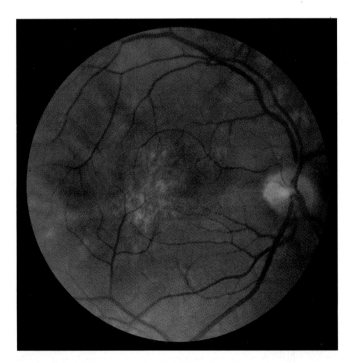

Fig. 365. Diffuse retinal epitheliopathy after several years of chronic progression. There is a diffuse conspicuous alteration of the pigment epithelium.

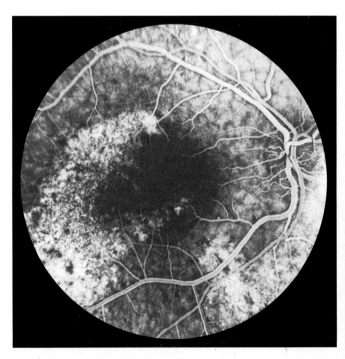

Fig. 366. Diffuse retinal epitheliopathy. Fluorescein angiogram of an extensive alteration of pigment epithelium.

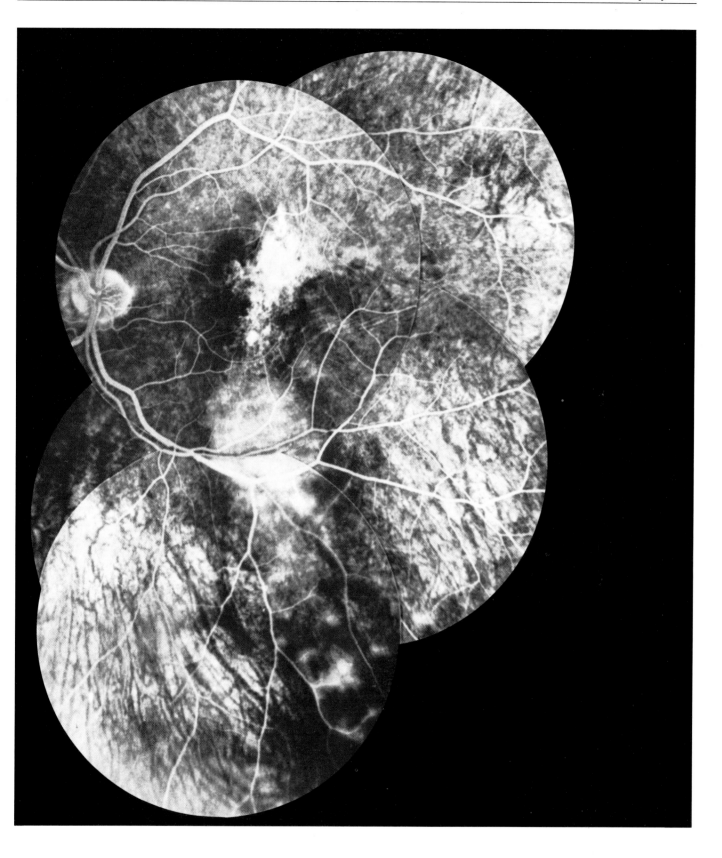

Fig. 367. Diffuse retinal epitheliopathy. Fluorescein angiogram. There are several foci of subretinal dye diffusion next to the macula; the exudation associated with the dystrophy of the pigment epithelium has a tendency to accumulate in the lower part following the force of gravity.

Chapter 7

Inflammations of the choroid and retina

RETINITIS, RETINOCHOROIDITIS, CHOROIDITIS AND CHORIORETINITIS

Endogenous inflammations involving the retina and the choroid only rarely remain localized in the tissue primarily affected but usually spill over into adjacent structures producing a uveo-retinitis. We call a retinochoroiditis an inflammation primarily involving the retina and only secondarily the underlying choroid; a chorioretinitis is a primary inflammation of the choroid secondarily affecting the retina. In the initial phases it is usually possible to determine the tissue primarily affected, whereas this is not so in the end-stage because every case will end in a chorioretinal scar.

When determining the diagnosis of a clinical picture the following factors are of special importance and usefulness: the area primarily affected by the inflammation, the clinical appearance and the topographic localization of the lesion.

From a clinical and morphological point of view uveoretinitis is classified into a *focal*, *disseminated* and *diffuse form*.

In the *focal form* the affected area can easily be distinguished from the surrounding normal tissue; the focus may be single or multiple and its size may vary. An active focus has blurred outlines, is elevated and grey or white-grey in color; it is sometimes surrounded by hemorrhages and produces signs of an inflammatory perivasculitis. With time the lesion flattens and the margins become more distinct, festooned and pigmented. The resulting chorioretinal scar represents a well demarcated atrophic area, which is more or less white, but shows pigment accumulation mainly at the margin; within it the choroidal vessels may be visible or the sclera is directly exposed.

The *disseminate form* has the characteristics of a multifocal uveoretinitis; the lesions are here more numerous and disseminated over the entire fundus, more or less scattered or crowded into one sector. The disseminated foci may either all be in the same stage of evolution or may be in different phases of development when this is a recurrent case.

In the *diffuse form* it is difficult to differentiate clearly between normal and pathologic areas. The fundus appears in the affected area edematous, thickened, grey-yellow, opaque and without reflexes.
In the cicatricial phase the retinal atrophy permits visualization of the choroidal vessels, whereas the thickening and proliferation of the retinal pigment epithelium, especially along the large vessels and at the equator, may produce the picture of an acquired pseudoretinits pigmentosa.

According to the location we distinguish: *macular*, *juxtapapillary*, *equatorial* and *peripheral forms*.

The macular form will obviously produce severe functional defects (central scotoma), whereas the peripheral form may often remain unrecognized due to the scarcity or absence of symptoms and the difficulty with which the diagnosis can be made except by binocular indirect ophthalmoscopy with scleral indentation or using the contact lens of Goldmann.
The juxtapapillary uveoretinitis (Jensen) involves also the optic nervehead by a papilledema affecting the nerve fibers and producing a corresponding and characteristic field defect (Jensen scotoma).

RETINITIS AND RETINOCHOROIDITIS

Characteristic for every retinitis are edema and exudation into the retinal layers. The affected retina appears ophthalmoscopically swollen, opaque, without reflexes, white (Figg. 368, 369 a), with indistinct margins and hemorrhages and exudates in the superficial layers and in front of the retinal vessels. The inflammatory reaction in the vitreous may be more or less severe and diffuse. This opacification prevents during the initial stages a detailed examination of the fundus and contributes to produce the phenomenon of "a headlight in the fog", i.e., shining bright light through the opaque vitreous produces a white, fluffy and blurred reflex (Fig. 370).

In the area of retinitis there will be signs of periphlebitis with vascular sheathing. This will disappear when the retinal inflammation has run its course (Figs. 369 a, b). These vascular changes are responsible for the hemorrhages around the lesion. If the inflammation also involves the superficial retinal layers then we may also see bright red retinal hemorrhages overlying the inflammatory focus which may enlarge and protrude into the vitreous.

The inflammatory reaction will inevitably also involve the pigment epithelium and the choriocapillaries therefore producing a retinochoroiditis and later a chorioretinal scar (Fig. 369 b). From a differential diagnostic point choroiditis and retinal vasculitis have to be considered. A focus of choroiditis differs from a retinitis by the absence of a cellular reaction in the vitreous and by the secondary signs of a retinal inflammation. The retina overlying the focus may indeed be thickened and swollen by the subretinal exudation, but the pigment epithelium is not necrotic nor are there retinal hemorrhages around the lesion.

In a primary retinal vasculitis the sheathing and constriction of the blood vessels are progressive and there are no accompanying signs of a retinitis; a vitreous reaction is rare or absent; sometimes it may be difficult to differentiate without the help of fluorescein angiography the ischemic lesions of a cotton-wool spot from a focus of acute retinitis. Pure retinitis is relatively rare and is mainly due to three types of infections which are transferred from the mother to the fetus: toxoplasmosis, rubella and cytomegalovirus disease. The most frequent type of retinochoroiditis is toxoplasmosis, followed by *Toxocara canis*, *Candida albicans* and cytomegalovirus disease. The last two types are mainly seen in patients with a compromised immune response. The bacterial form, the classical septic retinitis of Roth, has become quite rare.

Septic retinitis of Roth may be seen in some forms of bacterial infections, but is most often seen in subacute bacterial endocarditis. This condition is characterized by cotton-wool patches associated with small flame-shaped retinal hemorrhages that have a white center; they are mainly at the posterior pole and may be three-quarters of a disc diameter large. These disseminated retinal lesions change very slowly, but may resolve completely within a few months. We may also see small atrophic and pigmented

retroequatorial chorioretinal patches. The condition is always associated with a retinal perivasculitis.

The pathogenesis of Roth spots is uncertain; they are quite likely produced by a septic microembolus and a secondary vasculitis.

CHOROIDITIS AND CHORIORETINITIS

A focus of choroiditis appears as a pale, white-yellow or grey patch with blurred outlines over which the retinal vessels course undisturbed. These lesions are more or less deep and may be swollen depending upon the degree of edema and subretinal exudation; there is no inflammatory reaction in the vitreous provided the process remains confined to the choroid (Figs. 371, 372). An involvement of the retina is nearly always inevitable. It begins in the choriocapillaries and extends to the retinal epithelium (epithelitis); the retina will then appear thickened, edematous, without reflexes and without any signs of vasculitis or retinal necrosis. Fluorescein angiography may be useful in localizing the primary lesion (choroid, choriocapillaries and pigment epithelium). In cases of diffuse choroiditis, e.g., Vogt-Koyanagi-Harada disease or sympathetic ophthalmia, the subretinal choroidal exudation may be so massive that it produces an exudative retinal detachment. The process of scar formation causes choroidal atrophy and proliferation of the retinal pigment epithelium. The chorioretinal scars appear as white patches with sharp outlines and pigmentation in the form of variable pigment deposits within and around the lesion (Figs. 373-379).

The most frequently encountered forms of choroiditis and chorioretinitis are caused by microorganisms (tuberculosis, syphilis), by sarcoidosis, or represent presumed histoplasmosis, Vogt-Koyanagi-Harada disease and sympathetic ophthalmia.

A number of clinical entities have recently been described which affect predominantly the retinal pigment epithelium and the choriocapillaries. Their etiology is still unknown. It is quite likely that some of them are due to a viral infection. To this group belong: the acute posterior multifocal placoid pigment epitheliopathy, the helicoidal, geographic or serpiginous choroiditis, the "birdshot" choroidopathy and the pigment epithelitis of Deutman.

Fluorescein angiography is most useful in diagnosing all these clinical entities which have to be considered in the differential diagnosis of other types of choroiditis and chorioretinitis.

Fig. 368. Focus of parafoveal retinitis with moderate macular edema in a case of systemic toxoplasmosis involving the lymphnodes.

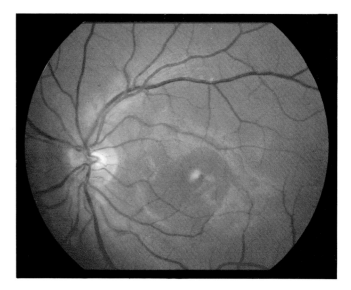

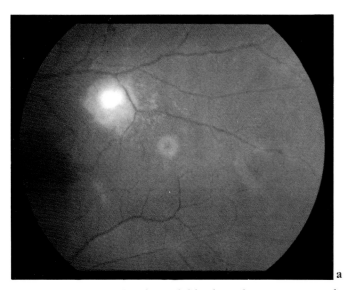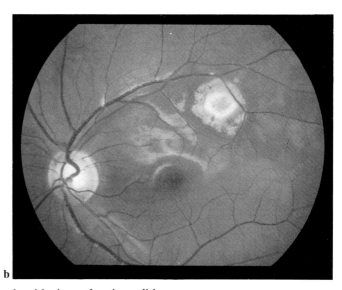

a   b

Fig. 369. **a)** Focus of active retinitis along the upper temporal arcade with signs of perivasculitis.
b) Cicatricial stage with a sharply demarcated focus and surrounding chorioretinal atrophy.

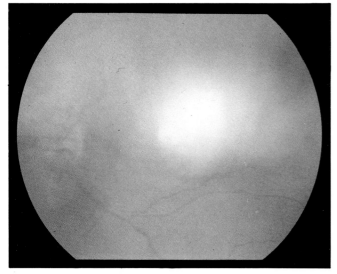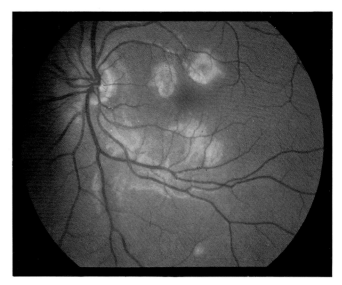

Fig. 370. Focus of active retinitis with marked vitreous exudates which prevent a detailed ophthalmoscopic examination (fog light phenomenon).

Fig. 371. Foci of active perimacular chorioretinitis.

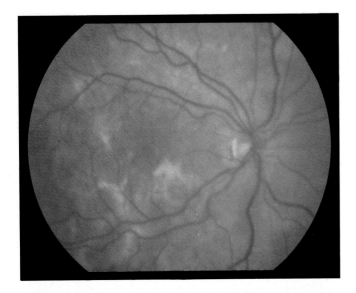

Fig. 372.   Disseminate choroiditis in an active phase.

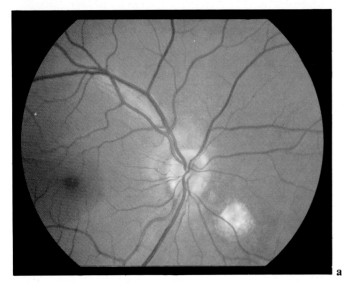 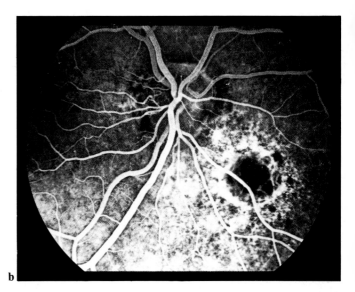

a   b

Fig. 373.   Focus of chorioretinitis in a phase of atrophic scar formation.
a) Fundus photo.
b) Fluorescein angiogram.

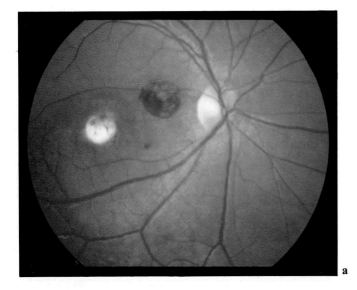 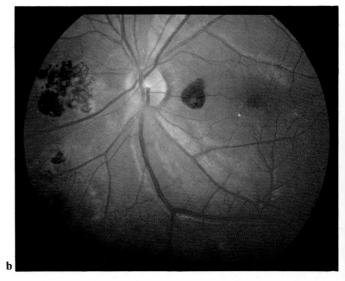

a   b

Fig. 374.   Bilateral chorioretinitis with multiple foci in the stage of scar formation; the foci are to a large extent pigmented and partly atrophic.
a) Right eye. **b)** Left eye.

Fig. 375. End result of a severe disseminate chorioretinitis. Numerous chorioretinal scars with scattered and varying pigmentation.

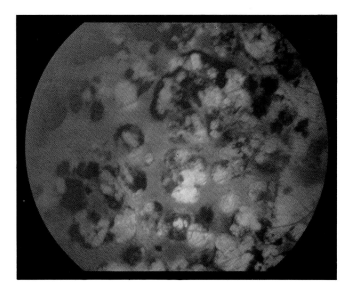

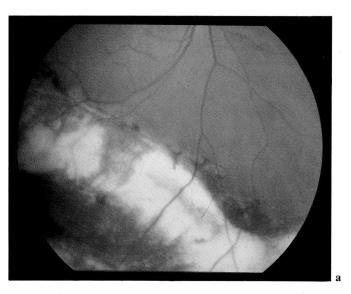

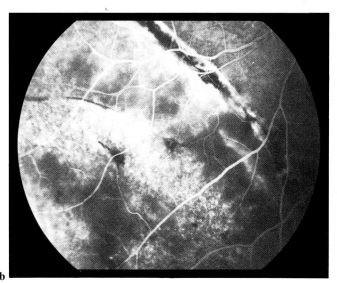

a b

Fig. 376. Cicatricial end stage of peripheral diffuse choroiditis in the lower segment progressing to a demarcated exudative retinal detachment. The fluorescein angiogram shows no break in the retina; there is pigment dissemination, the retinal vessels appear normal and a pigmented demarcation line surrounds the detachment.
a) Fundus photo.
b) Fluorescein angiogram.

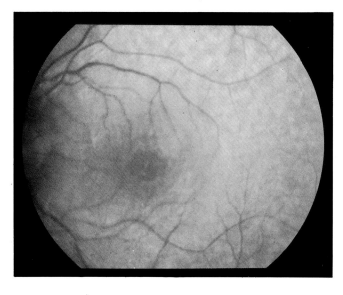

Fig. 377. End result of a diffuse choroiditis leading to pepper and salt fundus by severe changes in the retinal pigment epithelium; cystoid macular degeneration.

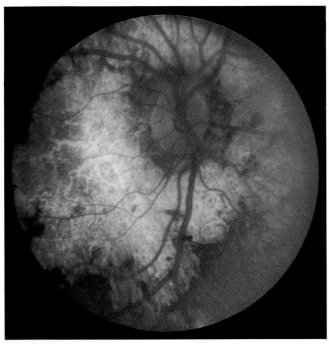

Fig. 378

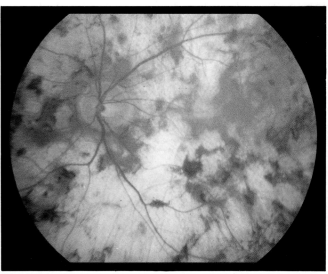

Fig. 379

Figs. 378, 379. End result of a severe diffuse chorioretinitis with marked atrophy of the retina and of the choriocapillaries allowing a visualization of the large choroidal vessels and of the sclera.

TUBERCULOSIS

Nearly all ocular structures may be involved by a tuberculous infection (conjunctiva, cornea, sclera, uvea, optic nerve). The disease has become rare, but the most frequently encountered ocular involvement concerns the uvea. An anterior uveitis may be observed in the course of a miliary tuberculosis; these are frequently resistant to therapy and may lead to a secondary involvement of the choroid and of the optic nerve in the framework of a progressive panuveitis. In some cases there may be an involvement of the posterior segment under the picture of a disseminated miliary choroidits. The latter is characterized by yellow-white choroidal nodules which vary in size from pinpoint to one disc diameter; they have blurred outlines, are disseminated over the fundus, more or less clustered or crowded into a certain sector of the ocular fundus. These foci develop into chorioretinal scars with varying amounts of pigmentation. These lesions usually constitute granulomatous inflammations consisting of epithelioid cells, lymphocytes and Langhans giant cells.

A tuberculous iridocyclitis and choroiditis may also be seen in the absence of clear-cut signs of systemic tuberculosis. In this case there may also develop a granulomatous reaction with multiple foci or the infection may be disseminated with the characteristic ophthalmoscopic signs described above (Figs. 380-383). For a long time it was assumed that the juxtapapillary choroiditis of Jensen was pathognomonic for a tuberculous etiology; actually this lesions does not have any etiologic significance and may be more frequently found in toxoplasmosis than in tuberculosis. More characteristic for tuberculosis are signs of a secondary retinal vasculitis, and especially a periphlebitis which may be either peripheral or affect mainly the large vessels.

In the past tuberculosis was a much more frequent infection. Nowadays we see usually choroidal or chorioretinal tuberculous scars in older patients. We have to keep in mind, however, that tuberculosis is still found as the etiologic factor in 3-5% of uveitis and that this incidence is probably underestimated. On the other hand, tuberculosis has nearly completely been eradicated in the industrialized countries. The clinical diagnosis is not always easy; the ocular tubercular manifestations are protean in nature and not specific. The tuberculin skin test does not definitely establish the diagnosis. On the other hand, this skin test may provoke an exacerbation of the ocular lesion (focal reaction).

The differential diagnosis is between other forms of chorioretinitis secondary to a granulomatous disease, e.g., sarcoidosis and syphilis.

A specific antituberculous treatment is indicated in well documented cases, though a successful treatment may be useful in establishing the correct diagnosis (therapeutic tests of isoniazid). Corticosteroids should be used only for short periods of time in severe progressive cases and should be given under the umbrella of an adequate antiobiotic protection (isoniazid, refampicin, etc.).

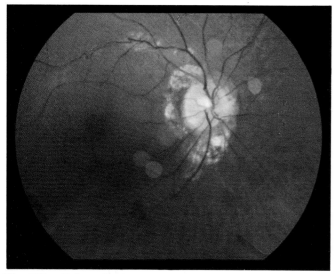

Fig. 380. Tuberculous chorioretinitis with multiple foci mostly juxtapapillary, retinal vasculitis with periphlebitis and neovascularization along the upper temporal arcade.

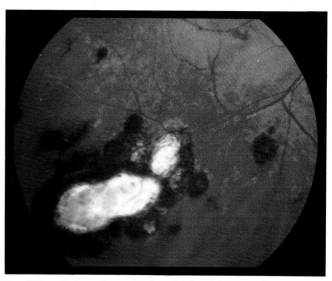

Fig. 381. Tuberculous chorioretinitis with disseminated foci; cicatricial stage with marked pigmentation within and around the lesions.

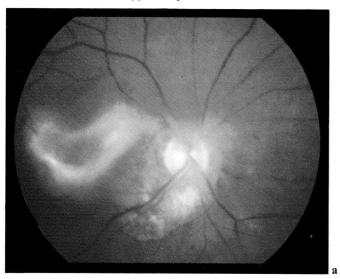

a   b

Fig. 382. Recurrent tuberculous juxtapapillary chorioretinitis.
a) Cicatricial foci below and nasal from the disc; one active focus over the papillomacular bundle; marked exudation into the vitreous above the active lesion.
b) Cicatricial stage of the papillo-macular focus partly obscured by a proliferating membrane; partial optic atrophy.

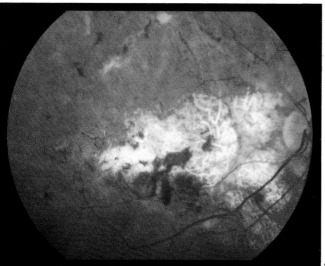
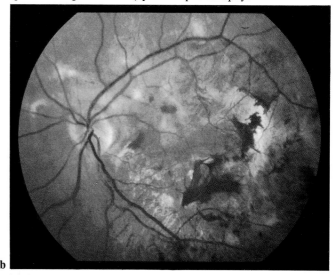

a   b

Fig. 383. Bilateral disseminate tuberculous chorioretinitis in the cicatricial stage. Cicatricial foci of various forms and size with massive accumulation of pigment and formation of geographic lesions.
a) Right eye.
b) Left eye.

SYPHILIS

There has been an increase in the prevalence of syphilis in all industrialized countries after the infection had nearly disappeared following the discovery of penicillin. Nevertheless, ocular involvement remains rare in the western countries, but this diagnosis should be kept in mind for the differential diagnosis of anterior and posterior uveitis. In tropical and subtropical countries, on the other hand, syphilis still represents one of the most frequent causes of uveitis.

The most characteristic ocular manifestations of **congenital syphilis** are interstitial keratitis, iridocyclitis, chorioretinitis with salt and pepper fundus and optic neuritis. About 5% of patients with congenital syphilis will show optic nerve involvement (papillitis) which evolves into a secondary optic atrophy; about 14% of these patients will develop uveoretinitis and many more show interstitial keratitis, whether acute or healed.

The chorioretinitis usually begins in infancy but is often diagnosed only in its late stage. The acute phase is difficult to observe. The typical salt and pepper fundus is nearly always bilateral and involves mainly the peripheral and equatorial region of the fundus. It is the end result of a diffuse choroiditis with secondary involvement of the pigment epithelium. Characteristic are small pigmented, grey-brown deposits disseminated over a red-yellow, pale background; sometimes this may be associated with a sector-shaped pseudoretinitis pigmentosa (Figs. 384 a, b). The visual function will not be affected unless there is an involvement of the optic nerve.

Characteristic for congenital syphilis are also disseminated or multifocal chorioretinitis in which atrophic areas alternate with pigmented scars. These conditions are often associated with endo and perivasculitis and a subsequent sclerosis of choroidal and retinal vessels. In these cases the visual acuity will be reduced and the visual field restricted. The congenital specific chorioretinitis and neuroretinitis, whether early or late in onset, may recur in adulthood.

Acquired syphilis involves the eye most often during the secondary and tertiary stages. Iridocyclitis associated with cutaneous rash may be complicated by diffuse chorioretinitis, neuroretinitis and optic neuritis, finally leading to a panuveitis. Characteristic is also a primary choroidal inflammation with secondary retinal involvement, vasculitis (especially periphlebitis) and retinal hemorrhages. Choroiditis may appear under various aspects and forms. It may be uni- or bilateral. The diffuse form manifests itself with a considerable choroidal edema evolving into a cicatricial chorioretinitis, vascular sclerosis and intensive pigment migration. There may also be disseminated chorioretinitis (Fig. 385), while focal forms are rare. The optic nerve (primarily or secondarily) is frequently affected. Important for the diagnosis are specific serologic tests, e.g., VDRL, TPI, FTA-ABS, which also can be obtained from the cerebrospinal fluid.

The therapy consists of a prolonged administration of penicillin.

Fig. 384. Congenital syphilis (Hutchinson triad). Bilateral pepper and salt chorioretinitis with papillitis, retinal vasculitis and cystoid macular degeneration during a reactivation in adulthood. The right eye (**a**) also shows a pseudoretinitis pigmentosa in the upper nasal segment.
a) Right eye.
b) Left eye.

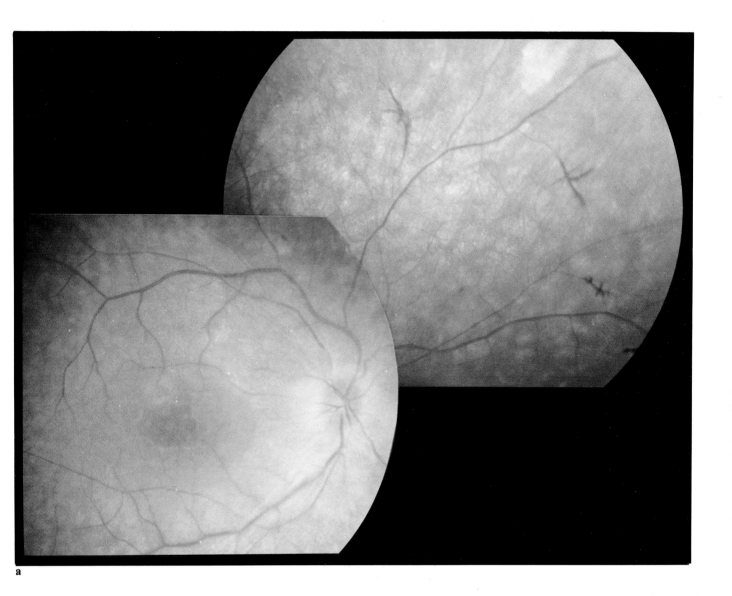

a

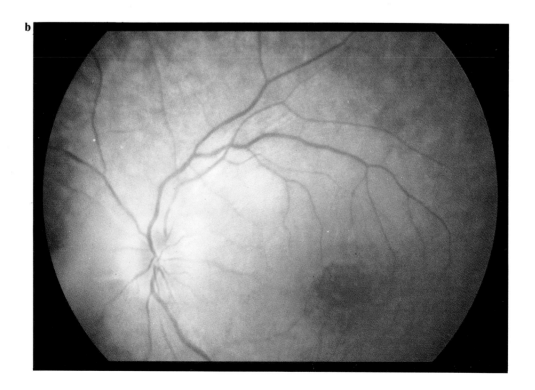

b

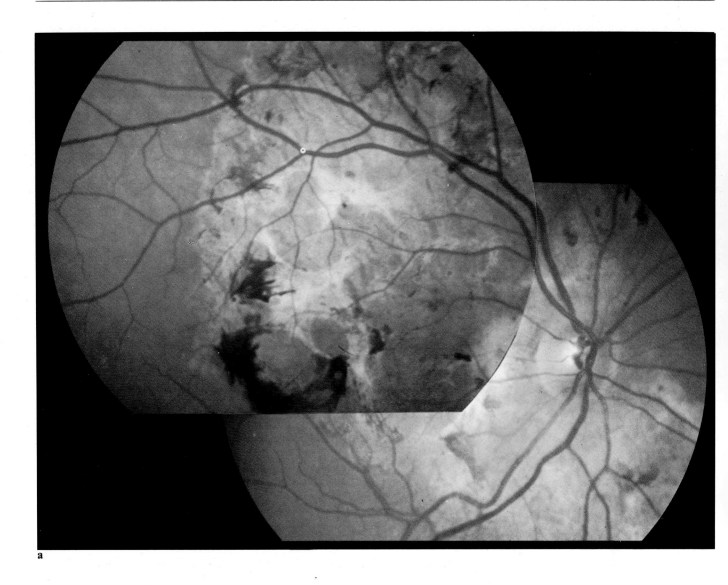

a

b

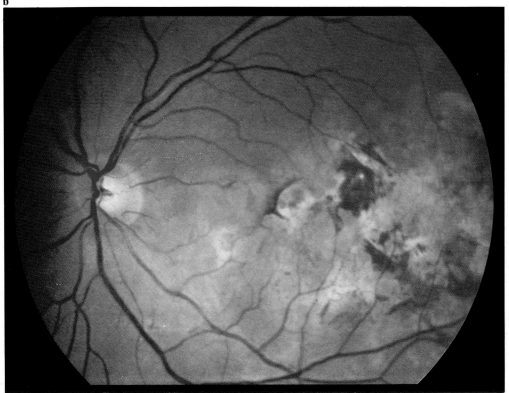

Fig. 385. Bilateral disseminate syphilitic chorioretinitis in the cicatricial phase with marked and severe pigmentary changes.
a) Right eye.
b) Left eye.

TOXOPLASMIC RETINOCHOROIDITIS

Toxoplasmosis is the most frequent cause of posterior segment inflammations, representing about 30-50% of all cases of posterior uveitis in the western world. The disease is caused by *Toxoplasma gondii*, an obligatory intracellular protozoon with special affinity to the retinal and cerebral tissue. The natural host is the cat; man can be infected by eating raw meat or other contaminated food. Only 1% of the patients who contract the disease in adulthood will develop ocular lesions; most cases of ocular toxoplasmosis are a manifestation of an infection which occurred during fetal life. Even toxoplasmosis encountered in adults may more likely be a late recurrence of a latent or subclinical congenital infection.

The diagnosis is based on the ophthalmoscopic picture associated with positive serologic tests (immunofluorescence, agglutination, dye test, ELISA, etc.). There is, however, no correlation between the antibody titer in the serum and the degree of activity or severity of the ocular disease.

Ocular toxoplasmosis is characterized by an exudative retinitis, which may be uni- or multifocal, and a secondary choroiditis. The lesion is usually behind the equator and mainly found in the macula. It is often bilateral. In general these retinochoroidal lesions heal within two to six months leaving atrophic scars with pigment proliferation at the border.

In the **congenital forms** we distinguished the cicatricial lesion from acute and recurrent lesions.

The *cicatricial chorioretinitis* is often found incidentally on a routine eye examination. The scars may be of any form and size and are usually situated behind the equator, with a predilection for the macular area, in at least one eye; peripheral locations are, however, not rare. The cicatricial lesion is characterized by a large white chorioretinal atrophy which develops in the area of the original inflammation (macular pseudocoloboma) (Figs. 386, 387). The scar is surrounded by polymorphic pigmented lines due to the destruction and proliferation of the retinal pigment epithelium (Fig. 388). In some cases there may be a proliferation of glial and subretinal connective tissue producing a grey-blue prominance, i.e., vascularized tumefaction surrounded by a zone of pigment (jellyfish lesion) (Figs. 389, 390). These chorioretinal lesions may remain inactive for life. They are the expression of a fetal retinitis which developed before or immediately after birth or of a post-natal retinitis which had remained undiagnosed and developed without any evident clinical signs or symptoms. If the macula is involved there will be severe and irreversible reduction of visual acuity with subsequent strabismus or nystagmus.

Another characteristic manifestation of congenital ocular toxoplasmosis is the *chorioretinal scar with satellite lesions*. Such reactivations of the retinitis may occur at any time during the first year of life up to adulthood; they occur most frequently during the second and third decade. In general the active lesion is a single focus in one eye, but there may be several recurrences. The ophthalmoscopic picture is characterized by the presence of one focus of active, grey-yellow retinitis with blurred margins lying adjacent to the chorioretinal scar (Figs. 391, 392). There is always an overlying cellular reaction in the fundus which, when marked, may obstruct a precise visualization of the ocular fundus and may produce the picture of a "headlight in the fog", characteristic for many cases of active retinitis (Fig. 370). The adjacent retinal vessels often show perivasculitis which will resolve together with the primary retinal lesions without leaving any ischemic damages. The focus of retinitis may vary in size; it is usually at the posterior pole and therefore produces permanent severe loss of central vision. A juxtapapillary location may simulate during the acute phase a primary optic neuritis and may appear under the classical clinical picture of a Jensen chorioretinitis (Figs. 391, 392). The evolution from a granulomatous to an atrophic lesion is quite slow and cicatricization takes on an average three to six months (Figs. 393, 394). A recurrence of the retinitis is accompanied by inflammatory signs in the anterior segment, by marked vitreous exudations, sometimes by edema and atrophy of the optic nervehead. In rare cases the intraocular inflammation may progress to a marked retraction of the vitreous causing a total retinal detachment and producing the clinical picture of a pseudoglioma (leukokoria).

The **acquired form** of toxoplasmic retinochoroiditis is ophthalmoscopically also characterized by an area of acute retinitis, white-yellow in color, involving the nerve fiber layer and the blood vessels, with blurred margins and surrounding hemorrhages; the lesion may be one to two disc diameters in size and is localized behind the equator, mainly in the macula or next to the disc. Characteristically there is no chorioretinal scar next to the active focus. The vitreous exudates are conspicuous and often associated with a reactive inflammation of the anterior segment; both factors may make it difficult to examine the fundus.

The evolution toward a scar is slow and pigment appears after 4-6 weeks. The so-called acquired toxoplasmic retinochoroiditis resembling the classical congenital type is frequently unilateral and has a strong tendency to recur. Repeated recurrences may cause an endophthalmitis with massive vitreous hemorrhage and retinal detachment. A retinopathy associated with systemic toxoplasmosis is more often found in those patients in whom the central nervous system and the lungs are involved; it is less frequent in the lymphoglandular form; nevertheless this is a rare event (1-2% of the cases) (Fig. 368).

The acute phase of ocular toxoplasmosis is treated with pyrimethamine and trisulfapyrimidine, combined with corticosteroids if the lesion is in or close to the macula requiring an intensive anti-inflammatory treatment in order to limit, as much as possible, damage to central vision and to the papillomacular bundle. Any kind of corticosteroid treatment has to be supplemented with specific antitoxoplasmic medications in order to avoid reactivation of a localized toxoplasmic infection which may lead to exudative and necrotic paravascular lesions. Clindamycin is indicated for massive lesions at the posterior pole not responding to the conventional treatment. On the other hand, no treatment whatsoever is needed for peripheral lesions with a moderate inflammatory reaction as these foci of retinochoroiditis have a strong tendency to heal spontaneously.

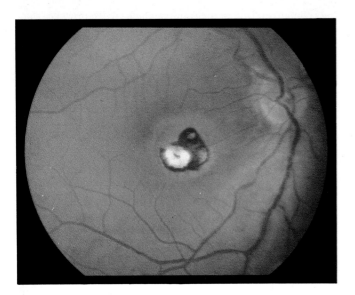

Fig. 386

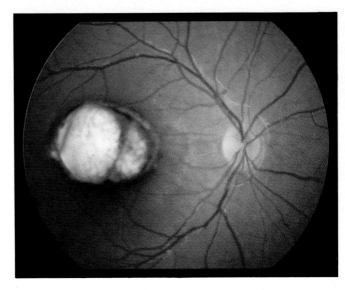

Fig. 387

Figs. 386, 387.   Congenital ocular toxoplasmosis. Examples of a macular chorioretinal scar (macular pseudocoloboma).

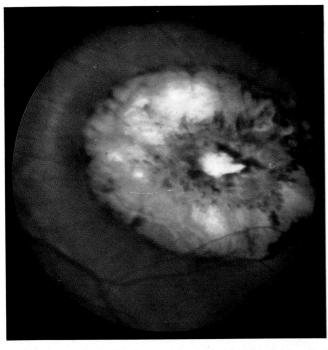

Fig. 388.   Congenital ocular toxoplasmosis. Macular chorioretinal scar resembling "a wheel" or "a rosette".

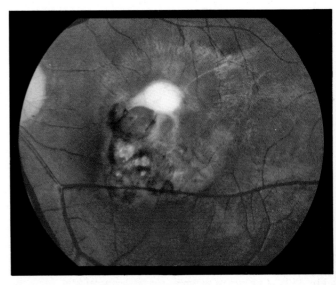

Fig. 389.   Congenital ocular toxoplasmosis. Macular chorioretinal scar with glial proliferation (resembling "a medusa head" or "jellyfish lesion").

Fig. 390. Congenital ocular toxoplasmosis. Macular chorioretinal scar with central proliferation.

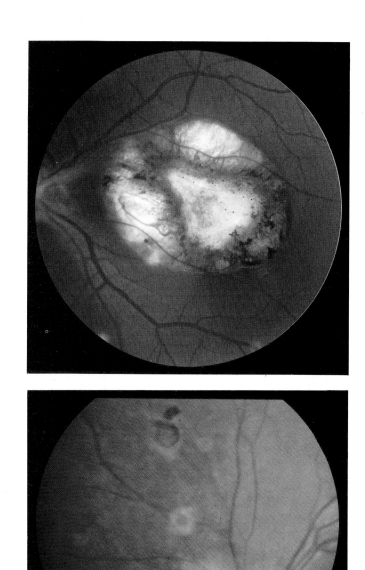

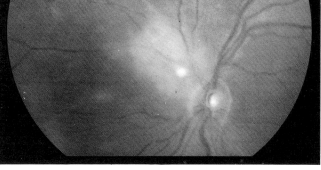

a   b

Fig. 391. Congenital toxoplasmic retinochoroiditis.
a) Focus of active juxtapapillary retinitis, a satellite of a heavily pigmented chorioretinal scar in the upper temporal segment; evidence of reactive perivasculitis around the active lesion.
b) The juxtapapillary focus has developed into a scar the margins of which are moderately pigmented; the retinal vasculitis has resolved.

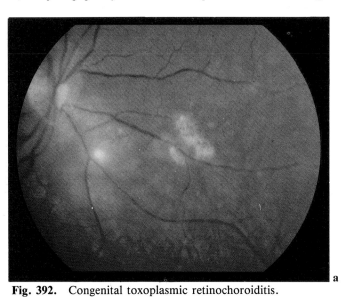

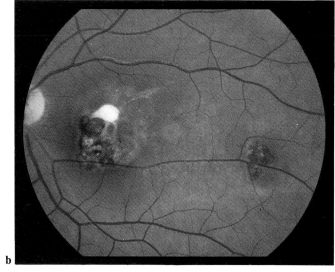

a   b

Fig. 392. Congenital toxoplasmic retinochoroiditis.
a) Right eye: focus of juxtapapillary active retinitis in the lower nasal segment, satellite to two small atrophic barely pigmented chorioretinal scars.
b) Left eye: characteristic chorioretinal scars at the posterior pole (same as Fig. 389 at lower magnification).

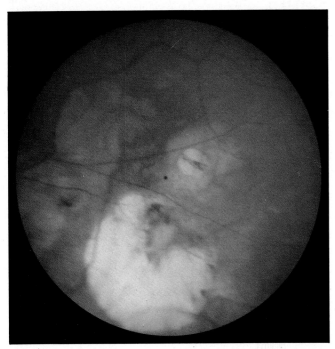

Fig. 393. Toxoplasmic retinochoroiditis. Peripheral atrophic chorioretinal scars with a small satellite focus becoming atrophic.

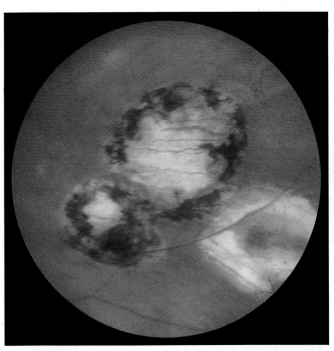

394. Toxoplasmic retinochoroiditis. Multiple chorioretinal scars in different degrees of atrophy and pigmentation, expression of several episodes of recurrences of the peripheral toxoplasmic retinochoroiditis.

OCULAR INFESTATION WITH TOXOCARA

This infestation is caused by *Toxocara canis* or *Toxocara cati*, parasitic ascaris, commonly found in dogs and cats in which they also complete their life cycle.

Man is infected by eating dirt or food contaminated with the egg of the parasite. These eggs develop in the intestinal tract to larvae which penetrate the vessel walls and are then disseminated into various organs, especially the liver, lungs, eyes, brain and skin. The systemic manifestation of toxocariasis (visceral larva migrans) appear usually in infancy and are rarely associated with ocular manifestations. The eye involvement is mostly found in children and young adults, frequently between the ages of 3 and 14.

The ocular infestation is nearly always unilateral and may cause an *endophthalmitis* with vitreous opacities, thick cyclitic membranes, retinal detachment and cataracta complicata. Often there is a *granulomatous chorioretinitis* in the macula or in the periphery. The macular location is more frequent and manifests itself as a granulomatous chorioretinitis of the posterior pole characterized by a mass of an elevated, white tumefaction of one to two disc diameters in size and accompanied by subretinal hemorrhages and a serous detachment of the surrounding retina (Figs. 395, 396). There is usually a mild cellular reaction in the vitreous. The differential diagnosis with toxoplasmosis is relatively easy.

There is a marked irreversible visual field defect.

The peripheral lesions are more often found in young adults than in children. The peripheral chorioretinal granuloma is always anterior to the equator, often multiple and has the same characteristics as the macular lesion. It is complicated by membranes and vitreous bands which by traction may distort and drag the macula and the optic nervehead (Fig. 397) leading eventually to a secondary retinal detachment. There is usually no inflammatory reaction in the anterior segment or in the vitreous, but snow banks may be observed as in pars planitis. The differential diagnosis encompasses congenital retinal folds and retinopathy of prematurity.

Histologically the lesions represent a granulomatous reaction containing eosinophilic and neutrophilic leukocytes, epithelioid cells and occasional giant cells. The infiltrate surrounds the *Toxocara* larva.

The diagnosis can often be made clinically and is substantiated by an esosinophilia and by a positive ELISA test (which is still difficult to obtain in many countries). There is no specific therapy and the usual antihelmintic medications are here not effective. Systemic and periocular corticosteroids may be applied in cases of active inflammatory involvement of the macula.

Fig. 395. Toxocariasis. Acute macular chorioretinal granuloma with serous detachment of the surrounding retina, edema along the upper and lower temporal arcade.

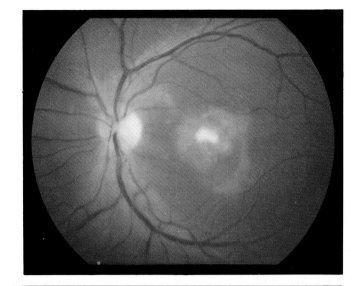

Fig. 396. Toxocariasis.
a) Active macular chorioretinal granuloma with hemorrhage below the overlying retina.
b) Evolution of the chorioretinal granuloma which now appears as a circumscribed elevated round yellow mass; the blood absorbed after four months.

a   b

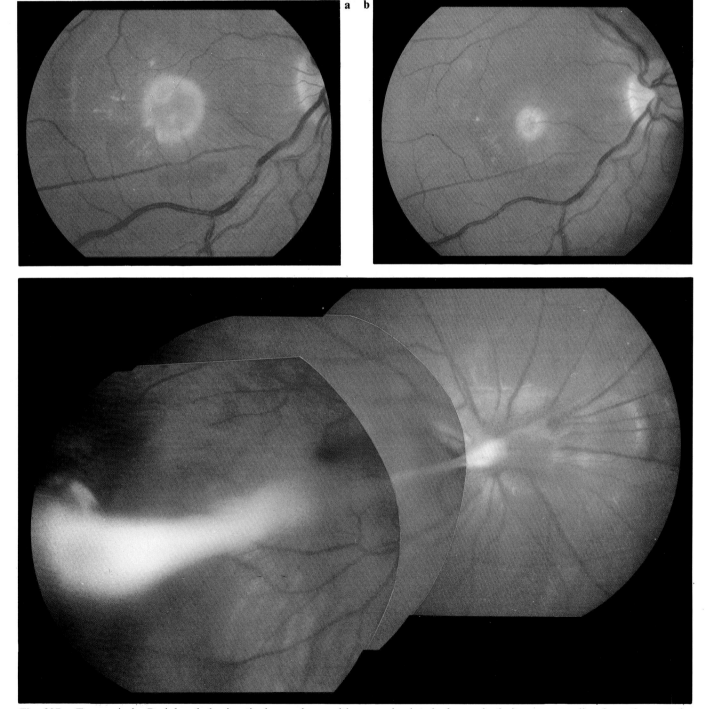

Fig. 397. Toxocariasis. Peripheral chorioretinal granuloma with a massive band of organized vitreous extending from the posterior pole to the optic nervehead distorting the vessels on the disc.

OCULAR CYSTICERCOSIS

Human infestation with a tape worm may cause an ocular disease if the larva migrates from the intestinal tract against the bloodstream to the eye. Man is the intermediate host of the parasite and the primary source of infection are hogs and cattle.

Various species of *Taenia* may invade the posterior segment, but the cysticercosis cellulosa (larva of *Taenia solium*) is the most frequently encountered tapeworm. The disease is usually unilateral and affects children in the first or second year of infancy. The larva reaches the choroid via the posterior ciliary arteries and from there migrates into the subretinal space producing a retinal detachment. Ophthalmoscopically there may also be a grey cystoid tumefaction with a dense white center corresponding to the more or less uncinated scolex. The larva may then migrate through a retinal hole into the subhyaloid space and then into the vitreous. There it appears as a round preretinal cyst measuring one to two disc diameters, yellowish—with a bilobed protruberance or scolex (Fig. 398). Undulating movements of the larva or to and from movements of the scolex (Fig. 399) may be noted on repeated and prolonged observation. Cysticercus is better tolerated in the vitreous than in the retina; the larva may survive for one to five years and a chronic infestation will cause a diffuse progressive chorioretinitis due to a hypersensitivity reaction mediated by IgE; finally a preretinal gliosis, retinal detachment and atrophy of the globe may ensue.

The characteristic ophthalmoscopic picture should be sufficient for a diagnosis; useful is also eosinophilia and a positive ELISA test for the specific antibodies of the various types of *Taenia*. The echographic examination reveals the cyst when a close examination of the fundus is impossible because of opaque media.

The treatment is exclusively surgical.

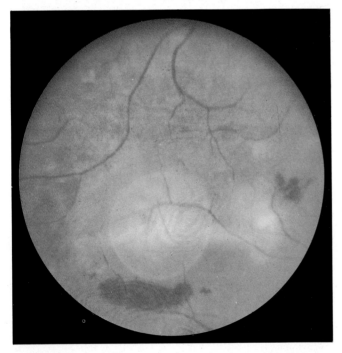

Fig. 398. Ocular cysticercosis. Subretinal grey-yellow cyst of irregular round shape with expanding hemorrhages and surrounding edema.

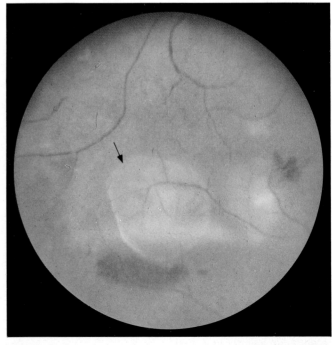

Fig. 399. Ocular cysticercosis. Later fundus photo of Fig. 398: the light stimulus (flash) has changed the form of this cyst by making the larva move (arrow).

PRESUMED OCULAR HISTOPLASMOSIS

Histoplasmosis is an infection which is common to man and animals. It is caused by inhaling the saprophytic fungus of the soil, *Histoplasma capsulatum*. The disease is endemic in the United States, especially in the Missisipi, Ohio and Missouri river beds. It has been absent from Europe for a long time. After inhalation the fungus causes a pulmonary disease which is often asymptomatic. Granulomas may develop in the liver, spleen, lymphnodes and bone marrow. The pulmonary and spleen lesions may calcify and can then be seen on x-ray. During the systemic manifestations of the disease ocular involvement is rare; it appears as an endophthalmitis and the fungus can be found in the ocular tissues.

Presumed ocular histoplasmosis, on the other hand, is a disease of young adults withouth any systemic or local signs of an inflammation; histoplasma capsulatum has never been found in any of these choroidal granulomas; it is probably the sequel of a benign systemic histoplasmosis of infancy which passed unobserved and healed completely. The clinical picture is characterized by:

— typical disciform lesion in or close to the macula;
— peripheral yellow small areas of choroidal and pigment epithelial atrophy; they are disseminated in both eyes just behind the equator;
— more or less pigmented chorioretinal scar around the optic nervehead;
— no inflammatory reaction in the vitreous.

The ocular disease becomes clinically evident after a period of 10-20 years when a subretinal neovascularization develops at the macular or juxtapapillary scar. The pathogenesis of this new-formation is still unknown. Such neovascularization may cause a serous and hemorrhagic detachment of the macula, paramacular area or around the optic nervehead.

Ophthalmoscopically we see at the posterior pole a grey-green, dark, circular or semilunar area around an old scar or a recent subretinal hemorrhage. The grey ring associated with a disciform macular lesion is an unmistakable sign of subretinal neovascularization. Occasionally the subretinal hemorrhage may appear quite dark because the overlying pigment epithelium is intact.

The symptoms are connected with the location of the lesion which is the origin of the neovascular membrane. Active lesions may regress with partial functional recovery, but episodes of recurrent subretinal exudation are frequent. The macular involvement seems to be associated with the histocompatibility antigens HLA-B7 and HLA-DR2.

In endemic areas the diagnosis can be made from the characteristic fundus lesions and the absence of any similar reaction in the vitreous. Fluorescein angiography is also useful revealing the peripheral hypofluorescent histo-spots and the subretinal neovascularization.

The complement fixation test is positive in only one third of the patients, whereas the histoplasmine skin test is positive in 90% of the cases.

The true efficacy of laser therapy to the subretinal neovascular membrane is still unknown. This phototreatment is usually contraindicated as a prophylactic measure for asymptomatic perimacular scars and active foveal lesions.

An intensive, early, corticosteroid treatment may be indicated for the disciform maculopathy.

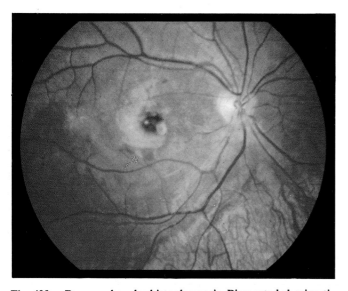

Fig. 400. Presumed ocular histoplasmosis. Pigmented chorioretinal scar in the macula surrounded by a semilunar grey-green area of subretinal neovascularization; small subretinal hemorrhages around the lesion.

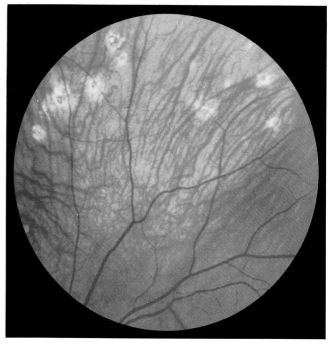

Fig. 401. Presumed ocular histoplasmosis. Multiple atrophic chorioretinal scars behind the equator (histospots).

MYCOTIC RETINITIS

During the last years the incidence of mycotic retinitis and endopthalmitis has significantly increased. These infections are quite often seen in drug abusers and in hospitalized patients undergoing a systemic prolonged treatment with antibiotics, corticosteroids or immunosuppressive drugs. The infection may also occur with parenteral alimentation through an intravenous route. In general, these infections are seen in immune compromised subjects and are produced by opportunistic agents. Infections with *Candida* are relatively frequent, whereas those with *Cryptococcus* and *Aspergillus* are quite rare. Retinitis may be the first manifestation of a systemic candidiasis, especially in drug abusers in which this condition can be differentiated from a retinopathy due to talc injection.

The ocular involvement appears as a multifocal retinochoroiditis localized mainly around the posterior pole evolving more or less rapidly toward an endophthalmitis (Fig. 402) with retinal necrosis, retinal detachment and atrophy of the globe. Both eyes are usually involved, though the intensity and severity of the disease may vary between the two.

The retinal foci are white-yellow lesions which are fluffy, have blurred outlines and are of varying size, up to several disc diameters; they grow slowly and finally invade the vitreous after rupturing the internal limiting membrane. In that event white fluffy, floating opacities appear in the vitreous (Figs. 403, 404). Characteristically the media remain clear and there is only minimal reaction of the anterior uvea, especially in the initial phases.

The ophthalmoscopic picture is typical and suffices for the diagnosis which probably will be confirmed by the microbiologic examination of the blood and of the vitreous. *Candida* retinitis differs from cytomegalic inclusion disease, which is also an opportunistic infection of an immunocompromised host, by the absence of retinal hemorrhages and the characteristic invasion of the vitreous.

Vitrectomy with aspiration of the fluffy exudates is not only of diagnostic, but also of therapeutic value. The treatment consists in the systemic application of amphotericin B (in special cases also by subconjunctival and intravitreal injection), flucytosine and miconazol.

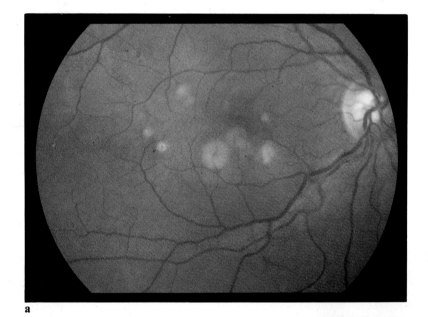

a

b

Fig. 402.   Bilateral candida retinitis.
a) Right eye: numerous small fluffy foci in and around the macula.
b) Left eye: endophthalmitis with characteristic grey-yellow pupillary reflex.

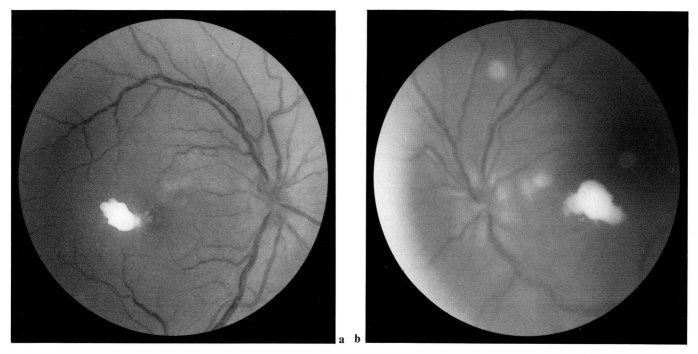

Fig. 403. Bilateral candida retinitis. Fluffy exudate at the posterior pole floating in the vitreous; secondary neuroretinitis.
a) Right eye.
b) Left eye.

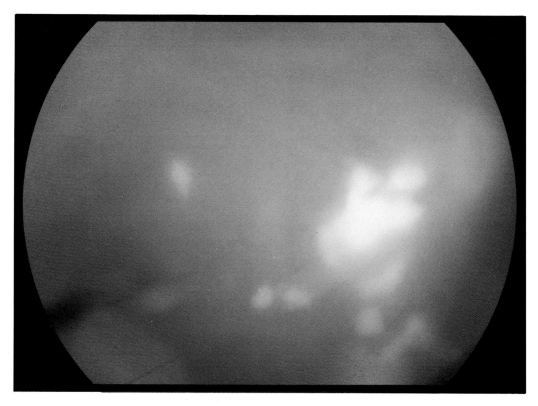

Fig. 404. *Candida* retinitis. White fluffy exudates invading the vitreous.

VIRAL RETINITIS

Congenital. Nearly any viral infection contracted by the mother, especially during the first two trimesters of pregnancy, may affect the retina of the fetus. This is usually a bilateral diffuse retinochoroiditis which already at birth or when diagnosed has developed to the typical "pepper and salt chorioretinitis" or the "pseudoretinitis pigmentosa" (Fig. 405). Visual acuity and electrophysiologic tests may remain normal.

Ophthalmoscopic examination reveals the typical pigment changes with small areas of atrophy intermingled with spots of hyperpigmentation. These patches are more numerous at the posterior pole. There may be an associated partial optic atrophy and some vitreous opacities.

In addition to the retinitis there may be other ocular involvements (microphthalmos, cataract) and systemic manifestations (heart defects, deafness, and encephalopathy).

The most frequent cause are *German measles* but other exanthematous diseases and congenital herpes may be responsible for retinitis in the newborn.

Acquired forms. Viral retinitis in an adult occurs mainly in immune compromised patients and leads to a necrotizing retinitis.

One exception is the chorioretinitis during a herpes simplex infection; the chicken-pox zoster virus may occasionally cause a diffuse chorioretinitis with perivasculitis and occlusive vasculitis, retinal hemorrhages, optic neuritis, and an exudative retinal detachment. An acute retinal epithelitis has also been described in the course of a German measles infection in adults.

The most frequently observed viral retinitis, both in adults and as a congenital form, is produced by the cytomegalic virus.

Cytomegalic viral retinitis. The cytomegalic virus (belonging to the group of herpes virus) produces both in the congenital form and in an adult an exudative necrotizing retinitis associated with occlusive retinal vasculitis and hemorrhages. The *congenital form*, seen not only in the newborn, but also in infants, produces systemic signs, e.g., fever, thrombocytopenia, pneumonia and hepatosplenomegaly. The ocular signs consist of peripheral and central bilateral disseminate chorioretinal scars with optic atrophy and cataract (Fig. 407). Exudative lesions occur frequently.

In the *adult*, on the other hand, the infection may only produce ocular changes with an acute necrotizing retinitis; this condition can be found in immunocompromised patients who suffer form a lymphoproliferative disease or neoplasm, are being treated by immunosuppressive medications for a kidney transport, or more recently, suffer from the acquired immunodeficiency syndrome (AIDS). This is, therefore, an opportunistic infection. Ophthalmoscopically we see cotton-wool patches coalescing to geographic lesions and retinal necrotic areas that appear as white spots with hemorrhages at the progressive margin of the lesion. The exudative retinitis is always associated with an occlusive vasculitis, perivascular sheathing and a reaction in the overlying vitreous (Fig. 406).

The ocular involvement is usually bilateral, but may be more marked in one eye than in the other. Occasionally there is a spontaneous regression; the retina will become atrophic and appear grey-brown. Histologically the retinal cells show the characteristic eosinophilic intranuclear and basophilic cytoplasmic inclusion bodies.

Treatment is problematic. If possible the immunosuppressive therapy should be reduced or discontinued. The newer antiviral drugs, e.g., acyclovir, and medications stimulating the immune response still have to be evaluated and tested.

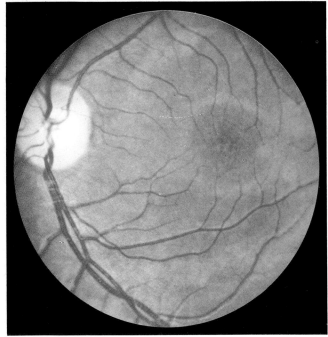

Fig. 405

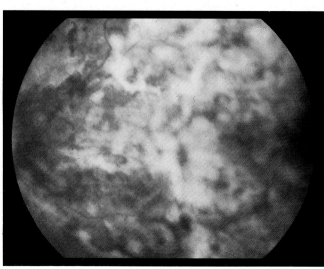

Fig. 406

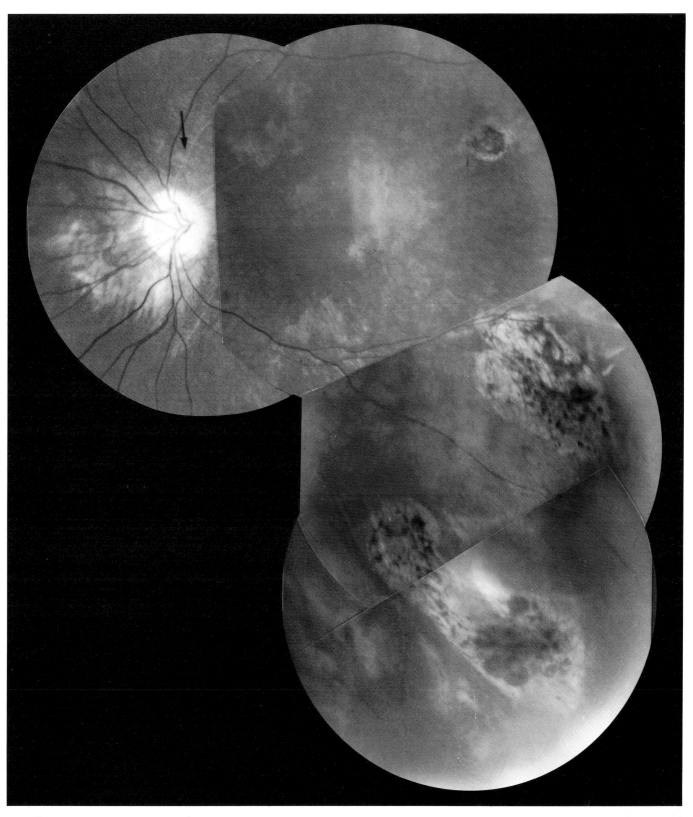

Fig. 407. Congenital cytomegalic retinitis. Disseminate focal chorioretinitis in the cicatricial stage, optic atrophy and retinal vasculitis (arrow).

Fig. 405. Macular pseudoretinitis pigmentosa secondary to congenital measles retinitis (clinical appearance similar to Stargardt disease).

Fig. 406. Cytomegalic retinitis in acquired immunodeficiency syndrome (AIDS).
Coalescing geographic areas of retinal necrosis with extensive retinal hemorrage and occlusive vasculitis (like "catsup and cottage cheese").

SARCOIDOSIS

Sarcoidosis is a granulomatous inflammation affecting many organ systems with protean symptoms; it is of unknown etiology and responsible for 2-10% of all cases of endogenous uveitis. It affects more often women (2:1) and black patients. About 20-50% of the patients show ocular complications; the most frequent manifestation is iridocyclitis, but nearly all the ocular and extraocular structures may be involved. The chorioretinitis is a granulomatous inflammation with multiple foci at the posterior pole and a retinal perivasculitis (Figs. 408, 409).

Ophthalmoscopically we see round, multiple, yellow-grey spots, usually one disc diameter in size which evolve into a chorioretinal scar (Fig. 408). These lesions are accompanied by grey retinal exudates resembling "candle wax droppings" and by a nodular periphlebitis (Fig. 409).

In the periphery we may find signs of a periphlebitis with hemorrhages, neovascularization, and exudates at the vitreous base resembling snow banks or ant eggs producing the clinical picture of a pars planitis. This chronic uveoretinitis is frequently complicated by a cystoid macular edema. Optic neuritis usually develops when the central nervous system is involved (Fig. 409).

The diagnosis can be corrobated by an x-ray picture of the chest and by determining the angiotension conversion enzyme, nuclear magnetic imaging, negative skin tests for the usual antigens and above all by biopsying an accessible granuloma.

Corticosteroids are the treatment of choice for systemic and ocular sarcoidosis.

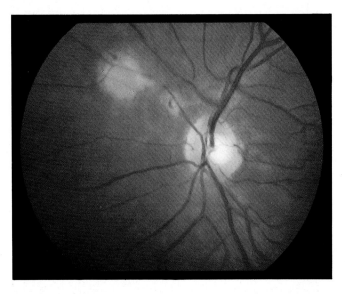

Fig. 408. Multiple foci of chorioretinitis in various stages of evolution with perivasculitis in a patient suffering from systemic sarcoidosis.

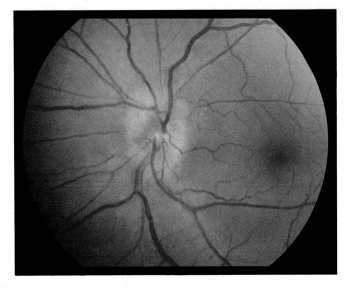

Fig. 409. Papillitis with small perivascular retinal exudates and diffuse vasculitis in a patient suffering from pulmonary sarcoidosis.

BEHÇET DISEASE

Behçet's disease presents a syndrome of unknown etiology consisting of oral and genital aphthous lesions, involvement of skin and eye, thrombophlebitis mainly of the gastrointestinal and central nervous systems. It occurs more often in men than women (4:1) and has a chronic progressive course with exacerbations.

Behçet's disease is usually regarded as one of the connective tissue disorders. An occlusive vasculitis occurs in all affected organs; immunocomplex systems circulate in the blood and produce the corresponding pathologic pictures and other immunologic, especially autoimmunologic, alterations.

The disease is more prevalent in Japan and in the Mediter-

ranean countries. This has suggested the possibility of an infection, especially with a slow virus, and a genetic predisposition underlined by the significant association with the histocompatibility antigen HLA-B5 (BW51).

In about 80% of the cases the eye is involved. This occurs more frequently in Japan where Behçet's disease represents 20% of all endogenous uveitis, and in the Mediterranean countries. The disease is rare in the anglo-saxon nations where the aphthous involvement of the mucous membranes with or without skin manifestations is more frequent. According to our material Behçet's disease represents 4% of all cases of uveitis.

The classical iridocyclitis with recurrent hypopyon (Fig. 410) is actually not that often seen and therefore not an indispensible prerequisite to establish the diagnosis.

More frequent is a recurrent exudative iridocyclitis and a *diffuse uveitis* predominantly involving the posterior segment (choroiditis, chorioretinitis, papillitis). The characteristic feature of this disease is the *retinal vasculitis* (Fig. 411), expression of an occlusive angiitis which histologically can be found in all involved organs.

The ophthalmoscopic picture varies a great deal and differs with the stage of the disease and the severity of a single acute attack. In the initial stages and during a moderately severe episode we may only see hyperemia of the optic nervehead associated with venous congestion, dilatation of the capillaries, and retinal edema, especially at the posterior pole. In hyper-acute cases the disc edema and the venous congestion become more conspicuous; the retinal edema is massive and there are white-yellow intraretinal exudates associated with hemorrhages producing a clinical picture similar to an occlusive disease (Fig. 412). Periphlebitis is often seen and may evolve toward true occlusions.

The hemorrhages and exudates occur most often at the posterior pole (Fig. 413), but may also be seen in the retinal periphery and along the vascular arcades.

Macular edema may after repeated attacks cause degenerative changes under the picture of a cystoid degeneration and in extreme cases true macular holes appear (Figs. 414, 415). The progressive vasculitis (peri- and endovasculitis) will produce sclerotic changes in the arteries and veins leading to a complete occlusion with subsequent optic atrophy and in the final stages to the appearance of the characteristic "fundus without vessels" (Figs. 416, 418). The relative, more or less diffuse avascularity of the retina will lead to degenerative lesions which are either ischemic (holes, neovascularization, etc.) or of the tapetoretinal type (Fig. 419).

The retinal neovascularization involves mainly the capillary bed and is associated with vitreo-retinal proliferations and hemorrhages.

Fluorescein angiography is most useful in establishing an early diagnosis during which it may demonstrate signs of retinal vasculitis and damage to the optic nervehead before these changes become evident ophthalmoscopically.

The ocular manifestations are always bilateral and represent the clinical manifestations of Behçet's disease which carry the poorest prognosis second only to the involvement of the cardiovascular and central nervous systems, which carry a poor prognosis as far as survival of the patient is concerned.

The recent introduction of immunosuppressive treatment combined with corticosteroids has considerably improved the visual prognosis.

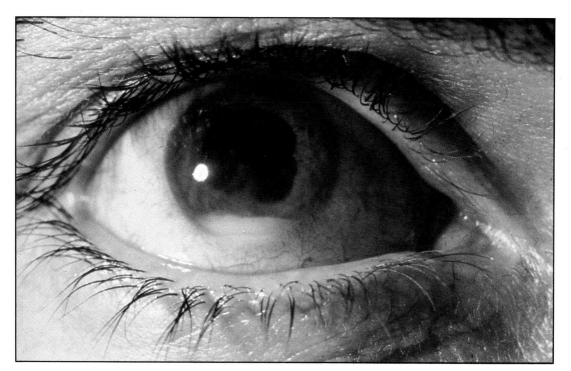

Fig. 410. Behçet disease. Hypopyon iridocyclitis.

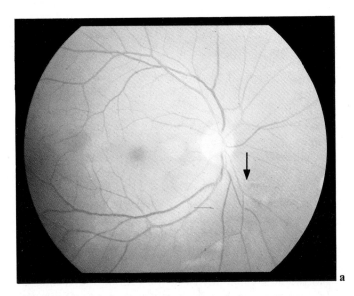

a

Fig. 411. Behçet disease.
a) Fundus photo: initial retinal vasculitis. Occlusion of a branch of the lower nasal vein (arrow).
b) Fluorescein angiograms: occlusion of a branch of the lower nasal vein (arrow) with large areas of non-perfusions and veno-venous capillary shunts and arterio-venous anastomoses in the area drained by that vein; diffuse segmental changes of vascular permeability indicating a vasculitis.

b

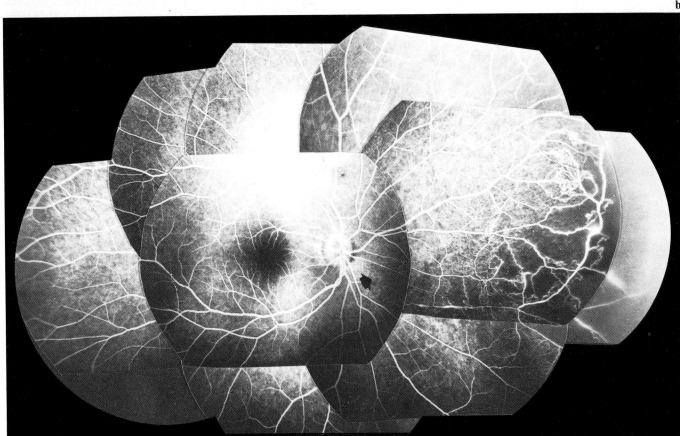

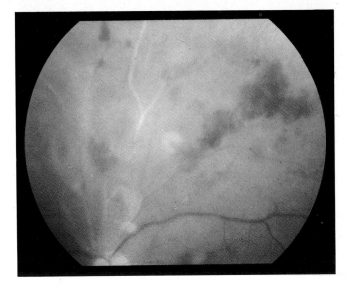

Fig. 412. Behçet disease. Vasculitis of the upper arcade leading to partial occlusions. Complete occlusion of the upper nasal vein and partial occlusion of the upper temporal branch; old retinal hemorrhages (the vitreous opacities prevent an exact examination of the details).

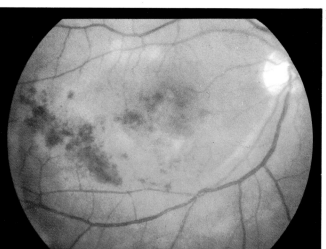

Fig. 413

Fig. 413. Behçet disease. Retinal edema, a few intraretinal hemorrhages of various shape and size, exudates at the posterior pole.

Fig. 414. Behçet disease. Partial ischemic optic atrophy, vasculitis of the large vessels with a tuft of proliferating tissue along the upper temporal venous branch; macular hole and chronic perimacular edema.

Fig. 415. Behçet disease (left eye of the same patient as in Fig. 414).
a) Fundus photo: temporal pallor of the optic nervehead, venous congestion, perivasculitis, cystoid macular degeneration.
b) Fluorescein angiogram: hyperfluorescence of the optic nervehead, cystoid macular edema, vasculitis of the upper and lower temporal veins with underlying hemorrhages.

Fig. 414

Fig. 415

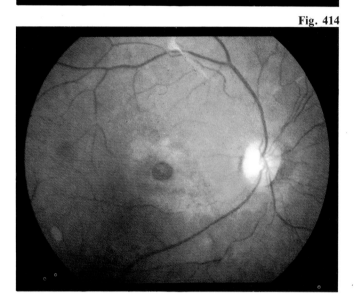

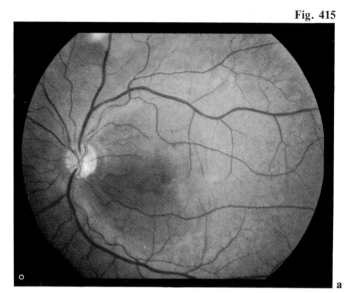

a

b

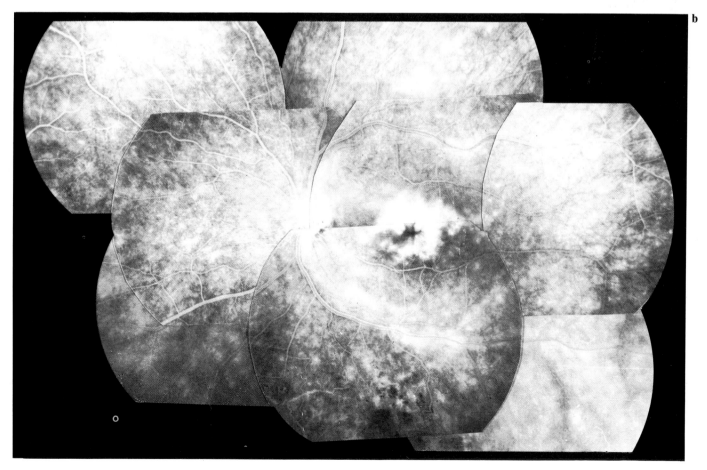

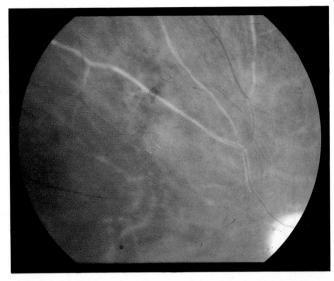

Fig. 416. Behçet disease. Optic atrophy, marked retinal vasculitis with blood vessels reduced to occluded bands (shadow vessels), perivenous sheathing, splashes of hemorrhages and signs of retinal ischemia.

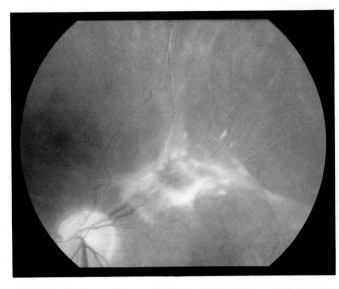

Fig. 417. Behçet disease. Perivasculitis with occlusions and neovascularization, proliferating connective tissue membrane involving the upper temporal arcade and the posterior pole.

Fig. 418. Behçet disease. Optic atrophy, the vascular tree is nearly completely occluded, capillary neovascularization around the disc with a few hemorrhages.

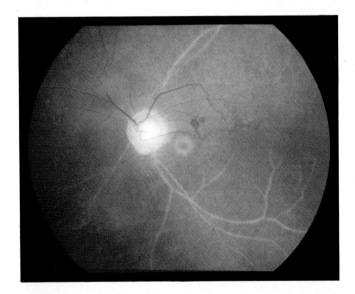

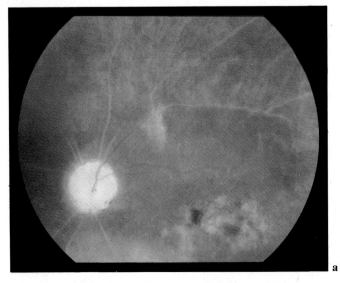

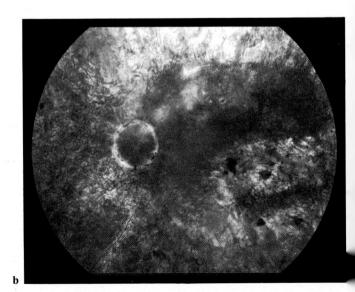

a   b

Fig. 419. Behçet disease. End stage of retinal vasculitis: optic atrophy, the vascular arcades are nearly completely occluded, diffuse chorioretinal degeneration and epiretinal membrane at the posterior pole (**a**). The lack of retinal blood vessels is even more evident on fluorescein angiography (**b**).

SYMPATHETIC OPHTHALMIA

This is a diffuse bilateral granulomatous uveitis which follows a perforating injury, accidental or surgical. The inflammation in the injured ("exciting") eye begins after a latency of variable duration, extending from 2-8 months up to many years. The disease has become quite rare, probably because of the modern treatment of ocular trauma using microsurgical techniques and because of the more efficatious anti-inflammatory treatment. It has been estimated that sympathetic ophtalmia occurs in 0.2 to 1% of all accidental perforating injuries and is 30-50 times more frequent after accidental trauma than after a surgical intervention.

The etiology of the disease remains unknown. A viral etiology has been proposed but not proven. Experimental studies support the hypothesis that this is an autoimmune inflammation perhaps connected with a polypeptide fraction of a soluble protein derived from the outer members of the photoreceptors (the S-antigen of the retina described by Wacker).

Clinically the disease appears as a severe anterior granulomatous uveitis which usually obscures the fundus and does not allow an ophthalmoscopic examination. In the course of time the posterior segment will be involved with a peripapillary choroiditis, cystoid macular edema (Fig. 420) and choroidal infiltrates or white-yellow subretinal exudates which are more numerous in the periphery (Fig. 421) and only sporadic at the posterior pole. These exudates may coalesce to large placoid masses rarely causing an exudative retinal detachment (Fig. 422).

Fluorescein angiography is most useful in establishing the diagnosis: characteristic are multiple foci which leak the dye into the choroid where it may accumulate in the subretinal space during the late phases of the angiogram. In the latest stages of the disease we see small multiple chorioretinal scars. These atrophic areas give the peripheral retina a moth eaten aspect (Fig. 423).

Histologically we see a typical granulomatous reaction with lymphocytes, epithelioid cells, giant cells and sometimes eosinophiles (Fig. 424); the choriocapillaries is usually spared. Characteristic for sympathetic ophthalmia is the phagocytosis of pigment by epithelioid cells and the proliferation of pigment epithelial cells forming the Dalen-Fuchs nodules, the histologic substrate of the above described subretinal exudations.

Occasionally systemic signs also appear, e.g., vitiligo, poliosis, alopecia, disturbances of the audio-vestibular apparatus, i.e., manifestations typical for Vogt-Koyanagi-Harada disease. These signs, together with the clinical picture and the fluorescein angiograms, prove the close relationship of the two conditions and make a differential diagnosis sometimes problematic.

In spite of effective therapy the long term prognosis of the disease is not good because of the tendency for recurrences. Anti-inflammatory treatment with corticosteroids and/or immuno-suppressors should be initiated early, given over a long period of time and at an adequate dose.

Enucleating the exciting (blind) eye may have a protective effect on the development of a sympathizing uveitis in the second eye, if it is done within two weeks after the injury.

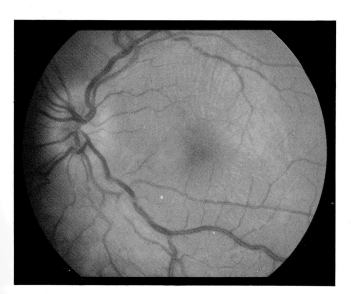

Fig. 420. Sympathetic ophthalmia. Papillitis and edema at the posterior pole.

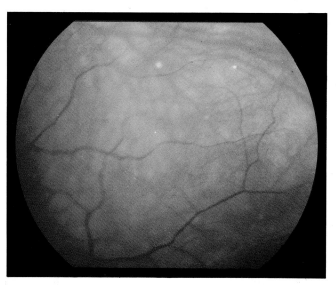

Fig. 421. Sympathetic ophthalmia. Moderate subretinal exudation with a few white-yellow infiltrates in mid periphery (same patient as in Fig. 420).

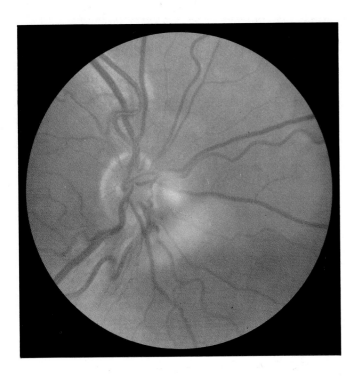

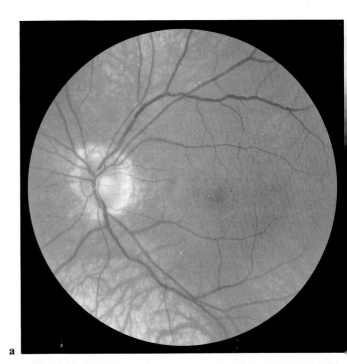

Fig. 422. Sympathetic ophthalmia. Hyperemia of the optic nervehead and subretinal edema below and nasal to the disc.

Fig. 423. Sympathetic ophthalmia. Cicatricial stage: atrophy of the optic nervehead and of the peripapillary choroid, pigmentary macular dystrophy (**a**) more conspicuous with red-free illumination (**b**); atrophic foci in mid-periphery (**c**).

a

b   c

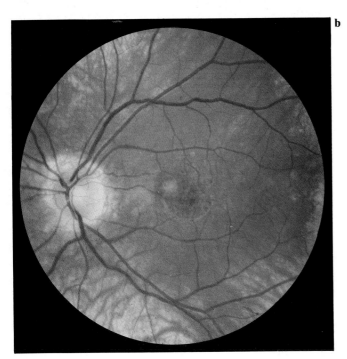

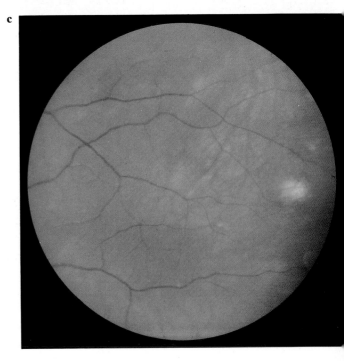

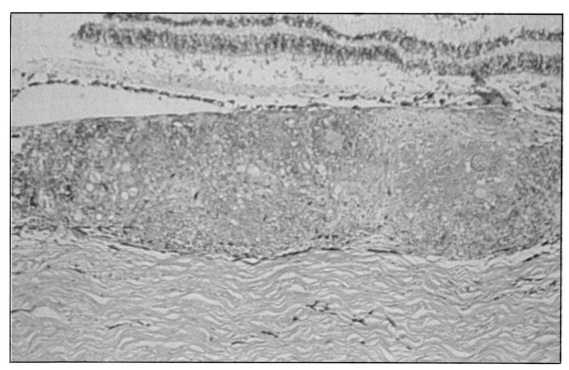

Fig. 424. Sympathetic ophthalmia. Histologic section (hematoxylin eosin). Diffuse granulomatous infiltration of the choroid; dark (lymphocytic) areas alternate with ligth (epithelioid cells) areas. Sclera and retina are within normal limits.

VOGT-KOYANAGI-HARADA DISEASE

This disease affects organs which contain melanocytes. It is of unknown etiology. The clinical picture varies, but is characterized by a diffuse bilateral granulomatous uveitis associated with vitiligo, poliosis, baldness, alopecia, loss of hearing and meningeal irritation (Fig. 425). For a long time Vogt-Koyanagi syndrome with anterior uveitis was differentiated from Harada disease in which the posterior uveitis with papillitis and bilateral exudative retinal detachment predominate.

The disease usually involves young adults in their third decade of life; women are more often affected than men. The prevalence shows geographic differences. The highest incidence has been reported in Japan where the condition represents 8% of all endogenous uveitis cases; it is rare in the western countries and seems to have a predilection for the pigmented races. In our own patient material the disease represents 2% of all uveitis cases.

The initial phase of the disease is usually acute and often follows an episode of an influenza-like disease with fever, malaise and rigidity of the neck (meningeal phase). These factors and the self-limiting aspect of the condition support an infectious etiology, especially a viral one. An autoimmune pathogenesis has been proposed based on the many clinical and histologic similarities between this condition and sympathetic ophthalmia. In addition there are multiple immunologic changes predominantly of the cell-mediated system concerning auto-antigens (uveo-retinal, connected with myelin and melanocytes). It seems to be established that VKH is part of a spectrum of inflammatory diseases, probably based on an autoimmune process and perhaps of

viral etiology; this spectrum extends from sympathetic ophthalmia to multiple sclerosis and it is quite probable that the acute posterior multiple placoid pigment epitheliopathy also belongs into this group.

Uveitis in VKH is always bilateral and begins at the posterior pole with a characteristic ophthalmoscopic picture. There is first hyperemia of the optic nervehead with disc edema and associated subretinal peripapillary edema (uveopapillitis) (Fig. 426). The accompanying massive diffuse choroiditis causes a multifocal subretinal exudation primarily at the posterior pole but progressing and producing localized exudative retinal detachments nearly always in the inferior segment of the fundus (Fig. 427). The ocular fundus acquires a piebald appearance with serous detachments in some and detachments of the pigment epithelium in other areas.

The exudative detachment of the lower segment may become extensive and bullous.

Fluorescein angiography shows multiple foci which leak the dye from the choroid into the subretinal space. In the acute phase the involvement of the anterior uvea may make the ophthalmoscopic evaluation difficult.

Two or three months after the onset the uveitis evolves into its cicatricial stage and is accompanied by depigmentation, not only in the eye but also in the skin and hair. The ocular fundus acquires the characteristic aspect of a "sunset glow fundus" with multiple focal chorioretinal scars, which are partly atrophic, partly heavily pigmented and are numerous in mid-periphery involving mainly the choriocapillaries and the retinal pigment epithelium (Figs. 428-431).

Characteristic is the pigment migration in the macular area which, however, does not compromise visual function (Fig. 429). In some cases there may be a nearly albinotic depigmentation of the fundus, whereas in others there may be organization of the subretinal fluid with the gross rearrangement of pigment in the area of the preceding exudative detachment. The papillitis will lead to disc pallor. Recurrences of the uveitis will generally spare the choriocapillaries.

Corticosteroid treatment has markedly modified the clinical course and the prognosis of VKH. An early adequate treatment will prevent progression of the disease, limit its duration and prevent involvement of the ear and the skin. Visual prognosis is good due to the effect of theraphy and the self-limiting tendency of the inflammation. According to recent statistics 70% of affected patients preserve a vision of more than 5-7/10.

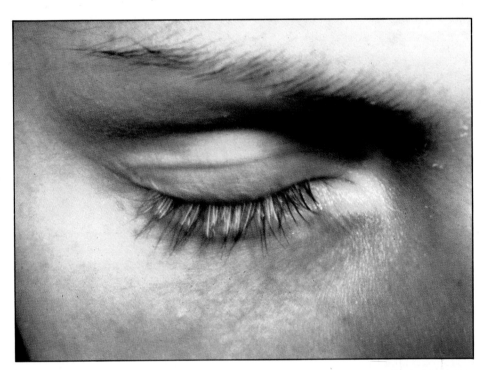

Fig. 425. Vogt-Koyanagi-Harada disease. Vitiligo around the eye with poliosis.

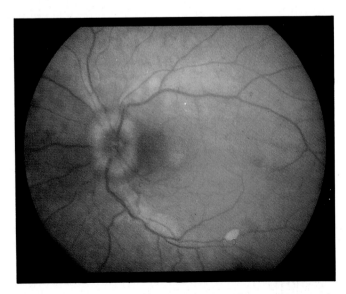

Fig. 426. Vogt-Koyanagi-Harada disease. Edema and hyperemia of the optic nervehead with beginning subretinal exudation around the disc.

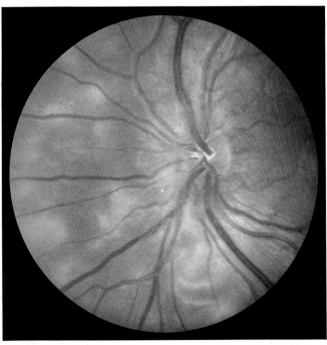

Fig. 427. Vogt-Koyanagi-Harada disease. Diffuse choroiditis with multifocal subretinal exudates (beginning exudative retinal detachment).

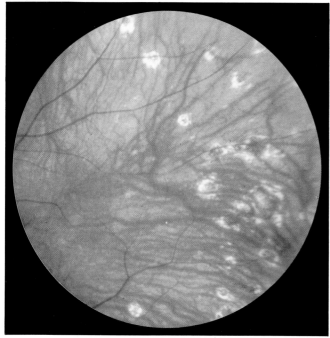

Fig. 428. Vogt-Koyanagi-Harada disease. Multiple chorioretinal scars with partly atrophic and partly pigmented foci in mid-periphery: atrophy of the pigment epithelium.

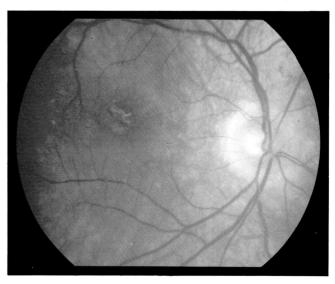

Fig. 429. Vogt-Koyanagi-Harada disease. Characteristic pigment migration in the macular area, pallor of the optic nervehead with chorioretinal atrophy around the disc.

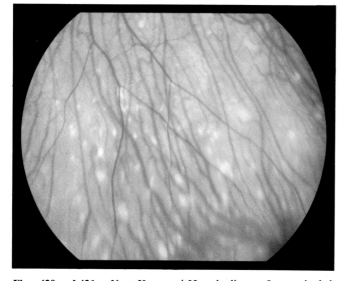

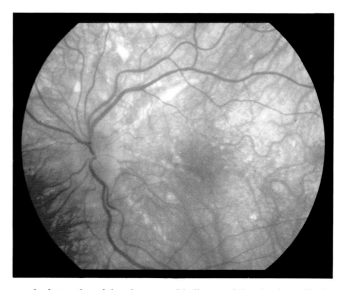

Figs. 430 and 431. Vogt-Koyanagi-Harada disease. Late retinal changes: marked atrophy of the pigment epithelium and the choriocapillaries with a characteristic "sunset glow fundus".

SERPIGINOUS OR GEOGRAPHIC CHOROIDITIS

This represents a chronic recurrent choroidopathy of unknown etiology characterized by inflammatory and atrophic changes of the choriocapillaries and pigment epithelium with involvement of the overlying external retinal layers.

It is a rare disease which is usually bilateral but may be asymmetrical; it is most often seen in patients in their fourth or fifth decade of life; there are no systemic manifestations. The process begins at the optic nervehead and then extends in a centrifugal fashion by sending out pseudopodes in all directions (helicoidal choroidopathy); the macula is involved early and progressively; the peripheral retina usually remains unaffected. The active lesions are characterized by grey edematous areas of the pigment epithelium which after weeks or months develop into serpiginous atrophic scars in which the pigment epithelium, the choriocapillaries and also the large choroidal vessels have been destroyed.

The diagnosis can usually be made when the lesions are involving the macular and perimacular area. Characteristic are the completely inactive atrophic areas around the optic nervehead. These are irregularly pigmented and associated with areas of active edematous margins progressing toward the posterior pole; these form the characteristic geographic configuration in the ocular fundus (Figs. 432, 433). There are sometimes also retinal hemorrhages, signs of a retinal vasculitis and of an anterior uveitis.

Fluorescein angiography shows the unmistakable primary involvement of the choriocapillaries and of the retinal pigment epithelium.

The pathogenesis of these chorioretinal lesions is still being debated, but the hypothesis of a viral infection seems more probable than assuming a vascular or degenerative etiology.

The prognosis for vision is not good because central vision will frequently be lost and occurs often early, at least in one eye. The slow and progressive natural history of this disease may arrest spontaneously after many months or years.

The efficacy of corticosteroid treatment is dubious, but the systemic and periocular application of such steroids seem to be indicated during the active phase.

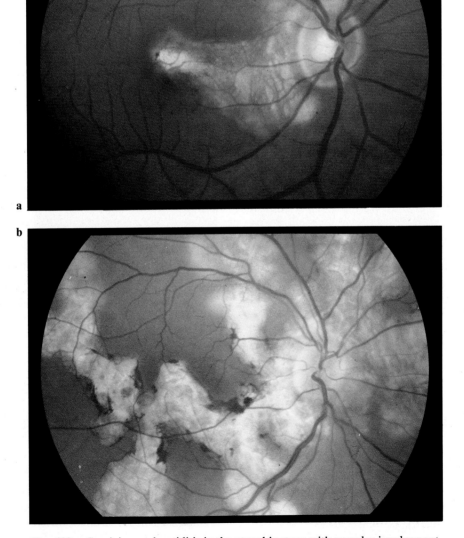

Fig. 432.   Serpiginous choroiditis in the atrophic stage with macular involvement.
a) The lesions involves the posterior pole.
b) The chorioretinal atrophy seems to be more extensive and in a more advanced stage.

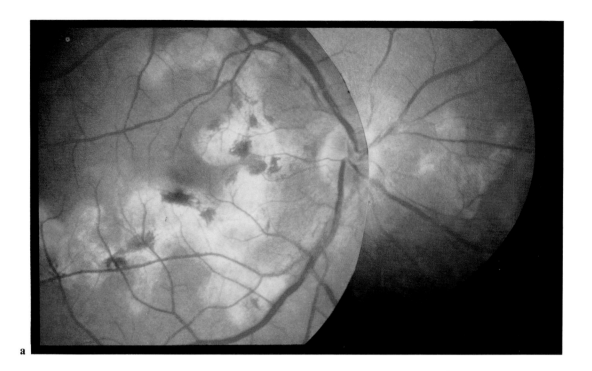

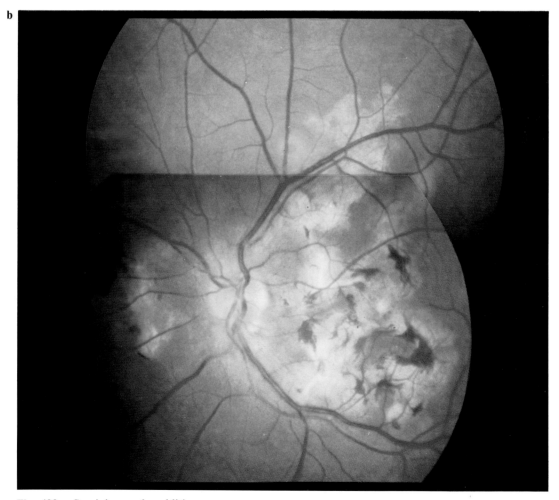

Fig. 433. Serpiginous choroiditis.
a) Right eye: atrophic and unevenly pigmented chorioretinal lesions extending from the optic nervehead to the macula; the margins around the macula are still edematous; signs of perivasculitis.
b) Left eye: atrophic, unevenly pigmented chorioretinal lesions, more extensive at the posterior pole.

"BIRDSHOT" CHORIORETINOPATHY

This condition was described in 1980 by Ryan and Maumenee (also referred to as vitiliginous choroiditis). It is a rare inflammatory (or pseudoinflammatory) bilateral disease which affects both sexes in middle age. It is characterized by:

— mild signs of an anterior uveitis with vitreous involvement which is sometimes marked, but without preretinal snow bank exudates or a cyclitic membrane;
— changes in the permeability of retinal vessels with subsequent retinal, macular and disc edema;
— multiple depigmented spots of the choriocapillaries and pigment epithelium.

These small cream colored foci (Fig. 434) are initially not conspicuous and are only seen by careful indirect ophthalmoscopic examination or on fluorescein angiograms; these foci evolve slowly (over ten years); they increase in number and extend from the posterior pole toward the periphery without becoming pigmented or acquiring the characteristic feature of histo-spots.

The prognosis as far as vision is concerned is poor because the vascular lesions and subsequent cystoid macular edema with optic atrophy will progress.

The etiology is completely unknown; a viral infection has been assumed.

The differential diagnosis encompasses acute posterior multifocal placoid pigment-epitheliopathy, serpiginous choroiditis and Vogt-Koyanagi-Harada disease.

Because of the inflammatory character and the progressive cystoid macular edema systemic and periocular corticosteroid treatment in high dosage are indicated even though the results may be unsatisfactory and sometimes zero.

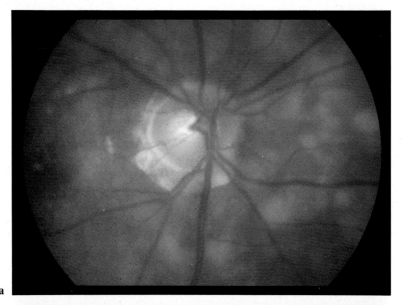

a

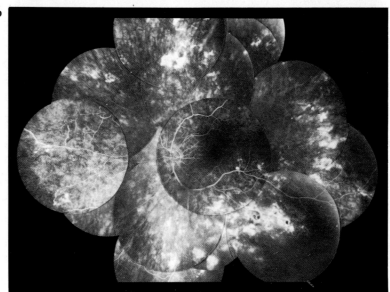

b

Fig. 434. Birdshot chorioretinopathy. Pallor of the optic nervehead; numerous small cream-colored coalescing spots at the posterior pole **(a)** and in the periphery (collage of fluorescein angiograms) **(b)**.

Chapter 8

Diseases of the choroid

CHOROIDAL DEGENERATIONS

Hereditary choroidal degenerations constitute an important group among choroidal diseases.

They include the excrescences (drusen) of Bruch's membrane, the colloid degeneration, angioid streaks, choroidal sclerosis, choroideremia, gyrate atrophy, and the pseudo-inflammatory dystrophy of Sorsby. The first two conditions have already been discussed in other chapters (see Chapters 2 and 6).

ANGIOID STREAKS

The ophthalmoscopic findings justify the term. The streaks which extend from the optic nervehead and anastomose with each other resemble the vascular tree.

In reality we are here dealing with a degeneration of the elastic part of Bruch's membrane involving often men after the fourth decade of life. The condition is transmitted as a recessive or incomplete dominant factor.

The angioid streaks may be isolated phenomena, but are more often an expression of a pathologic process in the elastic tissue in general (essential or hereditary elastosis). The streaks can be found in the Grönblad-Strandberg syndrome associated with pseudoxanthoma elasticum of Darier, in Ehlers-Danlos disease, in systemic elastorrhexis of Touraine, in osteitis deformans of Paget, and finally in sickle cell disease.

The condition usually occurs in adults; the ocular lesions are usually bilateral and asymptomatic until they involve the macula.

On ophthalmoscopic examination the streaks appear like a series of undulating lines of various diameter, usually not larger than a blood vessel; the borders are sharp and irregular; they course in a curved manner beneath the retinal vessels and above the choroidal vasculature.

They anastomose with each other forming a kind of ring around the disc. They extend toward the equator tapering off toward the periphery without branching; sometimes they end abruptly. They are red-brown or slategrey in color and are often lined by pigment (lacquer cracks); they are better visible with red-free illumination (Figs. 435-437).

In the advanced stages we see degenerative lesions at the posterior pole, usually preceded by retinal hemorrhages. These changes are characterized by tufts and plaques of scar tissue, deposition of coarse pigment clumps which makes the fundus look like an orange peel. There are zones of atrophy and sclerosis of the choroid and finally a disciform macular degeneration (Figs. 436-438); (see Chapter 6 the degenerative maculopathies).

Histologically we find breaks and gaps in the elastic part of Bruch's membrane. The membrane becomes basophilic and sometimes calcified. There is a glial reaction with fibrovascular proliferation from the choroid. The choroidal vessels become sclerotic and thickened (choroidal elastosis). On fluorescein angiography these lesions show hyperfluorescence.

Angioid streaks have a tendency to progress. Initially they do not cause any functional defects (sometimes it is difficult to establish exactly the onset of the lesions); later they produce a progressive and severe disturbance of visual acuity, mainly due to the hemorrhages and retinal exudates which are found in 50-78% of the patients in the macula; finally there is a central areolar choroidal atrophy.

The long-term prognosis for vision is not good because no mode of therapy, including attempts of photocoagulation with argon laser, will arrest the progress of the condition.

CHOROIDAL SCLEROSIS

This may either be a primary condition transmitted as a recessive autosomal Mendelian factor or may be secondary to other diseases (colloid degeneration, Stargardt disease, etc.) (see Chapter 6). It may be limited to the posterior pole or involve the entire fundus.

In the central form the ophthalmoscopic examination shows an areolar atrophic zone through which the choroidal vessels are seen as white structures, apparently sclerotic. Two stages can be differentiated angiographically: atrophy of the pigment epithelium with a window effect of the underlying fluorescence and a stage of atrophy of the choriocapillaries where only the large choroidal vessels are visible and blood filled. Central vision is affected.

In the generalized form we see diffuse atrophy of the choriocapillaries and the pigment epithelium (Fig. 439). In some areas there is an accumulation of pigment. The ERG is normal or subnormal.

CHOROIDEREMIA

This condition is characterized by an early atrophy of the choroid and slow progression; it is connected to the X chromosome and therefore affects men to a much more debilitating degree than women who are carriers.

Ophthalmoscopically we distinguish four stages which initially appear in adolescence. By the age of 40 the end stage is usually reached:

— *first stage:* zones of depigmentation alternate with pigment accumulations in the fundus periphery;
— *second stage:* the atrophy of the pigment epithelium progresses toward the posterior pole;
— *third stage:* the atrophy of the choroid is complete; only the macular area remains intact (Figs. 440 a-c);
— *fourth stage:* the choroid disappears completely.

On fluorescein angiography the choroidal circulation is slower than normal and the vessels have lost their permeability for the dye. The retinal pigment epithelium shows intensive fluorescence and the retinal circulation also appears slow.

The first functional defect is night blindness; the patients then experience progressive constriction of the visual field until they finally become blind. The central visual acuity remains preserved for a considerable period of time as the macula is affected last. The ERG remains normal for a period until it finally is extinguished.

GYRATE CHOROIDAL ATROPHY

This is a rare choroidal disease which is transmitted as an autosomal recessive. It is perhaps an expression of an inborn metabolic error (hyperornithinemia). It is characterized by areas of chorioretinal atrophy at the equator; they may coalesce extending in a helicoidal manner toward the posterior pole (Figs. 441 a-c). Ninety percent of these patients also have high myopia frequently complicated by a posterior cupuliform cataract. The visual field is irregularly constricted. ERG and EOG are affected late in the course of the disease.

PSEUDO-INFLAMMATORY DYSTROPHY OF SORSBY

This disease is transmitted as an autosomal dominant. Initially the condition appears as a chorioretinitis with macular edema and some hemorrhages.

The cicatricial stage also resembles chorioretinitis that has ended in chorioretinal atrophy with pigment accumulation.

After a variable period of time, lasting weeks or months, the other eye will also be affected in a similar manner. The functional loss is considerable.

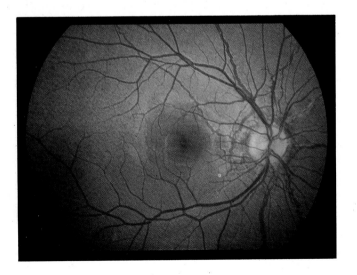

Fig. 435. Angioid streaks. The streaks seem to diverge from a peripapillary circle extending toward all quadrants of the fundus, but especially nasally.

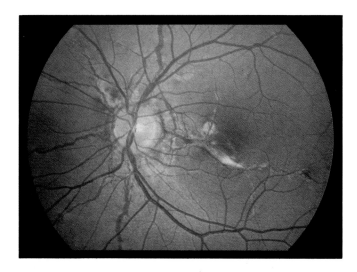

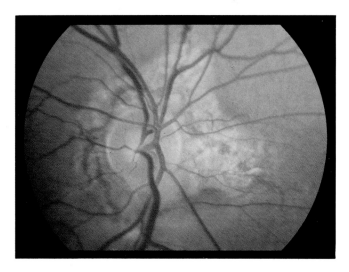

Fig. 436. Angioid streaks with a radial arrangement. The posterior pole is traversed by a large band of connective tissue with evidence of macular degeneration.

Fig. 437. Angioid streaks. Peripapillary edema more pronounced on the nasal side where there are some deep hemorrhages; conspicuous involvement and breakup of the retinal pigment epithelium.

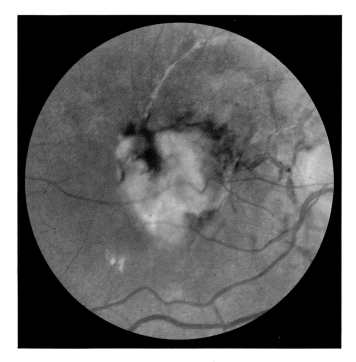

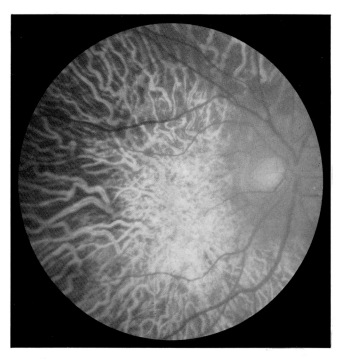

Fig. 438. Angioid streaks with disciform macular degeneration.

Fig. 439. Diffuse choroidal sclerosis. Pigment epithelium and choriocapillaries have disappeared.

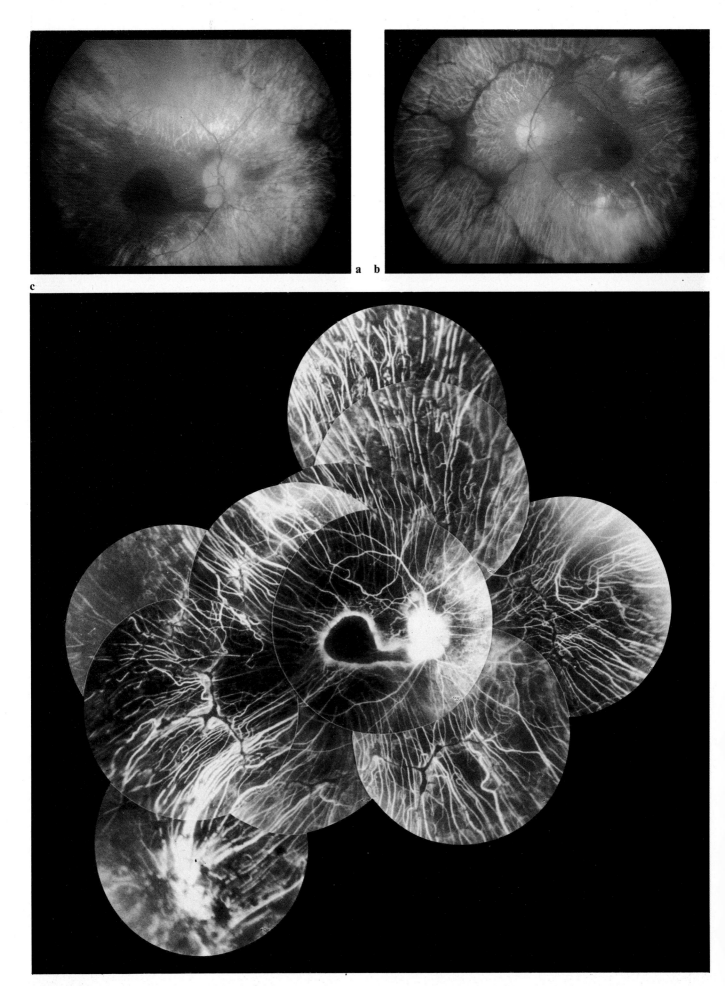

Fig. 440. Choroideremia. Nearly complete atrophy of the choroid; only the macular region is not yet affected.
a) Right eye.
b) Left eye.
c) Fluorescein angiography reveals complete lack of perfusion in the choriocapillaris.

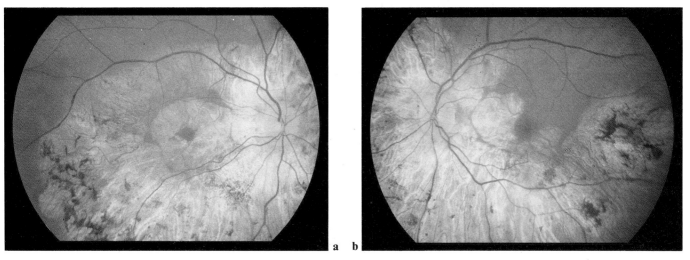

Fig. 441. Gyrate atrophy of the choroid. The areas of chorioretinal atrophy tend to coalesce toward the macular region.
a) Right eye.
b) Left eye.
c) Gyrate atrophy of choroid and retina in a patient with hyperornithinemia; the posterior pole is not involved. (*With the kind permission and cooperation of Prof. M.I. Kaiser-Kupfer*).

c

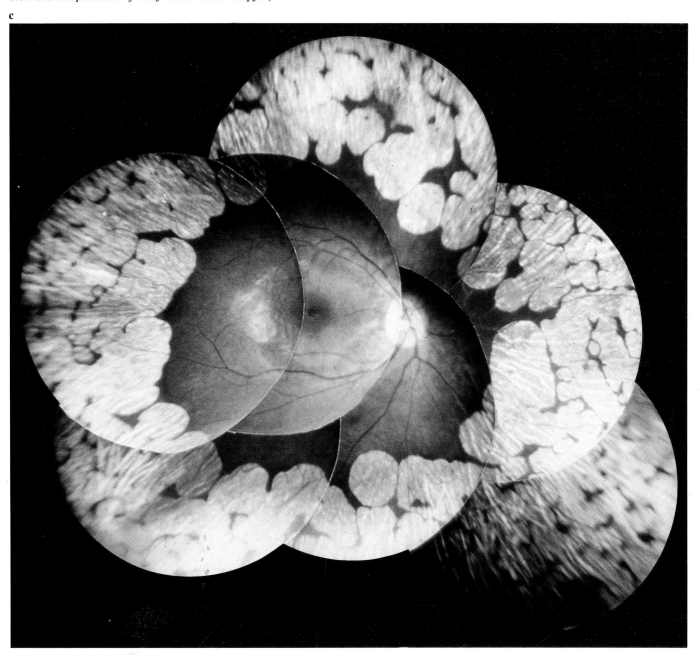

CHOROIDAL DETACHMENT

This is a serous swelling and edema of the choroid which elevates the retina toward the vitreous. This phenomenon begins in the area of the ciliary body. Because of the greater laxity of the tissues the elevation may there be bullous, whereas at the posterior pole the vascular connections between the sclera, choroid and retina keep the detachment rather flat.

Clinically we distinguish three types of choroidal detachment:

— inflammatory;
— traumatic;
— postoperative.

The **inflammatory type** is rare and includes the pseudotumoral exudative annular cyclitis, the idiopathic uveal effusion and the secondary inflammatory cilio-choroidal detachments (scleritis, iridocyclitis, chorioretinitis, sympathetic ophthalmia). With the ophthalmoscope we may be able to see the ora serrata and even ciliary processes without indenting the sclera. The cilio-choroidal detachment appears as an annular peripheral solid elevation which is grey-brown and sometimes lobulated. It may be more marked in certain areas than in others. It may be associated with a retinal detachment.

Traumatic choroidal detachment may be hemorrhagic and secondary to lesions of the large choroidal vessels or of the posterior ciliary arteries.

The most frequent type is the **postoperative form** which constitutes a complication of an intraocular operation and most frequently is seen after a cataract extraction, but may also develop after an antiglaucomatous procedure, retinal detachment operation, etc. In these cases the choroidal detachment is due to a transudate which forms secondary to the hypotony of the globe.

With the ophthalmoscope we see in the periphery greyish elevated areas which are more or less extensive and coalesce to form a ring shaped elevation in the ciliary area (Figs. 442-444). The choroidal detachment causes in these cases myopia (up to three-quarters of a diopter) because of the relaxation of the zonular fibers produced by the protrusion of the ciliary body. The functional deficit depends upon the extent and location of the detachment; the recovery depends upon the duration of the detachment.

A choroidal detachment can be suspected clinically when after a surgical intervention there is a shallowing of the anterior chamber, marked hypotony, a fistulating bleb (positive Seidel test), and persistent inflammatory signs. The treatment consists of bed rest, instillation of antiinflammatory medications and mydriasis. This will usually be successful. In some cases it is necessary to close the fistulating bleb surgically.

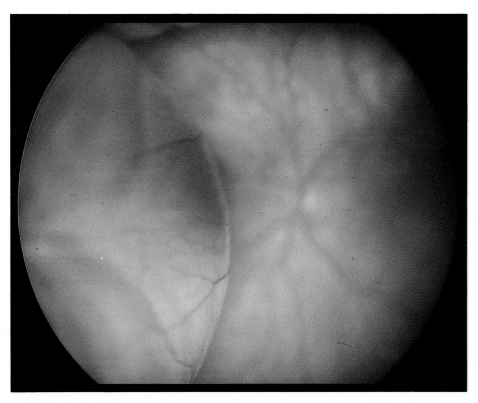

Fig. 442. Choroidal detachment secondary to an operation for a retinal detachment. The elevation is spherical and has a greyish color.

Fig. 443. Choroidal detachment secondary to laser photocoagulation in a patient with diabetic retinopathy.

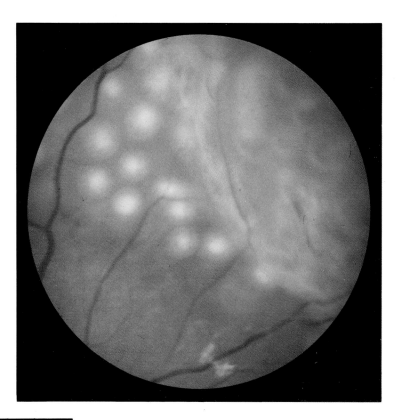

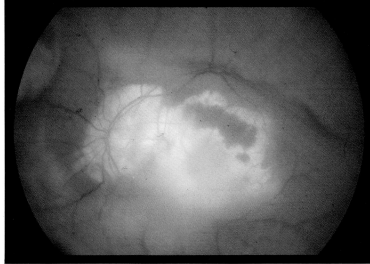

Fig. 444. Hemorrhagic choroidal detachment in a myopic and aphakic eye which had previously an operation for retinal detachment.

OCCLUSIONS OF THE POSTERIOR CILIARY ARTERIES: THE TRIANGULAR SYNDROME

Occlusions of the ciliary arteries may be due to trauma, inflammation, or vascular disease. They produce an ischemia of the retinal pigment epithelium and of the outer retinal layers. In the acute phase we see an ischemic edema of the external retina with an exudative retinal detachment which may be associated with a choroidal detachment.

In the more advanced cases there may be a permanent pigmentary rearrangement of the involved chorioretinal area (Fig. 445). This area is triangular in shape with the base toward the periphery. It corresponds to the area irrigated by the affected ciliary artery; the affected area may be extensive, if several or numerous ciliary arteries are involved (Fig. 446). During the early phase of fluorescein angiography we see an area of choroidal hypofluorescence which diminishes slowly as the entire choriocapillaries is filled; in the late phases the center of the triangle remains hypofluorescent whereas a certain diffusion of the dye can be noted at the margins of the lesion.

On perimetry we see a sector-like deficit corresponding to the chorioretinal scar.

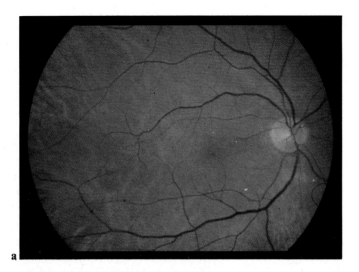

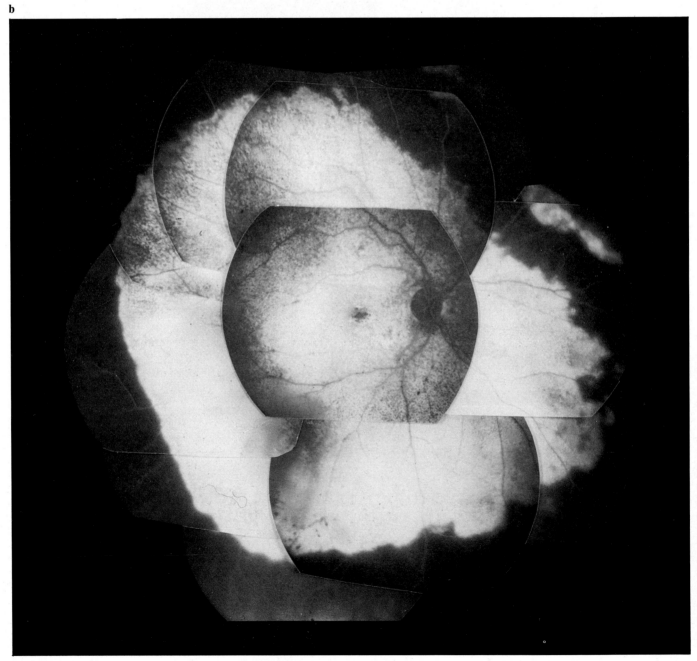

Fig. 445. Occlusion of the short posterior ciliary arteries after an operation for retinal detachment. The ophthalmoscopic picture (**a**) shows only a slight retinal pallor, whereas the fluorescein angiograms (**b**) reveal a marked alteration of the retinal pigment epithelium secondary to an occlusive accident.

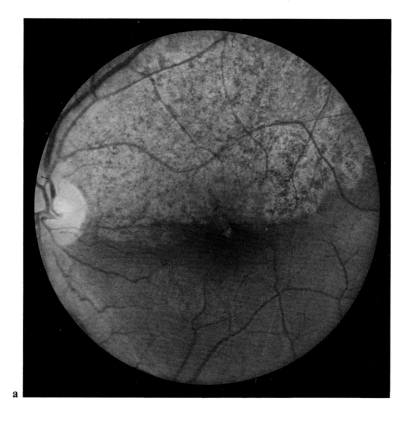

a

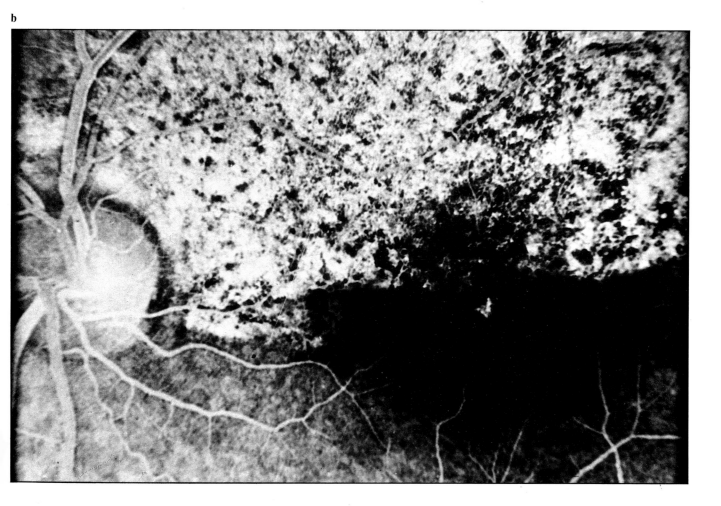

b

Fig. 446. End stage of a post-traumatic triangular syndrome.
a) Diffuse alteration of the retinal pigment epithelium.
b) The fluorescein angiogram shows much better the clear cut demarcation between healthy tissue and the area of occluded choriocapillaris.

Chapter 9

Diseases of the vitreous

ASTEROID HYALOSIS

In this condition we find numerous dot-like shiny opacities in the vitreous. These are either round or elongated and move within the framework of the vitreous together with the eye (Fig. 447). We distinguish an idiopathic form which is usually associated with advanced age, from a secondary form following trauma, inflammation, etc. The opacities are calcium salts of various lipids; the cause or their formation is unknown.

Usually vision remains unaffected though occasionally the patient may see floaters.

SYNCHISIS SCINTILLANS

In this condition the vitreous is liquified causing complete dyseresis. The condition is best appreciated with the slit lamp where we see optically empty vacuoles in the vitreous space together with punctiform or filamentous condensations. There may be many cholesterol deposits appearing as shiny crystals.

The deposits will be stirred up when the eye is moved and then sink down again. There is a complete posterior vitreous detachment, usually a spontaneous one. This type of synchisis may follow degenerative diseases (amyloidosis, senescence, myopia, Wagner disease, Marfan syndrome, retinopathy of prematurity), inflammatory (endophthalmitis, uveitis, parasitosis) (Fig. 448), hemorrhagic (trauma, diabetic retinopathy, retinal vasculitis, venous occlusion, sickle cell anemia, etc.) or neoplastic conditions. Visual acuity is not involved except in cases with particularly conspicuous condensations, but these are rare. The patient may notice superficial bright floaters.

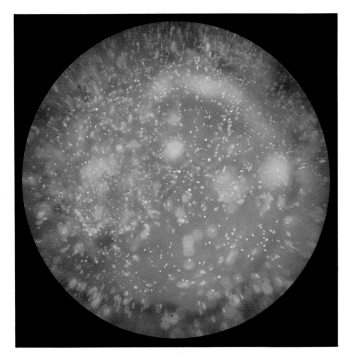

Fig. 447. Asteroid hyalosis.

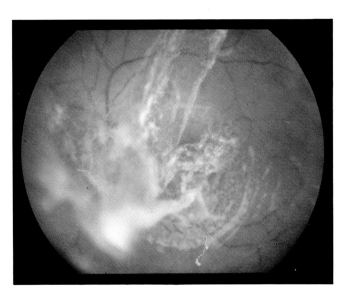

Fig. 448. Synchisis scintillans secondary to an inflammatory process in the vitreous.

Chapter 10

Tumors

RETINAL TUMORS

Primary retinal tumors occur nearly exclusively in children and infants. These tumors are congenital and hereditary; others may be associated with local or systemic pathologic changes.

Table 8.   Classification of retinal tumors.

Neuroectodermal neoplasms	Retinoblastoma Astrocytoma Glioneuroma Medulloepithelioma (or diktyoma)
Neoplasms of the ciliary epithelium	Pseudoadenomatous hyperplasia Adenoma Adenocarcinoma
Secondary neoplasms	Metastatic tumors Leukemia Lymphoma
Hamartomas (including the phakomatoses)	Angiomatosis (von Hippel Lindau, Coats disease) Neurogliomatosis (tuberous sclerosis, systemic neurofibromatosis)

NEUROECTODERMAL TUMORS

Retinoblastoma

This is the most frequent primary retinal tumor (80% of all retinal tumors) and represents one of the most frequent infantile neoplasms (one case per 25,000 live births).

About 25% of the cases are bilateral and familial. Spontaneous regression is the exception. The first diagnosis is usually made between the ages of 12-24 months in the hereditary and between 24-30 months in the sporadic form.

The tumor originates from immature retinal elements which may be present in the different stages of differentiation and which correspond to a different morphologic aspect. On macroscopic examination of a sectioned globe we see a white or yellow-red mass which is viscous, of irregular shape and friable. There are two types of growth: in the *exophytic type* the growth is directed toward the choroid and we therefore see ophthalmoscopically a solid retinal detachment; in the *endophytic type* the tumor grows toward the vitreous where it acquires the typical cauliflower shape. Frequently both types of growth are combined, but only rarely do we see only an infiltration of the retina. In general the tumor is located at the posterior pole but may occur in the far periphery and several independent tumor foci may exist.

The endophytic type can easily be seen clinically. We see in the vitreous a single lesion or, more rarely, multiple foci of a whitepink mass indented by normal retinal vessels which follow the convexity of the elevation; in addition there are new-formed vessels (Fig. 449). The neoplasm frequently occupies 1/4-1/2 of the vitreous cavity. The surface is usually irregular and lobulated; within the mass there may be zones of necrosis and calcification, the latter appear as brilliant white deposits. The exophytic type and late stages of the tumor will show vitreous hemorrhages and a secondary retinal detachment obscuring direct visualization of the neoplasm.

From a histopathological point of view we distinguish an undifferentiated from a differentiated form. The former consists of highly immature cells which hardly resemble the embryonal retinal cells from which they derive. They are arranged in a completely irregular pattern. The cell nuclei are large and hyperchromatic, situated at the base of the cell with dense chromatin, scarce cytoplasm, and frequent mitotic figures (Fig. 450). The differentiated form consists of more mature cells which frequently have a tendency to form rosettes or fleurettes (Fig. 451). These cells are cylindrical and arrange themselves around an empty lumen which is delineated by a membrane (Fig. 452). These tumors are usually well vascularized with areas of necrosis and calcification; the latter are nearly pathognomonic for retinoblastoma and important for establishing the diagnosis. With electron microscopy we see subcellular structures resembling those of retinal photoreceptors in a human fetus.

The tumor cells first invade into the vitreous and the aqueous humor. In a second stage when the choroid has been infiltrated they reach the systemic blood circulation. An infiltration of the optic nerve (Fig. 453) worsens the prognosis for survival down to 36% compared to 90% in cases in which the nerve is not involved. The tumor may also invade into the subarachnoidal space across the optic nerve and the cribriform plate. Metastases are most often seen in the central nervous system, the vertebral column, bones and lymphnodes. In addition the orbit may be involved directly.

The clinical course of retinoblastoma can be divided into four stages:

— *the early stage is asymptomatic* (but the diagnosis can be made with the ophthalmoscope);
— *in the next stage clinical signs appear*, e.g., a white pupillary reflex (leukokoria) or, if the tumor involves the macula, esotropia may develop;
— *the inflammatory* or *glaucomatous stage* in which there may be a secondary glaucoma with buphthalmus, mydriasis of the affected pupil, color changes of the iris due to neovascularization and tumor necrosis;
— *extraocular extension and hematogenous distant metastases.*

Early diagnosis is extremely important in order to initiate the appropriate therapy. In addition to ophthalmoscopy which assumes a pivotal importance, we may need transillumination, echography, xray pictures of the cranium and the orbits, CT scan and the concentration of lactic dehydrogenase in the aqueous, which may be elevated in eyes affected with retinoblastoma. A cytologic examination of the aqueous humor may confirm the presence of malignant cells in the anterior chamber. The diagnosis can also be confirmed by the P_{32} test. These tumors always show an increased uptake of radioactive phosphorus. An accurate evaluation of all these tests is necessary to differentiate this neoplasm from other diseases causing leukokoria (pseudoglioma), e.g., persistence and hyperplasia of the primary vitreous, retinopathy of prematurity, etc.

In general it is necessary to enucleate the affected eye. A long stump of the optic nerve should be excised at the same time. Small tumors (less than 1/4 of a disc diameter) and the less affected eye in bilateral cases may be treated with cryotherapy and/or photocoagulation and/or radiation therapy. Radiotherapy and chemotherapy, in addition to enucleation, are indicated when metastases are suspected, in advanced stages of the tumor or when there is extraocular extension.

The **prognosis** depends upon the local extent of the tumor, the degree of infiltration, the presence of metastases and of extraorbital extension.

Patients undergoing enucleation have a 95% chance of a five year survival if the tumor is a single lesion, well delineated and not infiltrating deeper structures; the survival rate is only 30% in patients with orbital involvement and there is nearly 100% mortality (and the survival is less than one year) in cases of metastases.

Astrocytoma

This is a rare tumor mostly seen in children; it is clinically indistinguishable from a retinoblastoma though in contrast to this neoplasma an astrocytoma may be observed in a microphthalmic eye. It is always a unilateral lesion.

Ophthalmoscopically the tumor appears as a white mass with elevated margins, richly vascularized, sometimes surrounded by retinal edema. It usually is located at the temporal disc margin; its size may reach or exceed one disc diameter. Histologically it resembles cerebellar tumors of the same type; according to the degree of cellular differentiation we distinguish four grades of astrocytoma:

— *Grade I:* small round cells disseminated in a dense fibrillar network with few vessels; there is a tendency for spontaneous regression and pseudocysts may form;
— *Grade II:* spindle shaped cells arranged around blood vessels forming pseudo-rosettes (astroblastoma);
— *Grade III:* the cells elongate and have a tendency for palisading (polar spongioblastoma);
— *Grade IV:* glioblastoma multiforme, with polymorphic, sometimes multi-nucleated cells and areas of necrosis and thrombosis within the lesion.

Glioneuroma

This is a rare congenital tumor often associated with other ocular anomalies, e.g., choroidal coloboma and persistence and hyperplasia of the primary vitreous. A frequent clinical sign is increase in intraocular pressure due to tumor infiltration of the chamber angle.

Histologically this lesion consists of mature cerebral tissue and is composed of glial and neural cells in the ciliary epithelium.

With the ophthalmoscope and the slit lamp the tumor appears as a white mass which often involves the adjacent iris stroma and may extend to the equator. Endophytic growth of the tumor may cause a dislocation of the crystalline lens in the opposite direction. The lens may also become cataractous.

Medulloepithelioma

This is an embryonal tumor localized in the non-pigmented ciliary epithelium. With the ophthalmoscope and the slit lamp it appears as a mass of varying size, grey-pink in color with some dark areas; it is little elevated and grows on the surface of the ciliary body with a tendency to infiltrate the iris stroma. More rarely it extends toward the vitreous cavity and into the retina reaching even the optic nerve. Histologically we see a polymorphic structure in which the stromal and epithelial elements form a network (therefore the old term "diktyoma"): the cells are small with a large nucleus and sparse cytoplasm. They have a tendency to form cystic cavities and rest on a basement membrane. The stroma is rich in acid mucopolysaccharides. In the teratoid form we find heteroplastic foci (cartilage, bone, striated muscle, glia and mesenchymal structures).

This tumor has a relatively good prognosis and is only moderately invasive; metastases are rare. A frequent complication is secondary glaucoma due to tumor invasion of the trabecular meshwork.

NEOPLASMS OF THE CILIARY EPITHELIUM

Pseudoadenomatous Hyperplasia (Fuchs Adenoma)

This is a senile lesion or may occur secondary to trauma or inflammation. It presents as a roundish tumor mass, white-grey in color and localized at the ciliary body. The size of the tumor may vary from small nodules to large masses which involve the iris and may invade the vitreous cavity (Fig. 454). Histologically the lesion consists of hyperplastic epithelial cells, which are amelanotic in small lesions, but may be pigmented in the more voluminous tumefactions (Fig. 455). The pseudoadenomatous proliferation may give rise to a large pigmented plaque.

Adenoma

This tumor stems from the non-pigmented epithelium of the ciliary processes. Its structure resembles a gland. It is formed of cords and strands in which an eosinophilic mucoid material is deposited. The material is probably produced by the epithelial cells. In general the lesion is not capsulated. On slit lamp examination it appears as a pigmented small mass, round in shape and localized at the ciliary processes.

Adenocarcinoma

This is rarely a spontaneous, more often a secondary lesion following chronic localized inflammations. It shows alveolar arrangement of the cells depending upon the degree of differentiation and of cellular proliferation. These are epithelial cuboidal cells surrounding a cavity which may be empty or contain pigment granules or an eosinophilic material. The prognosis depends upon the degree of cellular differentiation.

These three types of epithelial neoplasms have to be differentiated from a melanoma of the ciliary body.

SECONDARY NEOPLASM

Metastatic tumors to the retina are extremely rare; this may be due to the acute angle of the origin of the central retinal artery from the ophthalmic artery. The retina is more often involved in systemic lymphoma and leukemia (acute lymphoid and monocytic leukemia). In these cases we find ophthalmoscopically hemmorhages of varying size, often with a white fluffy center. The retinal veins are dilated and tortuous. If there is a leukemic intracranial infiltration a disc edema, especially in children, may appear (see Chapter 6).

Angiomatosis retinae and **neurofibromatosis** are discussed in Chapter 6, the Congenital retinopathies on page 149 and following.

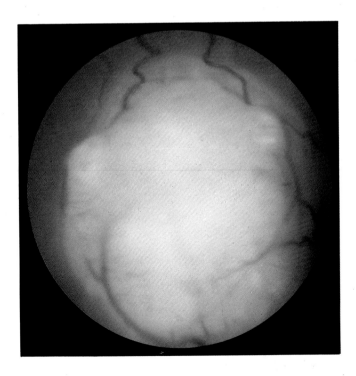

Fig. 449. Retinoblastoma. Large white mass protruding into the vitreous space. There is no red reflex in that area and the normal morphology of the retina has been lost.

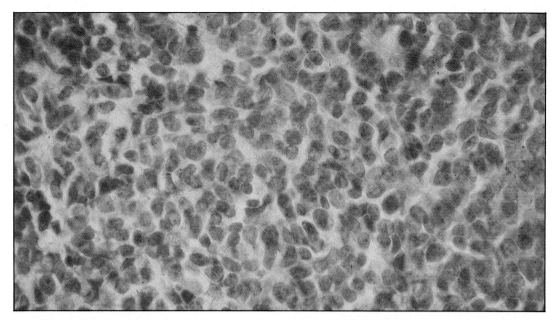

Fig. 450. Undifferentiated retinoblastoma (histologic section). Absence of any characteristic structures.

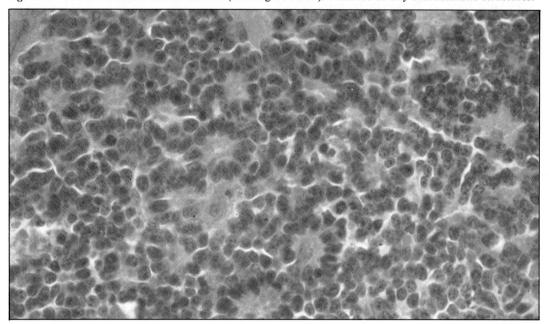

Fig. 451. Well differentiated retinoblastoma (histologic specimen). Numerous rosettes and feurettes.

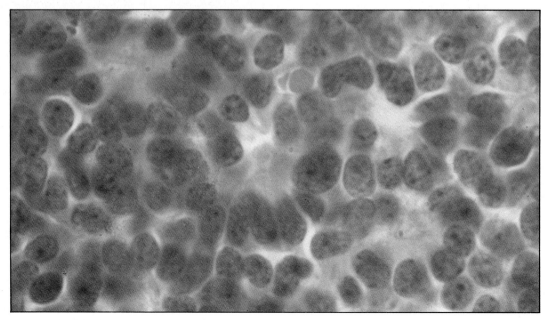

Fig. 452. Retinoblastoma (histologic section). Detail from Fig. 451 in higher magnification.

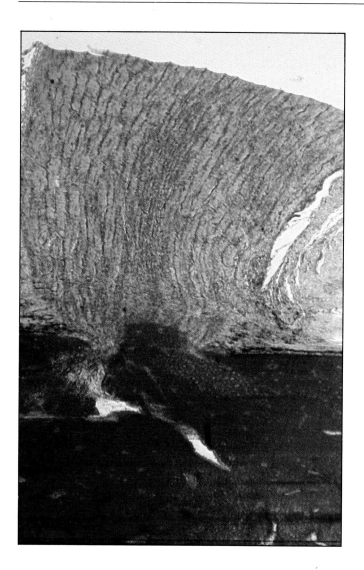

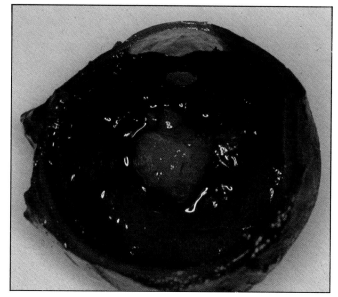

Fig. 453. Retinoblastoma (histologic section). Infiltration of the optic nerve.

Fig. 454. Pseudoadenomatous hyperplasia of the ciliary epithelium (cross section of the globe). The large round retrolenticular tissue mass is well visible.

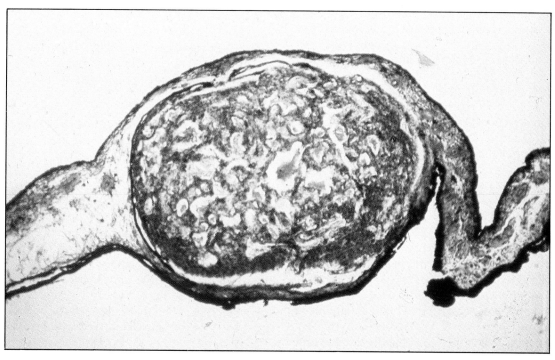

Fig. 455. Pseudoadenomatous hyperplasia of the ciliary epithelium (histologic section). Cords of pigmented and non-pigmented cells delineating pseudoadenomatous acini which contain amorphous material.

CHOROIDAL TUMORS

Choroidal tumors encompass numerous neoplams of various derivations which may involve predominantly the anterior or the posterior choroid, or both.

Table 9.   Classification of choroidal tumors.

Pigmented tumors	Melanocytosis oculi Localized hyperpigmentation Nevus Melanocytoma (magnocellular nevus) Melanoma
Vascular tumors	Hemangioma Hemangioendothelioma
Epithelial tumors	Epithelial cysts Pseudoadenomatous hyperplasia Adenoma Adenocarcinoma Medulloepithelioma (diktyoma)
Myogenic tumors	Leiomyoma Leiomyosarcoma
Neurogenic tumors	Neurofibroma Schwannoma (neurilemmoma)
Lymphoma	Benign Malignant
Leukemia	
Metastatic tumors	

PIGMENTED TUMORS

Melanocytosis Oculi, Hyperpigmentation, Nevi, Melanocytoma

These lesions are derived from the neural crest but originate in stromal melanocytes and in Schwann cells. They are benign lesions and encompass a gamut of alterations with varying degree of differentiation. They are congenital, but may only become apparent during puberty or pregnancy. The cells in melanocytosis and in hyperpigmentation are morphologically similar to normal uveal melanocytes. Nevi, on the other, hand show changes in the form and volume of the cells. Three types of cells can be observed: polyhedric, fusiform and dendritic cells. It has not been definitely established how often these lesions become malignant. That this does occur is supported by the fact that nevi are more frequently seen in eyes with a melanoma, that in about 70% of the melanomas we find nevus cells at the margin and nevi and melanomas share the same predilection for certain sites.

In *melanosis* there is a generalized *excessive pigmentation* of ocular tissues; in segmental hyperpigmentations these changes are localized.

The *nevi* appear as brown or greyish areas, have a smooth surface and sharp margins, and may vary in size from one to several disc diameters. They are usually located posterior to the equator. They are slightly elevated and above them the retinal vessels take a normal course (Figs. 456-462).

Melanocytomas are usually found in the optic nervehead and are only rarely seen in the uvea, where they usually involve the iris.

Melanoma

This is the most frequent malignant intraocular tumor in caucasians (71% of all malignat choroidal tumors); it affects both sexes and is most often encountered between the ages of 50 and 60. Bilateral cases are extremely rare and familial incidence is also unusual.

There are two hypotheses on the histogenesis of melanoma: the first one assumes a malignant degeneration of a nevus. Indeed we find in 70% of these tumors nevus cells in or around the melanoma. The second hypothesis assumes that these cells derive from Schwann cells, which also come from the neural crest.

Nearly 93% of uveal melanomas occur in the choroid, 4% in the ciliary body and 3 in the iris.

Ophthalmoscopically we see a brown, elevated, vascularized mass covered by the usually degenerated retina.

In the initial stages the lesion may be indistinguishable from a choroidal nevus. Some aspects, however, may allow a differential diagnosis: a nevus has usually a smooth surface, uniform color and sharp margins; a melanoma often has a corrugated surface, an uneven color because of new-formed blood vessels, hemorrhages and/or macroaneurysms; its margins are often blurred. Eventually the melanoma will grow in all directions and may break through Bruch's membrane. It then assumes the typical mushroom shape, growing into the vitreous and causing a progressive solid retinal detachment which may also have a serous component (Figs. 463-470). The ophthalmoscopic examination may be difficult because of opacities in the media or because of a vitreous hemorrhage which occurs mainly in the late stages. The symptoms vary. We usually assume four stages of development: asymptomatic (from one to several years), secondary glaucoma, extraocular extension and metastases.

Histologically these tumors show an extremely variable picture; the classification takes into consideration the morphologic aspects of the tumor cells which are important for the prognosis.

We distinguish four cells types:

— *Spindle cell A* (the spindle cell type A is the predominant cell), slender spindle shaped cell with a small nucleus. There is no nucleolus and often no melanin pigment (Fig. 471). This is the least malignant type with a mortality of 5% after 15 years.
— *Spindle cell B* (the spindle cell type B is the predominant cell) is more frequently seen than the first type; the cells are larger, the nuclei voluminous and a nucleolus is present (Fig. 472); there is a 25% mortality after 15 years.
— *Mixed type, grade I* (the spindle cell type B is the predominant component), this represents more than

half of all cases of choroidal melanoma and has a mortality of 30-60% after 15 years (Fig. 473).
— *Mixed cell type, grade II* (the epithelioid cell is the predominant cell), consists mainly of large round cells of varying size with a voluminous nucleus and conspicuous nucleolus; mitotic figures are frequent and there are areas of necrosis and hemorrhage; this is the most malignant type with a mortality of 60-70% after 15 years.

In addition to the cell type other prognostic factors are the volume of the neoplasm, the presence of stromal tissue, especially of reticulum fibers, which is higher in the more benign lesions, and the degree of pigmentation which increases with malignancy. The same applies for necrotic areas. Factors which worsen the prognosis are obviously the infiltration of adjacent structures, a break through Bruch's membrane, or an invasion of the sclera. Metastases occur via the blood stream, but may remain latent for a long time due to immunologic inhibition. The most frequently affected organs are: liver, lungs, brain and G.I. tract. In the more advanced stages the melanoma may be complicated by uveitis, serous retinal detachment, macular hole, rubeosis iridis or secondary glaucoma.
The diagnosis can be corroborated by transillumination, echography, fluorescein angiography, the P_{32} test and a cytologic examination of the aqueous humor.
A small circumscribed tumor (not larger than 10 mm in diameter) can be treated by photocoagulation (Fig. 465), various radiation treatments or by a segmental surgical excision; larger tumors require an enucleation. If there is an extraocular extension exenteration of the orbit will be necessary. Chemotherapy may be given before or after the surgical procedure, alone or combined with radiation therapy.

VASCULAR TUMORS

Hemangioma

This is the only intraocular tumor which is certainly not of neuroectodermal origin. It could be classified as hamartoma and often is part of a more widespread syndrome, e.g., Sturge-Weber or Von Hippel-Lindau (page 150). The tumor is usually found close to the optic nervehead on the temporal side where it produces a retinal elevation.
Ophthalmoscopically it appears as a solid yellowish mass, slightly pigmented and elevated; the margins are usually sharply outlined and hyperpigmented. There are often changes in the pigment epithelium which will later becomes atrophic; in some cases there may be a cystoid retinal degeneration with gliosis.
Histologically we find a thickening of the choroid with blood spaces lined by a tenuous layer of endothelium (Fig. 474). The tumor does not have a capsule and Bruch's membrane is intact. The tumor may cause secondary glaucoma, which may be due to associated congenital malformation in the chamber angle, the increase in intraocular volume, compression of the vorticose veins and the venous drainage of the ciliary body, decrease in choroidal circulation due

to the increased number of choroidal vessels. In the Sturge-Weber syndrome there is an associated cutaneous hemangioma corresponding to the distribution of a branch of the trigeminal nerve, a meningeal hemangioma and an episcleral hemangioma which increases the pressure in the episcleral veins.

Hemangioendothelioma

This is a rare tumor which occurs in newborn and produces a retinal detachment. It is usually benign like the hemangioendothelioma of the lids in infants. Ophthalmoscopically we see a secondary non-characteristic retinal detachment.

MYOGENIC AND NEURAL TUMORS

Leiomyoma

This is a benign tumor which may come from the sphincter muscle of the pupil or from the ciliary muscle. It may be confused with a nonpigmented melanoma because the leiomyoma appears as a red-brown nodule, richly vascularized at the pupillary margin or over the ciliary body.
The histologic picture shows amelanotic spindle cells arranged in fascicles. The ciliary leiomyomas are rare and so are tumors from the smooth muscles of the choroidal vessels.
Ophthalmoscopically the lesion has to be differentiated from a melanoma.

Leiomyosarcoma

This lesion differs from the leiomyoma mainly by a different clinical course (tendency to invade, recur, etc.).

Neurilemmoma

This may be an isolated nodule in the iris or ciliary body, or may diffusely involve the entire choroid. It may be associated with neurofibromatosis (page 149). It is often indistinguishable from a leiomyoma; it has a similar morphologic structure, both macro- and micro-scopically.

LYMPHOMA AND LEUKEMIA

The uvea is frequently involved in systemic *lymphomas*. It may be either a nodular lesion or, more often, a diffuse infiltration (Fig. 475). The benign lymphoid hyperplasia contains numerous mature lymphoid cells. The malignant non-Hodgkin lymphomas can be divided according to increasing malignancy into the well differentiated to the poorly differentiated, into stem cell or histiocytic lymphoma.
In *leukemia* the choroid is the most frequently affected intraocular structure, especially in acute lymphoid leukemia of childhood. The ocular fundus appears colorless and grey, with multiple disseminated exudates of the "cotton-wool

patch'' type. The retina may undergo hemorrhagic necrosis (see Chapter 6).

METASTATIC TUMORS

These are usually found at the posterior pole, in the paramacular area and occur more often in the left than in the right eye. The most frequent primary tumor are cancer of the breast, the lungs, and the G.I. tract. The tumor cells reach the choroid via the short posterior ciliary arteries. Ophthalmoscopically the lesions appear opaque, yellow with more or less well defined margins of varying size, round and elevated (Figs. 476 a,b). There may be a single focus or numerous lesions. The tumors may cause a flat retinal detachment. The differential diagnosis from a choroidal melanoma may be clinically difficult, especially in the 20-30% of the cases in which there are no clinical signs of a primary tumor.

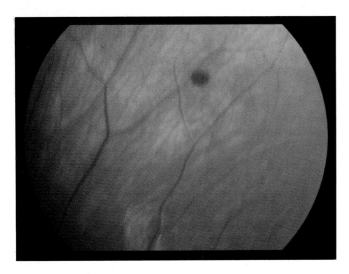

Fig. 456.   Small peripheral choroidal nevus.

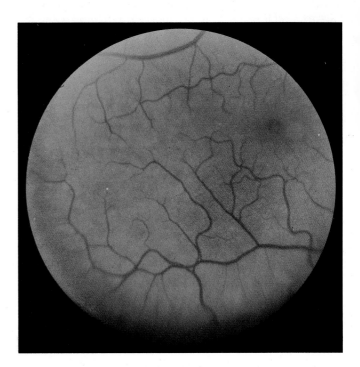

Fig. 457.   Slightly pigmented choroidal nevus at the posterior pole.

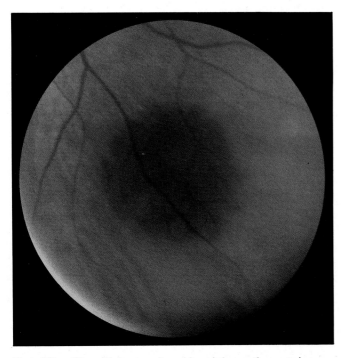

Fig. 458.   Choroidal nevus in mid-periphery; the margins are slightly blurred.

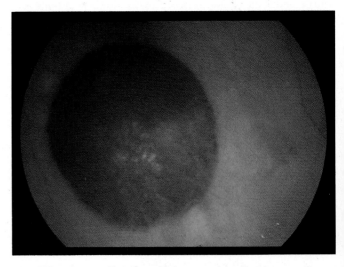

Fig. 459.   Large, flat choroidal nevus, heavily pigmented.

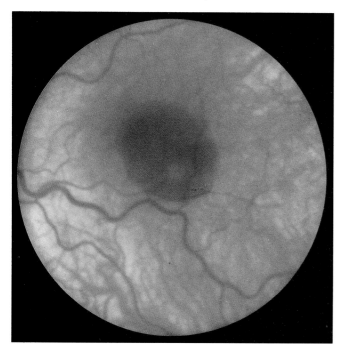

Fig. 460. Choroidal nevus with blurred outlines in an area with hardly any pigment in the epithelium. The choroidal vasculature is well visible.

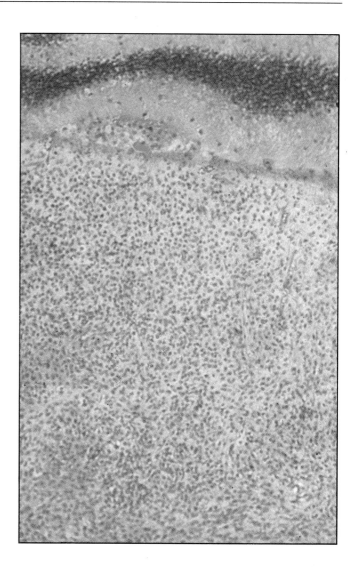

Fig. 461. Choroidal nevus (histologic section). Only minimal variations in size and shape of the cells.

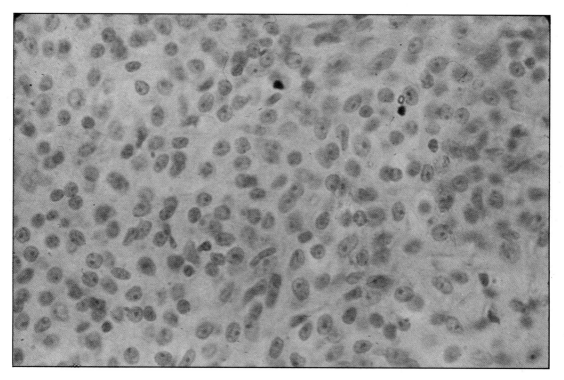

Fig. 462 Choroidal nevus (histologic section). Detail of Fig. 461 in higher magnification.

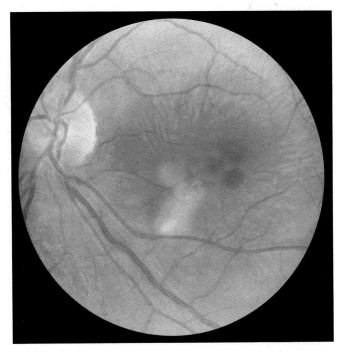

Fig. 463. Choroidal melanoma of moderate size at the posterior pole; beginning solid detachment. Hemorrhagic areas around the lesion.

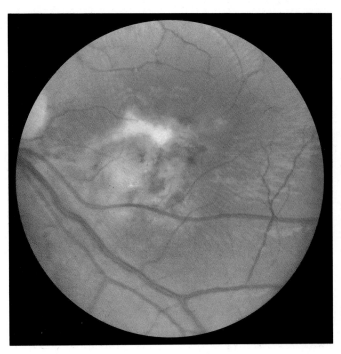

Fig. 464. Choroidal melanoma (same case as Fig. 463) after photocoagulation with argon laser. The neoplasm seems to be partially within a pigmented scar. The hemorrhages have become pigment deposits.

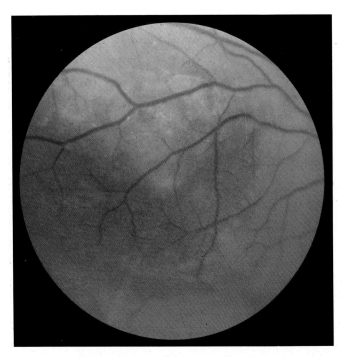

Fig. 465. Choroidal melanoma of considerable dimensions with beginning retinal elevation.

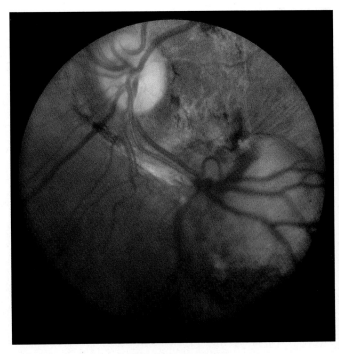

Fig. 466. Choroidal melanoma with solid retinal detachment. The large vessels deviate in their course; there is marked pigment dissemination around the lesion and around the optic nervehead.

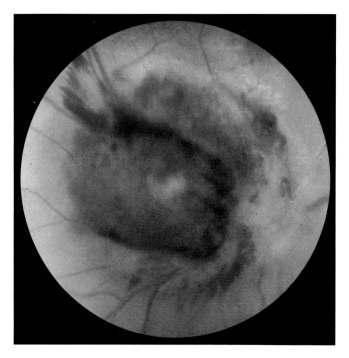

Fig. 467. Large pigmented choroidal melanoma above and next to the optic nervehead. Occlusion of the temporal and nasal retinal veins, marked disc edema and considerable retinal reaction around the lesion.

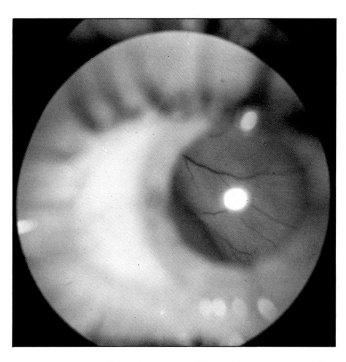

Fig. 468. Choroidal melanoma. Solid retinal detachment visible through the dilated pupil.

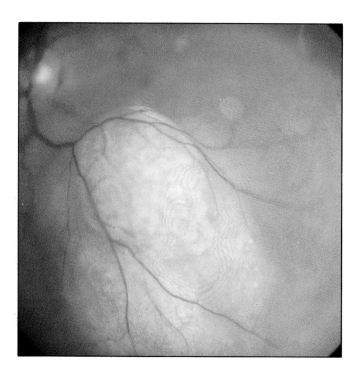

Fig. 469. Slightly pigmented choroidal melanoma.

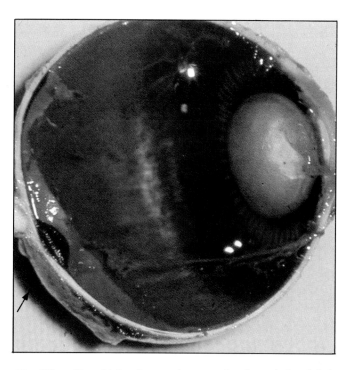

Fig. 470. Choroidal melanoma (cross section through the globe). There is a small tumor nodule next to the optic nervehead (arrow); difficult clinical diagnosis.

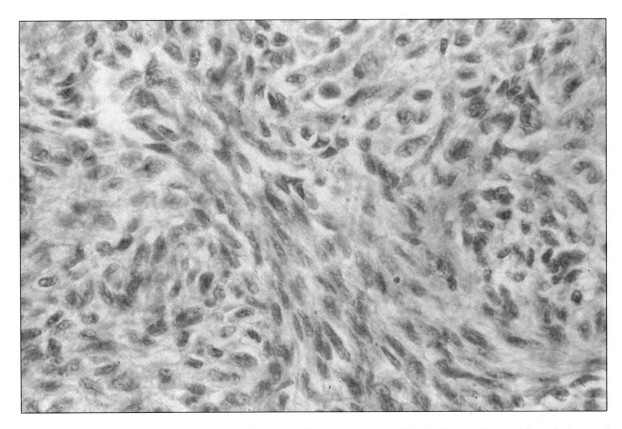

Fig. 471.   Choroidal melanoma of spindle cell type A (histologic section). The fusiform cells are thin and elongated with a small nucleus and no nucleolus.

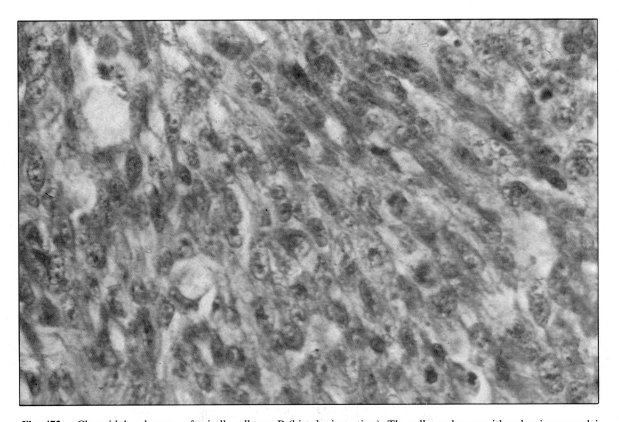

Fig. 472.   Choroidal melanoma of spindle cell type B (histologic section). The cells are larger with voluminous nuclei often containing a nucleolus.

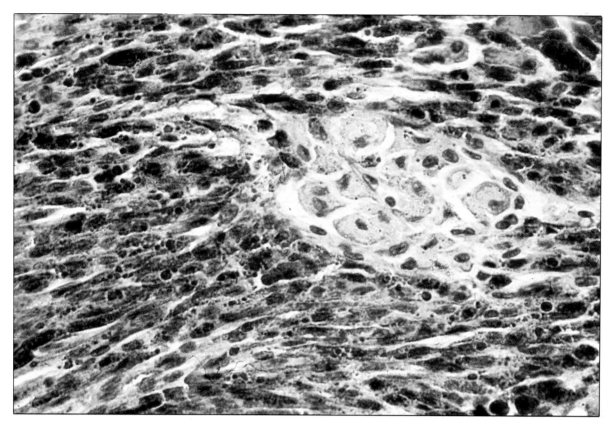

Fig. 473. Choroidal melanoma of the mixed type (histologic section). In addition to deeply pigmented spindle cells there is a nodule of non-pigmented epithelioid cells.

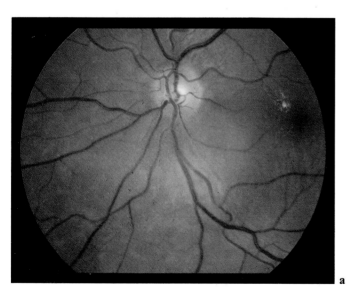

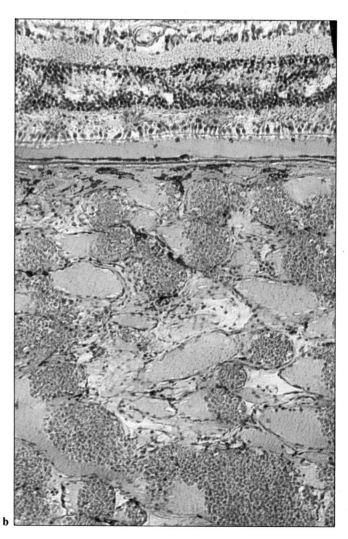

Fig. 474. Choroidal hemangioma.
a) Chorioretinal elevation below the optic nervehead. Hard exudates at the posterior pole.
b) Considerable thickening of the choroid; Bruch's membrane is intact (histologic section).

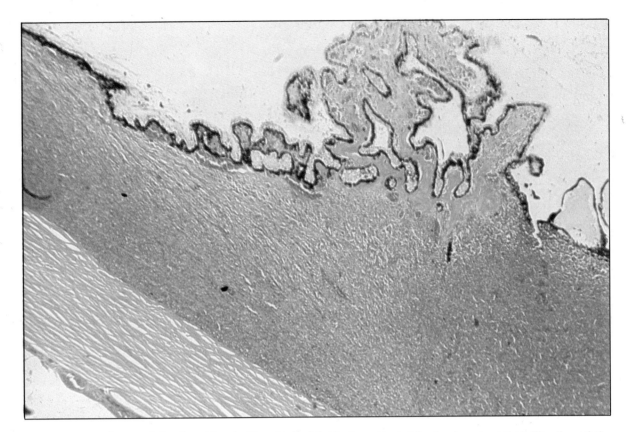

Fig. 475. Lymphoma of the choroid and ciliary body (histologic section). Massive lymphocytic infiltration of the choroid and ciliary body.

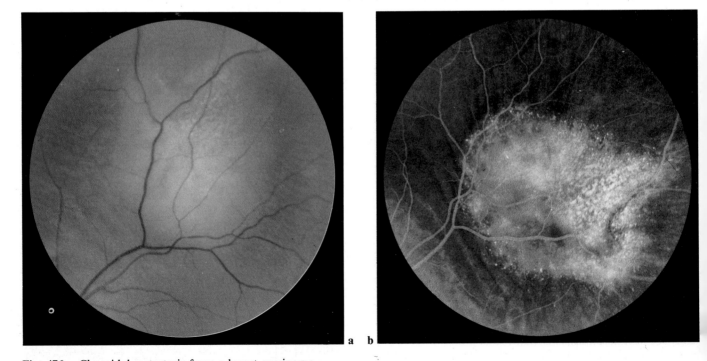

a   b

Fig. 476. Choroidal metastasis from a breast carcinoma.
a) Fundus photo.
b) Fluorescein angiogram.

TUMORS OF THE OPTIC NERVE

These tumors may be located at the disc, intraorbital or intracranial. Each site will cause characteristic clinical signs with different diagnostic approaches and therapeutic considerations.

Table 10. **Classification of optic nerve tumors.**

Primary	Optic nervehead:	Melanocytoma (neuroectodermal
	Orbital:	Glioma (neuroectodermal)
	Intracranial:	Meningioma (mesodermal)
Secondary	Retinoblastoma Melanoma Metastatic carcinoma Leukemia	

PRIMARY TUMORS

Melanocytoma

Melanocytoma of the optic nervehead is a neuroectodermal, benign, unilateral tumor which usually remains stationary or progresses very slowly. It consists of a dense accumulation of nevus cells which are heavily pigmented, polyhedral, of uniform shape with abundant cytoplasm and small nuclei. There are no mitotic figures, nor atypical cells. In contrast to the melanoma the melanocytoma is found in the pigmented races and is therefore often seen in blacks. For a long period of time this tumor will not cause any symptoms.
Ophthalmoscopically we see a black shiny mass localized predominantly in the lower temporal quadrant of the optic nervehead; the pigmentation may extend into the adjacent retina. The tumor is usually smaller than one disc diameter and its margins are blurred (Figs. 477-482). It usually does not require any treatment. The differential diagnosis with a juxtapapillary melanoma may be difficult.

Glioma

This is a neuroectodermal tumor which may derive from the astrocytes or from the oligodendrocytes of the optic nerve. It occurs in infancy and may be congenital; it is frequently associated with neurofibromatosis (Von Recklinghausen disease; 30-50% of the cases). The prognosis is good even though the visual loss may be pronounced.
The eye may often show nystagmus or a strabismus. This may bring the affected children to the physician and bring about the correct diagnosis. These signs are followed by exophthalmus and disturbances of ocular motility.

Ophthalmoscopically we may see disc edema, optic atrophy, when the tumor is localized more posteriorly, or an occlusion of the central retinal vein (see Chapter 5).
CT scan and x-ray pictures of the skull and the orbit may not only corroborate the diagnosis, but may also give prognostic clues: an enlargement of the optic canal indicates a possible endocranial extension, whereas a flattening of the sella turcica or erosion of the anterior clinoid processes may indicate an involvement of the chiasm.
Histologically the glioma is characterized by a proliferation of astrocytes producing a fusiform thickening of the optic nerve; there may be areas of pseudocystoid degeneration; the cystoid spaces contain a mucoid (Fig. 483).
There are two modalities of growth: one is around the nerve invading the sheaths, but not extending outside the dura; the other shows an intraneural infiltration and is seen in patients with systemic neurofibromatosis.
The astrocytic glioma of childhood has usually a good prognosis and is essentially a benign process, growing slowly and without metastases; the *glioblastoma of adulthood*, on the other hand, is extremely malignant (Fig. 484) with rapid growth and lethal outcome because of its extension to the hypothalamus and the cerebellum.
The first symptoms resemble those of an acute optic neuritis, with ocular pain, disc edema and loss of vision in one eye; as soon as the tumor has invaded the chiasm the controlateral optic nerve will be involved and the visual loss becomes bilateral.

Meningioma

This tumor stems from the arachnoidal endothelial cells and is most frequently seen in adults. The clinical symptoms and signs are mainly due to compression of the optic nerve and not so much to actual tumor infiltration. The tumor may be intraorbital or intracranial and the clinical aspects will therefore differ. In an orbital meningioma we find exophthalmus, disc edema, induced hypermetropia, reduced circulation (edema of the lids and conjunctiva, venous stenosis, retinal hemorrhages) and later defective ocular motility with unilateral fixed mydriasis. The intracranial meningioma on the other hand produces hemianopic field defects, optic disc edema in one and optic atrophy in the controlateral eye (Foster Kennedy syndrome) associated with anosmia.
The x-ray picture shows not only an enlargement of the optic canal and the sella turcica, but also calcifications characteristic for this type of neoplasm.
Ophthalmoscopically we observe disc edema which evolves into optic atrophy together with signs of an intracranial space occupying lesion (see Chapter 5).
The prognosis is theoretically good; we have to keep in mind, however, that these neoplasms may also involve the central nervous system.

SECONDARY TUMORS.

These may be divided into three types:

— the first group consists of intraocular tumors extending into the orbit (retinoblastoma or melanoma) (Figs. 467, 485);

— the second group consists of metastases from distant neoplasms;
— the third group are optic nerve involvements in the course of a diffuse leukemia.

In the latter group the ophthalmoscopic picture is quite typical: there is disc edema associated with retinal hemorrhages and a diffuse leukemic infiltration of the optic nervehead involving perivascular tissues.

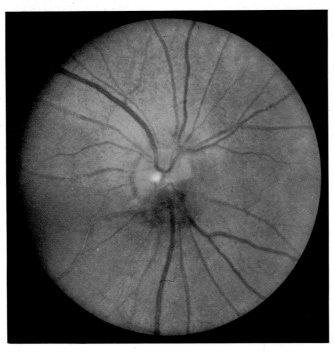

Fig. 477. Melanocytoma of the optic nerve. There is a massive lesion with blurred outlines, partly pigmented, infiltrating the lower half of the disc. Slight peripapillary pigment dispersion.

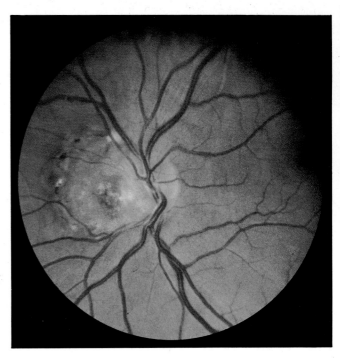

Fig. 478. Melanocytoma of the optic nerve. The tumor involves the nasal part of the disc and grows exophytically; it measures 1.6 disc diameters, is irregularly pigmented and has blurred margins.

Fig. 479. Melanocytoma of the optic nerve. Considerable pigmentation over the nasal half of the optic disc. The temporal disc margin appears blurred.

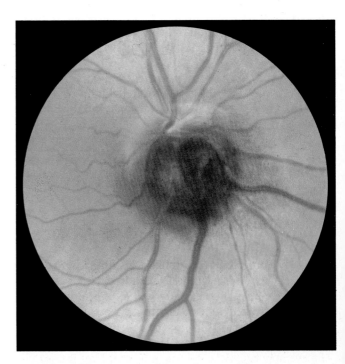

Fig. 480. Melanocytoma of the optic nerve. The optic nervehead is nearly completely obscured by the heavily pigmented tumor mass. The neoplasm markedly deviates the retinal vessels.

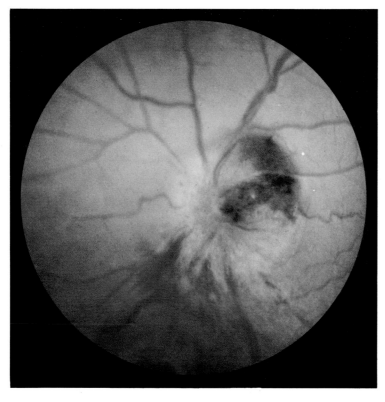

Fig. 481. Melanocytoma of the optic nerve. Small amount of pigment. Hemorrhagic areas along the lower nasal vessels.

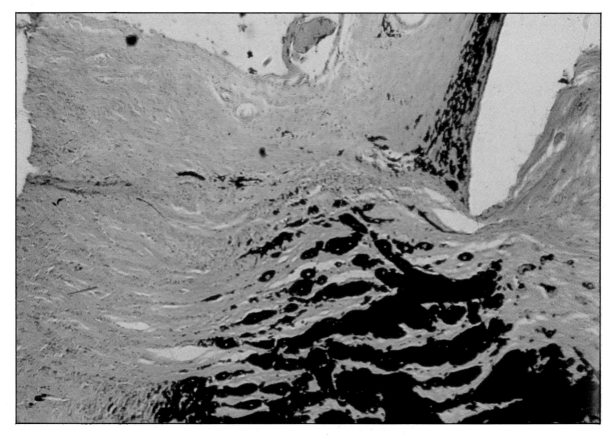

Fig. 482. Melanocytoma of the optic nerve (histologic section). Pigment streaks infiltrate the nerve fibers thereby obscuring the normal architecture.

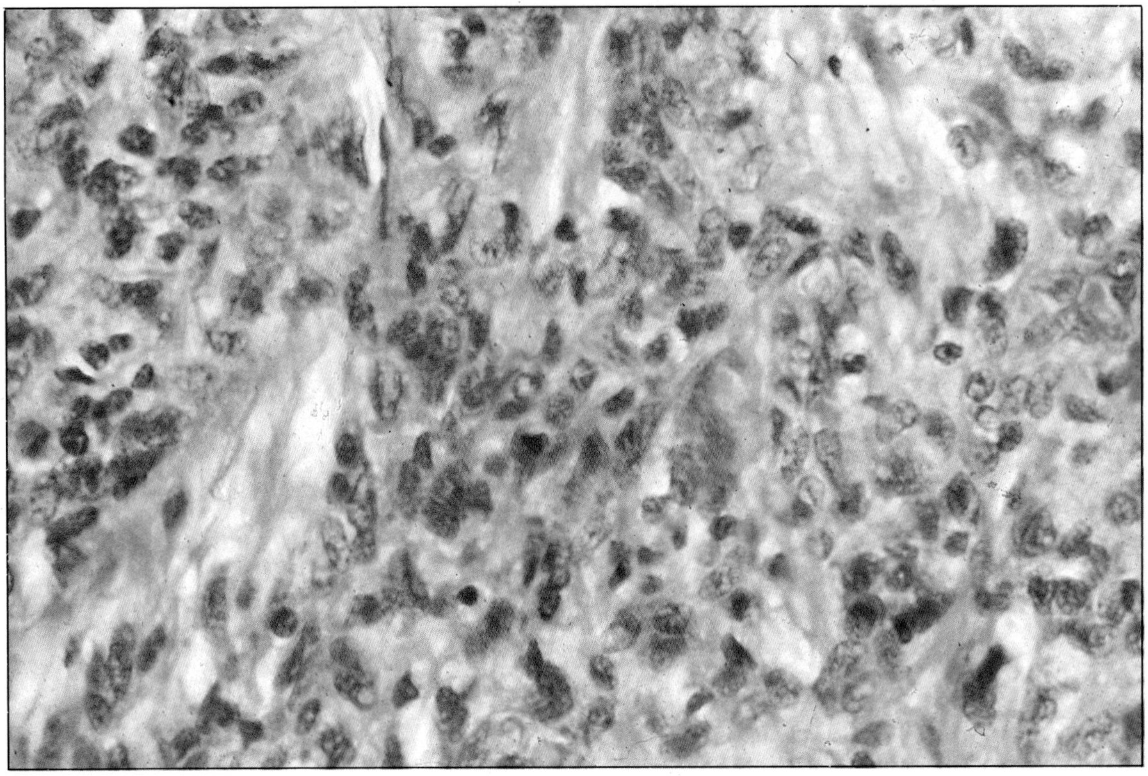

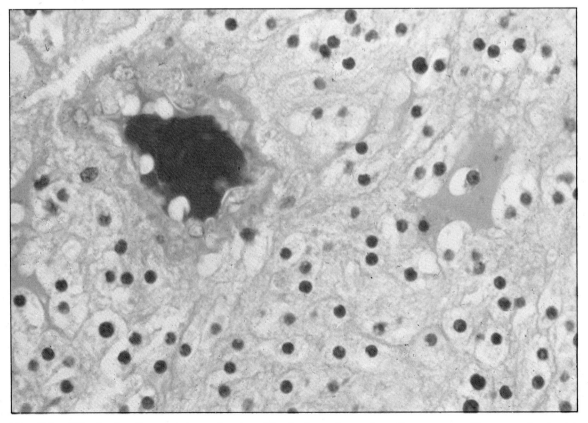

Fig. 483. Astrocytoma of the optic nerve (histologic section). The small neoplastic cells are immersed in a rich network of fibrils.

Fig. 484. Oligodendroglioma of the optic nerve (histologic section). The cells appear swollen, vacuolized, with a round and central nucleus.

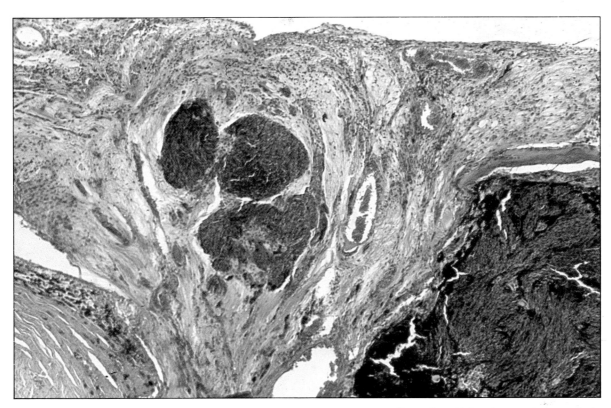

Fig. 485. Melanoma of the optic nerve (histologic section). The juxtapapillary choroidal melanoma has massively infiltrated the optic nervehead.

Chapter 11

Ocular trauma

RETINAL CONTUSIONS

Direct contusion of the globe (tennis ball, rock, champagne cork, etc.) and concussion from a distance may produce the syndrome of commotio retinae (Berlin edema), an expression of vascular changes in the choriocapillaries and in the retina. The initial vasoconstriction is followed by a vasodilatation with increased vascular permeability producing edema which begins about 24 hours after the trauma. Depending on the circumstances, there may be retino-vitreal hemorrhages, traumatic chorioretinitis and choroidal ruptures.

Berlin Edema

In severe cases the ophthalmoscopic picture is similar to an occlusion of the central retinal artery with a milky discoloration of the retina at the posterior pole and a cherry red spot in the macula (Figs. 486, 487). More often the retinal edema is less severe and reveals itself as a greyish discoloration of the affected area which also seems to be elevated, opaque and white striae and exaggerated retinal reflexes in the surrounding normal retina (Fig. 486).

The edema may extend along the retinal vessels producing a white perivascular halo. In the more common central localization the macula is always conspicuous by its dark red color which contrasts with a grey milky fundus. In a peripheral location of the edema, usually at the equator, the edematous ischemic area surrounded by hemorrhages has the form of a triangle, the base of which is peripheral. The margins are arcuate and delineated by retinal vessels (Fig. 488).

The edema disappears in the majority of cases within a few days and leaves no sequelae. When hemorrhages and chorioretinitis are present the course is less benign. The unfavorable outcome of the central type of edema is due to pigment changes and atrophy (Fig. 489) which may lead to a macular hole (Fig. 497). The peripheral lesions of chorio-retinal atrophy may lead to retinal breaks or a pseudo-disinsertion of the retina.

Retinal hemorrhages

Direct or indirect trauma to the globe may lead to all kinds of hemorrhages: intraretinal, preretinal and subretinal (see Chapter 2).

Small superficial intraretinal hemorrhages are frequent. They lie at the periphery of the edematous area in sectors which are not involved by the swelling, e.g. peripapillary hemorrhages which are arranged like a crescent around the optic disc and stem from the capillaries around the optic nerve. The macular involvement will obviously cause severe loss of visual acuity and may ophthalmoscopically simulate a macular pseudohole (Fig. 490).

Lesions of the posterior ciliary arteries may produce a hemorrhagic infarct around the optic nervehead which on resolving will leave a peripapillary area of choroidal atrophy. There may also be preretinal and subretinal hemorrhages, usually at the posterior pole which may coalesce to a bullous roundish retinal elevation which is well delineated against the retina normal and protrudes over the retinal surface.

In the depth of the hemorrhage there may be blood cells and a serous supernatant (Fig. 491). In general these hemorrhages absorb completely in spite of the fact that they may be quite extensive. They leave degenerative changes which give the posterior pole a greyish aspect, forming a star figure (Fig. 492). Sometimes these bleedings may extend into the vitreous causing a massive hemorrhage.

Choroidal hemorrhages are dark blue in color and may resemble a choroidal rupture (Fig. 493). (See below, Choroidal ruptures).

Traumatic chorioretinitis

The traumatic chorioretinitis of Hutchinson-Siegrist is characterized by one or several geographic, white-yellow foci and hemorrhages which are usually situated in the papillo-macular area. These develop into atrophic grey chorioretinal scars with pigment proliferation that may be condensed into numerous round deposits (Figs. 494-496). The proliferative type of traumatic chorioretinitis is rare. Here the scars are conspicuous black pigmentations and connective tissue organized into white bands and membranes (Fig. 497).

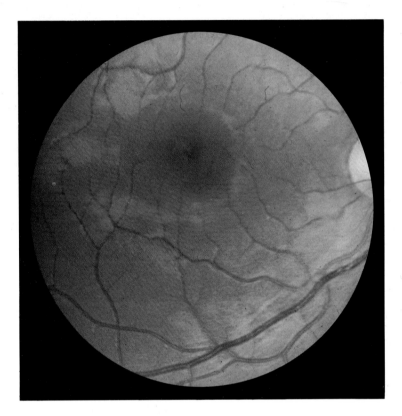

Fig. 486.   Commotio retinae. Berlin's edema in the macula.

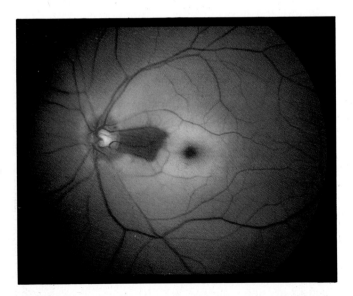

Fig. 487.   Commotio retinae. Marked edema of the posterior pole with cherry red spot of the macula (a picture similar to a central retinal artery occlusion), hyperemia of the disc and juxtapapillary hemorrhage.

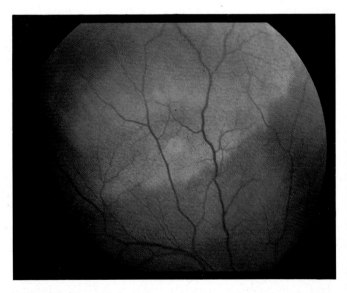

Fig. 488.   Commotio retinae. Ischemic edema at the equator.

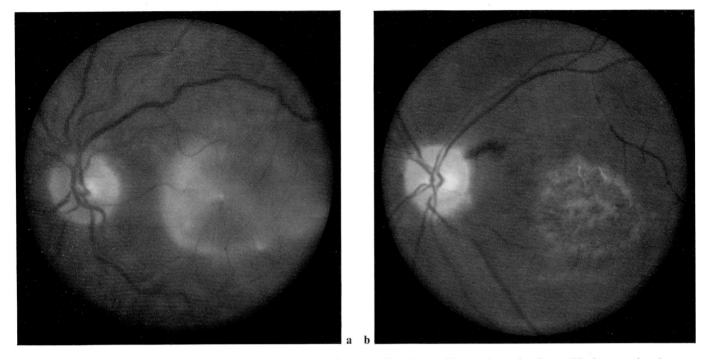

a   b

Fig. 489. **a)** and **b)** Commotio retinae. Deleterious evolution of the macular edema with a tendency for dystrophic degenerative changes.

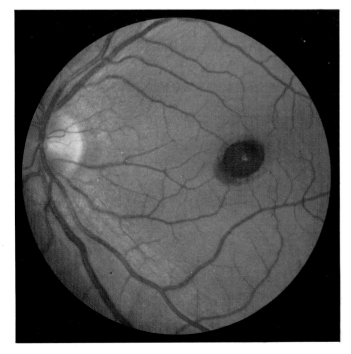

Fig. 490. Retinal contusion. Post-traumatic macular hemorrhage.

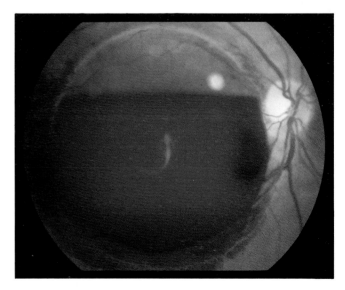

Fig. 491. Post-traumatic extensive preretinal (subhyaloid) hemorrhage at the posterior pole.

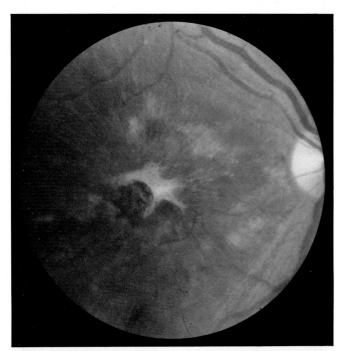

Fig. 492. End result of a post-traumatic preretinal hemorrhage. Chorioretinal degeneration in the macula associated with a preretinal retracting membrane (cellophane retinopathy).

Fig. 493. Retinal contusion. Post-traumatic elevation of the pigment epithelium secondary to a choroidal hemorrhage.
a) Fundus photo.
b) Fluorescein angiogram.

Fig. 493 a

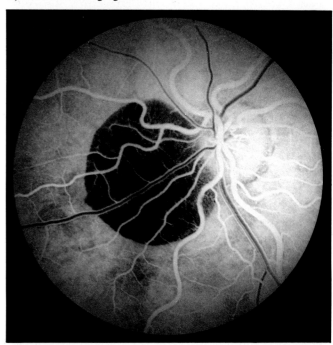

Fig. 493 b

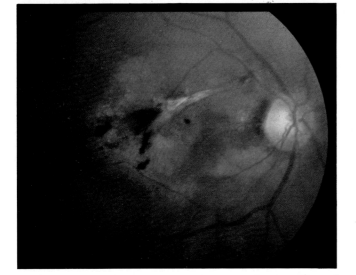

Fig. 494. Central post-traumatic chorioretinitis. Traction exerted by the proliferating and disorganized pigment masses.

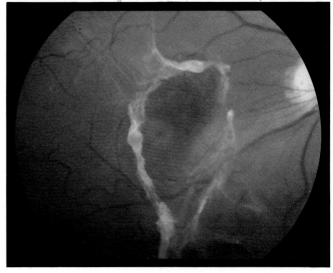

Fig. 495. Central post-traumatic chorioretinitis. A membrane of proliferating tissue causing distortion of the blood vessels.

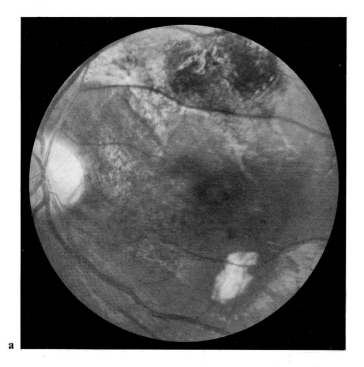

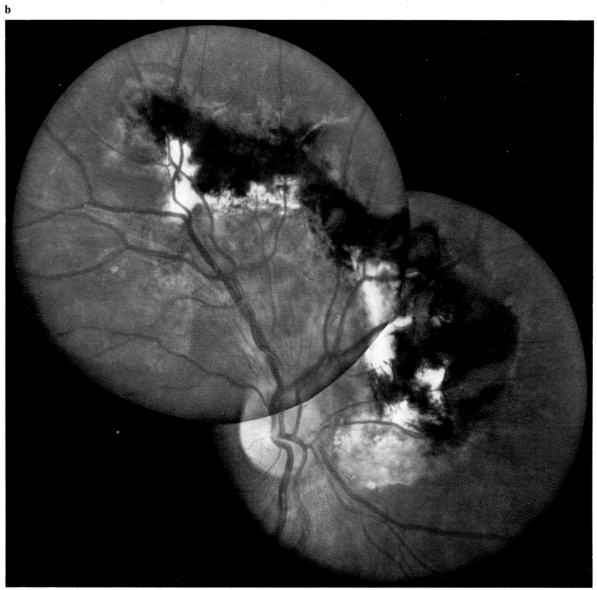

Fig. 496. **a)** and **b)** Post-traumatic chorioretinitis (Hutchinson-Siegrist). Cicatricial stage with marked pigment proliferation and scars arranged in a geographic pattern.

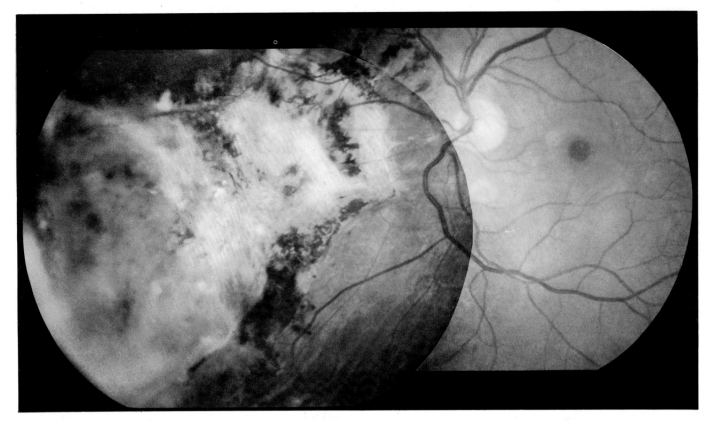

Fig. 497.   End result of a severe post-traumatic chorioretinitis. Marked chorioretinal degeneration of the nasal segment with conspicuous pigment deposition and connective tissue proliferation; macular hole.

PURTSCHER'S RETINOPATHY

The retinal traumatic angiopathy of Purtscher is usually bilateral and is found after severe compression or crush injury to the thorax. A unilateral retinopathy may follow a severe commotio cerebri.

The pathogenesis of this traumatic retinopathy is still under discussion. The venous stasis secondary to the abrupt increase of pressure in the jugular veins certainly plays an important pathogenetic role. The retinal changes develop within 24 hours after the trauma and lead to a sudden and severe diminution of visual acuity.

Ophthalmoscopically we see an ischemic retinal edema with cotton-wool patches accumulating at the posterior pole with festooned outlines resembling the contour of the brain (Fig. 498). There are flame-shaped hemorrhages. The veins are dilated and tortuous with hemorrhages into their walls, whereas the arteries appear normal. Within a variable period of time, lasting one to three months, the exudates and hemorrhages are completely absorbed. There may remain a more or less intensive pigment disturbance in the macula, but more often the retina assumes a slate-grey color and there is a partial optic atrophy.

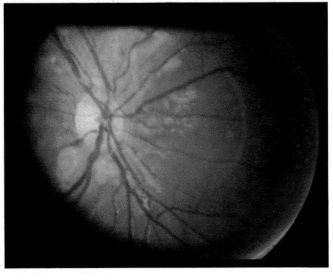

Fig. 498.   Purtscher's retinophaty. Cotton-wool patches disseminated over the posterior pole.

SOLAR RETINOPATY

This lesion is often caused by intensive light damage to the retina, e.g., by observing a partial sun eclipse. It is a central angiospastic retinopathy which is seen in young adults or in aphakic eyes either after observing the sun or in psychopathic persons or drug addicts who voluntarily or unconsciously expose themselves for a long time to solar radiation.

The patients complain first of glare accompanied by metaphorphopsia, scotomas, photophobia and chromatopsia; after two or three weeks these symptoms usually regress completely. A photophobia may, however, remain even for years after the photic trauma.

The ophthalmoscopic picture is initially characterized by a more or less pronounced diffuse edema at the posterior pole with accentuation of the red foveolar reflex (Figs. 499-500). In severe cases there are small hemorrhages and yellow foveal exudates. In time these lesions usually absorb completely and there only remains a fine foveal and parafoveal pigmentation (Fig. 501). In severe cases there may be degenerative changes in the macula leading to a lamellar macular hole with severe reduction of central vision.

A *foveal retinopathy* resembling solar retinopathy clinically and in its angiospastic pathogenesis may be rarely observed in plants engaged in the production of laser devices or may occur accidentally during laser photocoagulation of a maculopathy of a different origin (Fig. 502).

There are also idiopathic forms of this retinopathy due to a pure angiospasm.

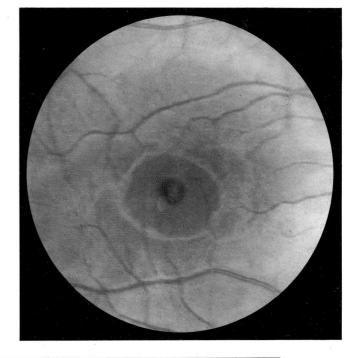

Fig. 499. Solar retinopathy. Macular edema with marked accentuation of the foveolar reflex.

Fig. 500. Solar retinopathy. Detail of the macular edema in higher magnification.

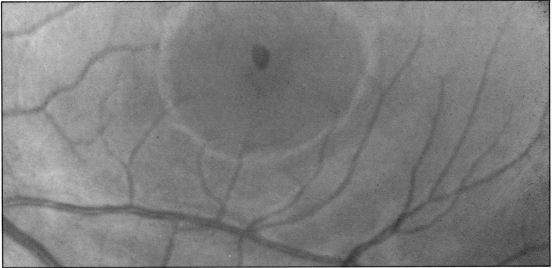

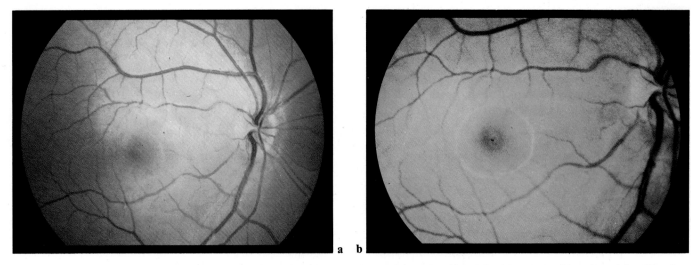

a   b

Fig. 501.   Cicatricial endstage of a solar retinopathy. Fine pigmentation and foveolar dystrophy **(a)**, more evident in red-free illumination **(b)**.

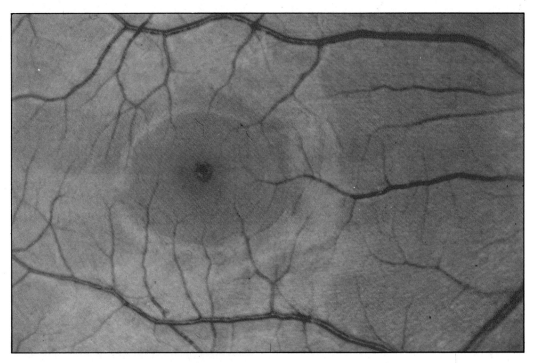

Fig. 502.   Foveal retinopathy.

RETINAL BREAKS

Retinal breaks may be caused by a blunt contusion or by a perforating injury. The first is most frequently seen in patients in whom the retina is already damaged by degenerative changes, e.g., myopia and senile changes, which act as predisposing factors.

The break may be situated in the area of the trauma or may be at the opposite side as an expression of contre coup. A break at the ora presents as a large retinal disinsertion. Lesions close to the disc are rare.

Ophthalmoscopically the traumatic tears or holes have the same characteristics as those described in Chapter 6 (Holes and tears of the retina, page 185); they may acquire the form and size of a typical horseshoe tear, a large dialysis or look like large holes in necrotic areas (Figs. 503, 504).

A macular hole is frequently the end result of a Berlin contusion edema and is visible as a dark red spot, localized in the foveola and usually is smaller than one disc diameter. It is typically round and there is retinal edema, sometimes retinal folds, around it (Figs. 497, 505).

All these lesions may lead to a retinal detachment; 80% of the traction detachments will develop within about two years after the trauma.

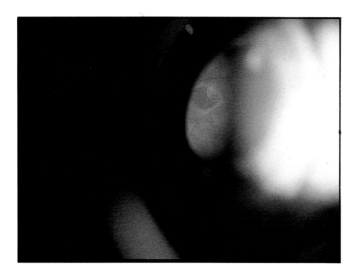

Fig. 503. Open traumatic giant retinal tear (slit lamp picture). The retinal flap is retracted by the vitreous.

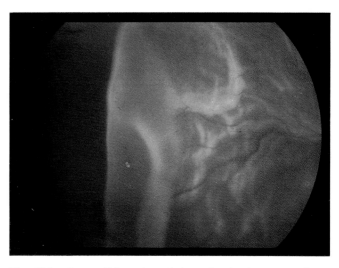

Fig. 504. Large disinsertion of the retina in the temporal segment with inversion of the flap and retinal detachment. The red color of the underlying choroid is visible.

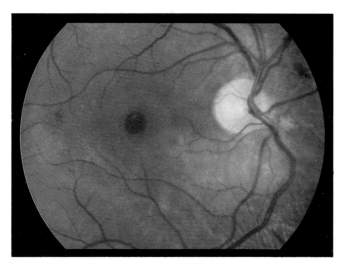

Fig. 505. Postcontusion macular hole.

CHOROIDAL RUPTURES

These are usually due to a severe contusion or a contre coup injury. They may also be caused by post-traumatic tissue necrosis.

Initially the ruptures are obscured by retinal edema and hemorrhages. Ophthalmoscopically they appear as brown-yellow, arcuate striae of varying width. They later become white because sclera is visible at the depth of the rupture. They have sharp outlines and are pigmented at the border. Retinal vessels course over them. The peripheral ruptures are usually the result of direct trauma and are rather irregular; the ruptures due to indirect trauma are at the posterior pole, often in the temporal half of the fundus and may involve the macula (Fig. 506). They are elongated, arcuate and concentric with the nervehead. They may be single or multiple. We may in these cases assume a disposition for such ruptures. They may extend over two or three disc diameters (Fig. 507). Radial ruptures are rare. The lesion is permanent. The overlying retina may show pigment proliferation and atrophy. Corresponding arcuate scotomas can be found on visual field testing; if the lesion involves the macula there will be a severe loss of central vision. In time there may be subretinal neovascularization corresponding to the area of the choroidal rupture which may cause an exudative retinal detachment.

Chorioretinitis sclopetaria consists of a rupture of the choroid and the retina whereby the sclera remains usually intact. It is due to a severe contusion, e.g., a bullet traversing the orbit. When the vitreous hemorrhage has cleared we see ophthalmoscopically the destroyed retina associated with marked fibrosis which nevertheless may prevent a retinal detachment.

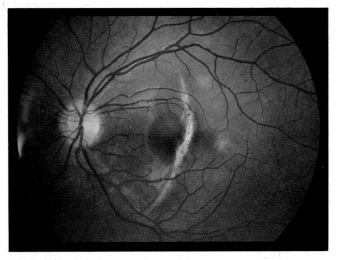

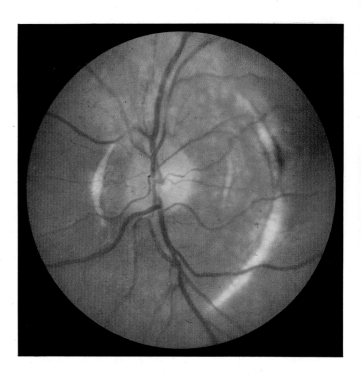

Fig. 506. Arcuate choroidal rupture at the posterior pole with involvement of the macula.

Fig. 507. Multiple choroidal ruptures. The arcuate white striae are well visible. They are concentric to the disc. Along the margins of the major rupture (on the temporal side) is a pigment accumulation.

INTRAOCULAR FOREIGN BODIES

In about 30-40% of eyes with a perforating injury there is also an intraocular foreign body.

The associated clinical problems are not only connected with the nature and location of the foreign body and its subsequent extraction, but above all with the intraocular complications, e.g., exudations, hemorrhages, inflammation, and subsequent scar tissue formation. The intraocular foreign bodies present indeed a severe danger to the anatomical and functional integrity of the eye, not only because of the penetration, but also because of the sequelae of the extraction.

These injuries are not easily classified because of the variety of lesions they produce and the multiplicity of clinical pictures they cause. Nevertheless, there are factors which influence the prognosis and indicate the mode of treatment necessary. The first factor determining the clinical couse is the chemical composition of the foreign body. Some substances, e.g., gold, silver, and platinum, are well tolerated. Other substances, e.g., stone, chalk, coal, or glass, produce a severe reaction, especially from the vitreous and the retina. Iron and copper containing foreign bodies cause the most severe intraocular reaction with a diffuse and progressive inflammatory response that occurs after varying intervals of time. All intraocular structures may be involved. The formation of iron oxide in siderosis and of copper salts in chalcosis will lead to a series of degenerative changes of the ocular structures which may lead to blindness. Other factors of prognostic importance are the entrance wound (corneal, limbal, scleral), the size of the foreign body, the severity of the impact and the location of the foreign body, the induced intraocular lesions and the interval between trauma and extraction.

The larger the volume of the foreign body the greater will be the lesions, on the other hand a small foreign body may have a greater chance to penetrate the ocular walls.

During the first days after trauma when the optic media are still transparent it is possible to recognize the course which the foreign body has followed inside the globe and occasionally to view it directly. If the foreign body lies in the vitreous — and this is most frequently the case — we may observe a rectilinear, slightly opaque streak similar to a white band, indicating the path of the foreign body. If the foreign body is visible and metallic it becomes quite conspicuous by its brilliant reflexes on a reddish background (Fig. 508). In most cases, however, a white exudate will after a few hours form around the foreign body thereby obscuring it, whereas the vitreous may become opaque and liquified. When the foreign body rests on the retina the surrounding tissue will be edematous and congested and show small hemorrhages. Later there will be a reactive pigmentary dispersion. If the foreign body remains lodged in the sclera its presence may be suspected by the circumscribed retinal edema, by localized hemorrhages and by opacification of the vitreous in the area of the lesion. In most instances, however, hyphema, traumatic cataract, vitreous hemorrhage and retinal detachment will not allow a visualization of the foreign body, but these are, on the other hand, signs which indicate its penetration into the eye. In these cases echography is especially important for the diagnosis (Fig. 509). The inflammatory reaction determines the progressive transformation of the vitreous into connective tissue with a secondary traction detachment of the retina. The inflammatory reactions may also be of a chemical nature, especially in cases of siderosis or chalcosis.

In **siderosis** the color of the iris and of the lens changes a few months after the trauma, becoming grey-green or brownred. There are associated severe retinal degenerations which end in optic atrophy. These alterations are due to a progressive impregnation of the ocular tissuese by iron containing granules.

In **chalcosis** we find purulent inflammatory reactions, not caused by microorganisms; the cataract shows here grey-green opacities with irridescent reflexes. There is retinal atrophy due to the deposition of small yellow particles which may be seen with the ophthalmoscope. These changes are due to the formation of copper salts.

The extraction of a foreign body is usually attempted as soon as possible. This may avoid or reduce the inflammatory or infectious complications, it may eliminate or attenuate the chemical reactions in the vitreous with the subsequent liquifaction and the formation of traction bands in the vitreous and on the retina. An early operation will also avoid the formation of reactive exudative fibrotic tissue which will envelop the foreign body and present an obstacle for its extraction (Fig. 510). The site of the foreign body will determine by which approach and by which technique the surgical procedure is performed.

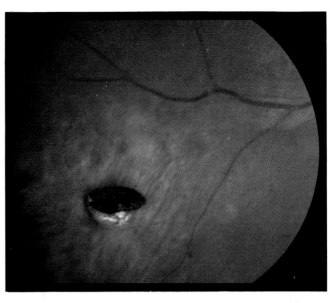

Fig. 508. Intraocular foreign body resting on the retinal surface. Underlying area of chorioretinal atrophy; the retina around the lesion shows a marked dystrophy of the pigment epithelium and large choroidal vessels are visible.

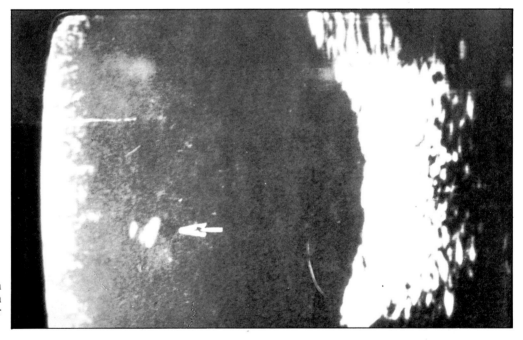

Fig. 509. B scan echogram reveals two intraocular foreign bodies situated in the anterior third of the vitreous (arrow).

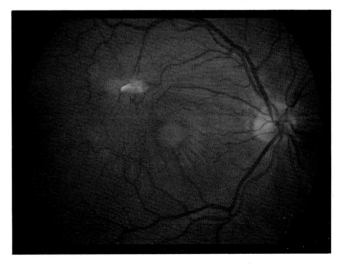

Fig. 510. End-result of a surgical extraction of an intraocular foreign body. Cicatricial vitreo-retinal retractions.

TRAUMA TO THE OPTIC NERVE

A direct contusion of the globe may lead to exudation and hemorrhage in the optic nerve sheaths, disc edema and more or less extensive hemorrhages around and in the area of the optic nervehead. Contusions or concussions to the cranium, especially in the area of the forehead, may damage the optic nerve on the same side by a pathogenic mechanism not yet understood. Characteristic is a type of blindness which does not produce any abnormal ophthalmoscopic signs. The descending optic atrophy becomes manifest only three to six weeks after the trauma (Fig. 511). A fracture of the optic canal or of the base of the skull can only be found in a minority of cases; in the majority the optic nerve lesion is probably due to a primary concussion necrosis or perhaps to injury to the small pial vessels or to intraneural hemorrhages caused by the severe compression of the nerve against the bony canal. Severe trauma of the cranial or facial bony structures with luxation and torsion of the globe or fire arm injuries may produce a partial or total severence of the optic nerve and its blood vessels. If the lesion is only partial then ophthalmoscopic picture resembles that of a central retinal artery occlusion with massive hemorrhagic retinal edema around the disc. This will result in optic atrophy with thread-like arteries and proliferative macular retinopathy. If the evulsion of the optic nervehead is complete we see on ophthalmoscopic examination instead of the disc a cavity which is deeper and wider than the optic nervehead. The cavity is grey-red and surrounded by coagulated blood (Fig. 512).

The subsequent connective tissue and glial proliferation lead to the formation of a white tendinous scar which is elevated, irregular in outlines, avascular and may occupy the entire posterior pole.

Fig. 511. Post-traumatic optic atrophy.

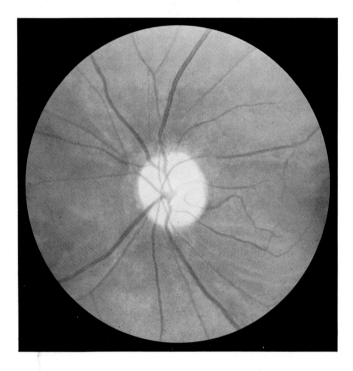

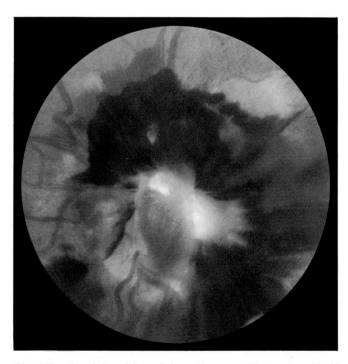

Fig. 512. Partial evulsion of the optic nerve. The temporal half of the optic nervehead is replaced by a grey-brown avascular cavity; massive hemorrhagic infarct around the disc.

References

BONAMOUR G. *Ophtalmologie Clinique*. Doin Ed., Paris, 1972.
DUKE ELDER W.S. *System of Ophthalmology*, vol. IX (1966), vol. X (1967), vol. XII (1971), vol. XIV 1972), Kimpton, London.
DUANE T. *Clinical Ophthalmology*. Harper and Row Pbl., Hagerstown, 1979.
DI MARZIO Q. *Fundus Oculi*, Ed. Salomone, Roma, 1937.
LARSEN H.W. *Manuel et Atlas du Fond d'Oeil normal et pathologique*. Masson ed., Paris, 1971.
JAEGER's *Atlas of Disease of the Ocular Fundus* by D.M. Albert. Saunders Co., Philadelphia, 1972.
MARCHESANI O. *Atlas des Augenhintergrundes*. Urban and Schwarzenberg, München, 1959.
MICHAELSON I.C. Textbook of the Fundus of the Eye. Livingston, Edimburg, 1980.
NOVER A. *Il Fondo dell'occhio*. Leonardo Ed., Roma, 1972.
PEYMAN G.A., SANDERS D.R., GOLDBERG M.F. *Principles and Practis of Ophthalmology*. W. B. Saunders, Philadelphia, 1980.
SAUTTER H., STRAUB W., TURSS R., ROSSMANN H. *Atlas of the Ocular Fundus*. Urban and Schwarzenberg, Baltimore, 1984.
SCHEIE H.G., ALBERT D.M. *Textbook of Ophthalmology*. W.B. Saunders, Philadelphia, 1977.
SORSBY A. *Disease of the Fundus Oculi*. Butterworths, London, 1975.
THIEL R. *Atlas of Disease of the Eye*. Elsevier Pbl.Co., Amsterdam, 1963.

Chapter 1

THE NORMAL OCULAR FUNDS

ARCHER D. B., DEUTMAN A., ERNEST J. T., KRILL A. E. *Arteriovenous communications of the retina*. Amer. J. Ophthal. 75, 224, 1973.
ASHTON N. *Observations on the choroidal circulation*. Br. J. Ophthal. 36, 465, 1952.
BEC P., RAVAULT M., ARNE' J. L., TREPSAT C. *La périphérie du fond d'oeil*. Soc. Franc. d'Opht. Masson, 1980.
BERNSTEIN M. N., HOLDENBER M. J. *Fine structure of the choriocapillaris and the retinal capillaries*. Invest. Ophthal. 4, 1016, 1965.
BIRD A. C., WEALE R. A. *On the retinal vasculature of the human fovea*. Exp. Eye Res. 10, 409, 1974.
BONAMOUR G. *Emergence et divisions anormales de l'artère centrale de la rétine*. Ann. d'Oculist. 203, 639, 1970.
CAGIANU T. *Tortuosité congénitale des petits vaisseaux rétiniens*. Ophthalmologica. 156, 322, 1968.
COGAN D. G. *The human retinal vasculature*. Trans. Ophthal. Soc. U.K. 83, 465, 1963.

DANIS P., TOUSSAINT P., VEREERSTRATEN P. *Etude du coefficient de densité vasculaire de la rétine humaine normale enfonction de l'éloignement de la papille*. Docum. Ophtalmol. 26, 31, 1969.
EISNER G. *Biomicroscopy of the Peripheral fundus*. Springer-Verlag, 1973.
FRIEDMAN E., SMITH T. R. *Senile changes of the choriocapillaris of the posterior pole*. Symposium macular disease. Trans. Am. Acad. Ophthalmol. Otolaryngol., 69, 652, 1965.
FRIEDMAN E., TS'O M. O. M. *The retinal pigment epithelium II. Histologic changes accounted with age*. Arch. Ophthalmol. (Chicago), 79, 315, 1968.
FRIEDMAN E., SMITH T., KUWABARA T. *Senile choroidal vascular patterns and drusen*. Arch. Ophthalmol. (Chicago), 69, 220, 1963.
GRIGNOLO A., SCHEPENS C. L., HEALTH P. *Cysts of the parsplana ciliaris. Ophthalmoscopic appearance and pathological description*. Arch. Ophthalmol. 58, 530, 1957.
HAYREH S. I.*Segmental nature of the choroidal vasculature*. Br. J. Ophthal. 59, 631, 1975.
KOBY E. *Le rôle du sang dans la production de la couleur rouge du fond de l'oeil éclairé à l'ophtalmoscope*. Ann. Oculist. (Paris), 160, 638, 1923.
KREY H. *Segmental vascular patterns of the choriocapillaris*. Am. J. Ophthal. 80, 198, 1975.
KUWABARA, T., COGAN D. G. *Studies of retinal vascular patterns. I. Normal architecture*. Arch. Ophthalmol. 64, 904, 1960.
LONN L.I., SMITH T.R. *Ora serrata pearls*. Arch. Ophthalmol. 77, 809, 1967.
MICHAELSON I. C. *Mode of development of the retinal vessels*. Trans. Ophthal. Soc. U.K. 68, 137, 1948.
MICHAELSON I. C. *Retinal Circulation in Man and Animals*. Thomas, Springfield, 1954.
MORONE G., TAZZI A., CARELLA G., GHISOLFI A. *The vascular system of the eye*. Ed. La Goliardica Pavese, Pavia, 1981.
RUTNIN U. *Fundus appearance in normal eyes. I. The choroid*. Am. J. Ophthalmol. 64, 821, 1967.
RUTNIN U., SCHEPENS C.L. *Fundus appearance in normal eyes. II. The standard peripheral fundus and development variations*. Am. J. Ophthalmol. 64, 840, 1967.
RUTNIN U., SCHEPENS C.L. *Fundus appearance in normal eyes. III. Peripheral degenerations*. Am. J. Ophthalmol. 64. 1040, 1967.
RUTNIN U., SCHEPENS C.L. *Fundus appearance in normal eyes. IV. Retinal breaks and other findings*. Am J. Ophthalmol. 64, 1063, 1967.
SCHEPENS C. L., BAHN G. C. *Examination of the ora serrata. Its importance in retinal detachment*. Arch. Ophthalmol. (Chicago), 44, 677, 1950.
URRETS-ZAVALIA A. *Le decollement de la retine*. Masson, Paris, 1968.
WERNER W., BENEDIKT O. *Trajet inhabituel d'un gros vaisseau rétinien dans la région maculaire*. Klin. Mbl. Augenheilk. 162, 387, 1973.

Chapter 2

BASIC CHANGES

AIBARA G. *Morphological studies on the retinal blood vessels in cases of hypertension.* Acta. Soc. Ophthal. Jap. 55, 1026, 1951.

ASHTON N., HARRY J. *The pathology of cotton wool spots and cytoid bodies in hypertensive retinopathy and other diseases.* Trans. Ophthal. Soc. U.K. 83, 91, 1963.

ASHTON N., DOLLERY C. T., HENKIND P., HILL D. W., PATERSON S. W., RAMALHO P. S., SHAKIB M. *Focal retinal ischaemia.* Br. J. Ophthal. 50, 281, 1966.

BALL C. J., HENKIND P. *Retinal arteriolar collaterals in man.* Br. J. Ophthal. 51, 688. 1967

BELL E.T. *Hypertension: A Symposium,* University of Minnesota Press, Minneapolis, 1950.

BJÖRK J. *Haemodynamic factors and retinal changes in hypertensive diseases.* Acta Med. Scand. Suppl. 175, 1, 1946.

BONAMOUR G., REGNAULT F. *Vasculopathies reteiniennes,* Masson, Paris, 1979.

BONNET M. *Les druses de la lame vitrée* Conf. Lyonn. d'Opht., 113, 1972.

BONNET M. *Les neovascularisations papillaires* Conf. Lyonn. d'Opht., 133, 1977.

COLLINS E. T. *Abiotrophy of the retinal neuro-epithelium.* Trans. Ophthal. Soc. U.K. 39, 165, 1919.

DOUBOIS-POULSEN A., MILLER H. A. *Etude comparative des modifications anatomiques et sphygmoscopiques rétiniennes dans l'hypertension artérielle.* XVI Int. Ophthal. Congr., London, 1, 381, 1950.

ELSCHNIG A. *Zur Anatomie des menschlichen Albinoauges.* Albrecht v. Graefes Arch. Ophthal. 84, 401, 1913.

FRIEDENWALD H. *Pathological changes in the retinal blood-vessels in arteriosclerosis and hypertension.* Trans. Ophthal. Soc. U.K. 50, 452, 1930.

GASS D. *Pathogenesis of disciform detachment of the neuroepithelium.* Am J. Ophthal. 63, 645, 1967.

GUNN M. R. *Ophthalmoscopic evidence of (1) Arterial changes associated with chronic renal disease and (2) of increased arterial tension.* Trans. Ophthal. Soc. U.K. 12, 124, 1892

GUNN M.R. *On ophthalmoscopic evidence of general arterial disease.* Trans. Ophthal. Soc. U.K. 18, 356, 1898.

GUNN M.R. *Note on vascular changes in retina.* Trans. Ophthal. Soc. U.K. 24, 118, 1904.

HILL D. W., DOLLERY C. T. *Calibre changes in retinal arterioles.* Trans. Ophthal. Soc. U.K. 83, 61, 1963.

HOUSTON W. L., WISE G. N. *Circinate retinopathy Parts I & II.* Arch. Ophthal., N. Y. 58, 777, 1957.

YANKO L., UNGAR H., MICHAELSON I. C. *The exudative lesions in diabetic retinopathy with special regard to the hard exudate.* Acta Ophtal. 52, 150, 1974.

KOHNER E. V. *Cotton wool spots in diabetic retinopathy.* Proc. Roy. Soc. Med. 62, 1269, 1969.

LEISHMAN R. *The eye in general vascular disease. Hypertension and arteriosclerosis* . Br. J. Ophthal. 41, 641, 1957.

LINDSAY A. *Retinal pigmentation due to choroidal melanomasarcoma with observations on congenital grouped pigmentation of the retina.* Brit. J. Ophthal. 39, 114, 1955.

MORONE G., TAZZI A., CARELLA G., GHISOLFI A. *The vascular system of the eye.* Ed. La Goliordica Pavese, Pavia, 1981.

MICHAELSON I. C. *The mode of development of the retinal vessels and some observations on its significance in certain retinal diseases.* Trans. Ophthal. Soc. U.K. 137, 68, 1948.

MICHAELSON I. C. *Intra-mural new vessels in an occluded retinal vein.* Brit. J. Ophthal. 32, 164. 1948.

MICHAELSON I. C. *Retinal Circulation in Man and Animals.* Thomas, Springfield, 1954.

ORZALESI N. *Le emorragie e gli essudati nella retina.* Atti 4° Corso di Aggiornamento A.P.I.M.O., 1982.

SALUS R. *Veränderungen der Netzhautvenen bei allgemeiner Blutdrucksteigerung.* Klin. Mbl. Augenheilk. 82, 471, 1929.

SALUS R. *Die ophthalmoscopische Diagnose der allgemeinen Blutdrucksteigerung.* Med. Klin. 31, 906, 1935.

SALUS R. *The fundus oculi in generalized hypertension and arteriosclerosis.* Arch. Ophthal. (Chicago), 21, 505, 1939.

SCULLICA L. *L'edema retinico.* Atti 4° Corso di Aggiornamento A.P.I.M.O., 1982.

SEITZ R. *The genesis and etiology of the crossing phenomenon and its significance for the diagnosis of diseases of the retinal blood vessels.* Klin. Mbl. Augenheilk. 139, 491, 1962.

STOKOE N. L., TURNER R. W. D. *Normal retinal vascular patterns. Arterio-venous ratio as measure of arterial calibre.* Br. J. Ophthal. 50, 21, 1966.

TLETERS V. W., BIRD A. C. *The development of neovascularisation of senile disciform macular degeneration.* Am. J. Ophthal, 76, 1, 1973.

VILLON J. C. *Les micro-aneurysmes retiniens.* Conf. Lyonn. d'Opth., 120, 1974.

WEINSTEIN P. *The problem of tortuositas vasorum retinae.* Am. J. Ophthal. 34, 721, 1951.

Chapter 3

CONGENITAL ANOMALIES AND MALFORMATION

DUKE-ELDER S. *System of Ophthalmology,* vol. III *Normal and abnormal devolopment.* Kimpton, London, 1964.

EDWARDS W. C., LAYDEN W. E. *Optic nerve hypoplasia.* Am. J. Ophthalmol. 70, 950, 1970.

MANN I. *Developmental abnormalities of the Eye.* British Med. Assoc., London, 1957.

MENCHINI U., CARNEVALINI A., PECE A., BRANCATO R. *Utilità e limiti della fotoresezione YAG laser in corso di cataratta secondaria a vitreo primitivo iperplastico: descrizione di un caso.* Clin. Oc. e Pat. Oculare, 3, 185, 1985.

MENCHINI U., PECE A., CAPOFERRI C., BRANCATO R.: *Cisti vitreale anteriore congenita, associata a piega falciforme retinica.* Clin. Oc. e Pat. Oculare, 2, 112, 1985.

PAGON P. A. *Ocular coloboma.* Surv. Ophthalmol. 25, 223, 1981.

PFAFFENBACH D.D., WALSH F.B. *Central pit of the optic disk* Am. J. Ophthalmol. 73, 102, 1972.

WALSH F. B., HOYT W. F. *Clinical Neuro-Ophthalmology,* Williams and Wilkins. Baltimore, 1969.

Chapter 5

DISEASES OF THE OPTIC NERVE

AMALRIC P. M., BESSOU P. *L'artérite temporale, cause fréquente de cécité chez les gens âgés.* Rev. O.N.O, 37, 240, 1965.

BARDELLI A. M.*Pseudo-papillites vasculaires.* Minerva Oftal., 6, 1, 1964.

BEHRMAN S. *Pathology of papilloedema.* Brain, 89, 1, 1966.

BETTELHEIM H. *Sur l'étiologie de l'oedème ischémique de la papille.* Ophthalmologica, 150, 241, 1965.

BIVON A. *Pseudo-oedème papillaire et tortuosité des vaisseaux rétiniens.* Ann. Otal. 91, 1294, 1965.

BONAMOUR G. *Les pseudo-papillites vasculaires.* Bull. Soc. Ophtal. Fr., 66, 846, 1966.

BONAMOUR G., BREGEAT P., BONNET M., JUGE P. *La papille optique.* Masson, Paris, 1968.

BONNET M., BOUDON C., DURAND L. *Névrite optique-oedémateuse bilatérale.* Bull. Soc. Ophtal. Fr. 1965.

BRÉGEAT P. *L'oedème papillaire.* Rapport Soc. Franc, Ophtal. Masson, Paris, 1956.

EAGLING E. M., SANDERS M. D., MILLER S. J. H. *Ischaemic papillopathy. Clinical and fluorescein angiographic study of forty cases.* Br. J. Ophthal. 58, 990, 1974.

FOULDS W. S., CHISHOLM I. A., PETTIGREW A. R. *The toxic optic neuropathies.* Br. J. Ophthal. 58, 386, 1974.

FRANÇOIS J. *Les pseudo-papillites vasculaires.* Rapport Soc. franç. Ophtal., Masson, Paris, 1956.

FRANÇOIS J. *Pseudo-névrites optiques oedémateuses d'origine vasculaire.* Ann. Oculist. 195, 830, 1962.

FRANÇOIS J., NEETENS A. *La vascularisation du nerf optique. Lamina cribrosa.* Brit. J. Ophthal. 38, 472, 1964.

HAMARD H., SAROUX H., BONNET M. *Ischemie aigue de la tête du nerf optique.* Bull. Soc. Opht. de France, 1977.

HENKIND P., CHARLES N. C., PEARSON J. *Histopathology of ischemic optic neuropathy*. Am. J. Ophthal. 69, 78, 1970.

HAYREH S. S. *Pathogenesis of oedema of the optic disc (papilloedema). A preliminary report*. Br. J. Ophthal 18, 522, 1964.

HAYREH S. S. *Blood supply of the optic nerve head and its role in optic atrophy, glaucoma and oedema of the optic disc*. Br. J. Ophthal 53, 721, 1969.

HAYREH S. S. *Pathogenesis of optic nerve damage and visual field defects in glaucoma*. Glaucoma Symposium, Amsterdam, 1979.

HAYREH S. S. *Anterior ischemic optic neuropathy*. Glaucoma Symposium, Amsterdam, 1979.

LANDOLT E. *Anatomie pathologique de la stase papillaire (Zur pathologischen Anatomie der Stauungspapille)*. Schweiz. Ophthal. Ges. Basel, 1960.

LEINFELDER P.J., PAUL W. D. *Papilledema in general diseases*. Arch. Ophthal. (Chicago), 28, 983, 1942.

MILLER G. R., SMITH J. L. *Ischaemic optic neuropathy*. Am. J. Ophthal. 62. 103, 1966.

MOBO F. *Pseudo-papillite vasculaire dans l'artérite temporale ignorée*. Atti. Soc. Oftal. Lombard., 18, 74, 1963.

MORONE G., TAZZI A., CARELLA G., GHISOLFI A. *Le système vasculaire perioptique: sa morphologie et ses implications physiopatologiques*. Bull. Soc. Ophtal. Fr., 90 année, 1978.

MORONE G., TAZZI A., CARELLA G., GHISOLFI A. *Uber die durchblutung des nervus opticus in hinblick auf die entestehung der glaukomatosen papillenexkavation*. Klin. Mbl. Augenheilk, 175, 741, 1979.

MORONE G., TAZZI A., CARELLA G., GHISOLFI A. *The vascular system of the eye*. Ed. La Goliardica Pavese, Pavia, 1981.

MORONE G., TAZZI A., CARELLA G., GHISOLFI A. *Microvascolarizzazione del nervo ottico e aspetti patogenetici di traumatologia papillare*. Atti del LXI congresso della S.O.I., Roma, 1981.

PAU H. *Differential diagnosis of eye disease*. Saunders, Philadelphia, 1970.

PEDERSEN E. *Papilloedema in encephalitis*. Arch. Neurol. 13, 403, 1965.

PONTE F. *La pseudo-papillite vasculaire artérioscléreuse*. G. Ital. Ottal. 17, 170, 1964.

PRIMROSE J. *Mécanisme de production d'un papilloedème (Mechanism of production of papilloedema)*. Brit. J. Ophthal., 48, 19, 1964.

SARAUX H., MURAT. *Les pseudo-papillites d'origine vasculaire*. Ann. Oculist. 200, 1, 1967.

SAMUELS B. *The histopathology of papilloedema*. Am. J. Ophthal. 21, 1242, 1938.

SANDERS M. D. *Ischaemic papillopathy*. Trans. Ophthal. Soc. U.K. 91, 369, 1971.

TRON E. *La stase papillaire compliquée. Die Komplirierte Stauungspapille (Cours de perfectionnement)*. Sächs. Thür, Ges, Augenheilk., dstch. Akademie für Aerzte Postbild., 16 oct. 1965, Leipzig. Klin. Mbl. Augenheilk., 1966, 149, 1, 108.

VENTURI G., SALVI G. *Pseudo-papillite vasculaire bilatérale à la suite de l'ablation d'une tumeur médullaire*. Ann. Ottal., 90, 737, 1965.

WIESER N. *Le pseudo-syndrome de Foster-Kennedy*. Ophthalmologica, 145, 362, 1963.

Chapter 6

RETINAL DISEASES

APPEN R. E., WRAY S. H., COGAN D. G.: *Central retinal artery occlusion*. Am. J. Ophthalmol. 79, 374, 1975.

ASHTON N. *The eye in malignant hypertension*. Trans. Am. Acad. Ophthalmol. Otolaryngol. 76, 17, 1972.

BALESTRAZZI E. *Anatomia ed istologia patologica oculare*. EMSI, Roma 1984.

BEC P., RAVAMET M., ARNE J. L., TREPSAT C. *La periphérie du fond d'oeil*. Masson, Paris 1980.

BONAMOUR G., REGNAULT F. *Vasculopathies retiniennes*. Masson, Paris, 1979.

BRANCATO R., MENCHINI U., SANTORO P., LA TORRE A. *Le sindromi vitreo-maculari*. Att. Soc. Oftalm. Lombarda 30, 19, 1975.

BRANCATO R., MENCHINI U. *La fotocoagulazione Argon laser nel trattamento della corioretinopatia sierosa centrale*. Corso teorico-pratico di fotocoagulazione Argon-laser. Roma, 1976.

BRANCATO R., MENCHINI U. *La prevenzione della retinopatia diabetica*. Riv. Oftalm. Sociale, 1, 8, 1978.

MENCHINI U., SCIALDONE A., CARNEVALINI A., PECE A., CHIRIACO G., BRANCATO R. *Evoluzione a lungo termine della corioretinopatia sierosa centrale*. Cl. Ocul. Pat. Ocul. 5,361,1983.

BRANCATO R. *Le angiomatosi retiniche*. La Clinique Ophtalmologique Ed. Lab. Martinet 1, 53, 1983.

BRANCATO R., MENCHINI U., PECE A. *Rétinoschisis maculaire idiopathique du sujet jeune associé à des néovaisseaux prérétiniens et prépapillaires*. J. Fr. Ophtalmol. 7, 685, 1984.

BUSACCA A., GOLDMANN H., SCHIFF-WERTHEIMER S. *Biomicroscopie du corp vitré et du fond d'oeil*. Masson, Paris, 1957.

CHUMBLEY L. C. *Ophthalmology in Internal Medicine*, W. B. Saunders, Philadelphia, 1981.

COSCAS G., DHERMY P. *Occlusions veineuses rétiniennes*. Masson, Paris, 1978.

CULLEN J. F., COLEIRO J.A *Ophthalmic complications of giant cell arteritis*. Surv. Ophthalmol. 20, 247, 1976.

FRANCESCHETTI A., FRANÇOIS J., BABEL J. *Les hérédodégenerescences chorio-retiniennes*. Masson, Paris, 1963.

GASS J. D. M. *Pathogenesis of disciform detachment of the neuroepithelium*. Am. J. Ophthalmol. 63. 573, 1967.

GASS J. D. M.*Acute posterior multifocal placoid pigment epitheliopathy*. Arch. Ophthal. 80, 177, 1968.

GOLD D. H., MORRIS D. A., HENKIND P. *Ocular findings in systemic lupus erythematosus*. Br. J. Ophthalmol. 56, 800, 1972.

HAVENER W. A., GLOECKNER S., *Atlas of diagnostic tecniques and treatment of retinal detachment*. Mosby, St. Louis, 1967.

HAYREH S. S. *Pathogenesis of occlusion of the central retinal vessels*. Am. J. Opthalmol. 72, 998, 1971.

HOGAN M. J., ZIMMERMAN L. E. *Ophthalmic Pathology. An atlas and textbook*. Saunders, Philadelphia, 1962.

KRILL A. E. *Hereditary retinal and choroidal disease*. Harper and Row, Hagerstown, 1977.

MAUSOL F.A. *The Eye and systemic disease*. C.V. Mosby, Louis, 1966.

NOBLE K. G., CARR R. E. *Pigmented paravenous chorioretinal atrophy*. Am. J. Ophthalmol. 96, 338, 1983.

PINERO BUSTAMANTE A. *La retina periferica*. Ed. Scriba, Barcelona, 1983.

POLYAK S. L. *The Retina*. University of Chicago. Press, Chicago, 1941.

RICCI B. VOLPI U. *L'apparato visivo del prematuro*. Ed. Verduci, 1983.

SCUDERI G. *Retinopatia diabetica e sua terapia*. Minerva Medica Ed., Torino, 1967.

SCUDERI G. *A classification of diabetic retinopathy*. Ann. Ophthalmol. 5, 411, 1973.

SCUDERI G., RECUPERO S. M., VALVO A. *Acute posterior multifocal placoid pigment epitheliopathy*. Ann. Ophthalmol. 9, 89, 1977.

SCUDERI G., RECUPERO S. M. *Retinite essudativa esterna diffusa benigna (epiteliopatia pigmentaria a placche multiple)*. Boll. Ocul. 59, 7, 1980.

SCUDERI G., PIVETTI PEZZI P., *Manifestazioni oculari nelle Malattie reumatiche e del collageno* in "Trattato Italiano di Medicina Interna. Progressi 1981-84". di P. Introzzi, USES, Firenze, 1984.

TOLENTINO F., SCHEPENS C. L., FREEMAN H., *Alterazioni vitreo-retiniche*. Cerretti, città, 1980.

URRETS-ZAVALIA Jr. A., *Le décollement de la retine*. Masson, Paris, 1968.

VENTURI G., BRANCATO R. *Le maculopatie dell'anziano*. Rel. 57° Congr. Soc. Oftal. Ital., Firenze, 1976.

WIRTH A., CAVALLACCI G. *Fisiopatologia e Clinica della retinite pigmentosa*. Relazione al 64° Cong. Soc. Oftal. Ital., Pacini Editore, Pisa, 1984.

YANOFF F. M., FIRE B. S. *Ocular Pathology. A text and Atlas.* Harper & Row, Hagerstown, 1975.

WOLFF S. M. *The ocular manifestations of congenital rubella.* Trans. Am. Ophthalmol. Soc. 70, 577, 1972.

Chapter 7

INFLAMMATIONS OF THE CHOROID AND RETINA

ANNERLEY W. H. Jr., SHILDS J. A., TOMER T., CHRISTOPHERSON K. *The Clinical Course of serpiginous choroidopathy.* Am. J. Ophthalmol 87, 133, 1979.

ARONSON S. *Clinical Methods in Uveitis.* C.V. Mosby, St. Louis, 1968.

CAMPINCHI R., FAURE J.P., BLOCH MICHAEL E., HANT J. *L'uvéite - Phenomenès immunologiques et allergiques.* Masson, Paris, 1970.

CAMPINCHI R., BRASUN C., TRABELSI S., DUFIER J. L. *Notions recentes sur la retino-choroidite toxoplasmique.* J. Fr. Ophtalmol. 1, 377, 1978.

CHUMBELY L. C., KEARNS T. P. *Retionopathy of sarcoidosis.* Am. J. Ophthalmol. 73, 123, 1972.

CHUMBLEY L. C., ROBERTSON D. M., SMITH T. F., CAMPBELL R. J. *Adult cytomegalovirus inclusion retino-uveitis.* Am. J. Opthalmol. 80, 807, 1975.

ELLIOTT J. H., O'DAY D. M., GUTOW G. S. *Mycotic endophthalmitis in drug abusers.* Am. J. Ophthalmol. 88, 66, 1978.

FRANÇOIS J., HAUSSEN S. *Endophtalmie chronique par Toxocara canis.* Bull. Soc. Belge Ophthalmol. 158, 445, 1971.

FREEMAN W. R., LERNER C. W., MINES J. A., LASH R. S. et al. *A prospective study of the ophthalmologic findings in the acquired immune deficiency syndrome.* Am. J. Ophthalmol. 97, 133, 1984.

FRIEDMAN A. H., LUNTZ M., HENLEY W. L. *Diagnosis and management of Uveitis. An Atlas Approach.* Williams and Wilkins, Baltimore, 1982.

GASS J. D. M., WILKINSON D. P. *Follow-up study of presumed ocular histoplasmosis.* Trans. Am. Acad. Ophthalm. Otolaryngol. 76, 672, 1972.

INABA G. *Behçet's Disease. Pathogenetic Mechanism and Clinical Future.* University of Tokyo Press, Tokyo, 1982.

KIMURA S. J., HOGAN M. J., THYGESON P. *Signs and symptoms of uveitis II. Classification of posterior uveitis.* Am. J. Opthalmol. 47, 171, 1959.

KRAUS-MACKIW E., O'CONNOR G. R. *Uveitis Pathophisiology and Therapy.* Thieme, Stratton Inc., New York, 1983.

MICHELSON J. B. *A colour Atlas of Uveitis Diagnosis.* Wolfe Medical Publ., Weert, 1984.

OHNO S., CHAR D. H., KIMURA S. J., O'CONNOR G. R. *Vogt-Koyanagi, Harada syndrome.* Am. J. Ophthalmol. 83, 735, 1977.

PIVETTI PEZZI P. *Etiologia delle uveiti: studio clinico di 1343 casi.* Boll. Ocul. 57, 193, 1978.

PIVETTI PEZZI P. *Le uveiti virali.* Atti SOI 1980, Cappelli Ed., Bologna 1982.

PIVETTI PEZZI P., SCUDERI G. *Malattia di Behçet, Malattia di Vogt-Koyanagi-Harada e sindromi correlate.* In *Allergia e Immunologia Oculare* di F. D'Ermo, Masson ed., Milano, 1982.

PIVETTI PEZZI P., GASPARRI G., DE LISO P., CATARINELLI G. *Prognosis in Behçet's disease.* Annals Ophthalmol. 17, 20, 1985.

RYAN S. J., MAUMENEE A. E. *Birdshot retinochoroidopathy.* Am. J. Ophthalmol. 98, 31, 1980.

SCHLAEGEL T. F. Jr. *Essentials of Uveitis.* Brown and Co., Boston, 1969.

SCHLAEGEL T. F. Jr. *Ocular toxoplasmosis and parsplanitis.* Grune and Stratton, New York, 1978.

SCHLAEGEL T. F., O'CONNOR G. R. *Tubercolosis and syphilis.* Arch. Ophthalmol. 99, 2206, 1981.

SCUDERI G., PIVETTI PEZZI P. *Manifestazioni oculari della toxoplasmosi congenita.* Atti Simposio Intern. Toxoplasmosi, Ed. Maccari, Parma, 1980.

SMITH R. E., NOZIK R. M. *Uveitis. A Clinical Approach to Diagnosis and Management.* Williams and Wilkins, Baltimore, 1983.

Chapter 8

DISEASES OF THE CHOROID

FRANCESCHETTI A., FRANÇOIS J., BABEL J. *Les hérédodégénérescences chorio-rétiniennes.* Rapport Soc. Fr. Ophtalmol., 1963, t. II.

FRANÇOIS P., BONNET M. *La macula.* Rapport Soc. Fr. Ophtamol. 1976.

KRILL A. E., ARCHER D. *Classification of the choroidal atrophies.* Am. J. Ophthalmol. 72, 562, 1971.

SARAUX H. *Maladies héréditaires de la choroide.* Clin. Opht. 5, 31, 1969.

VENTURI G., BRANCATO R. *Maculopatie nell'anziano.* Relazione 57° Congresso S.O.I. 1976.

Chapter 10

TUMORS

BALESTRAZZI E. *Anatomia ed istologia patologica oculare.* EMSI, Roma, 1984.

COGAN D. C. *Tumors of the optic nerve, in* VINKEN P.J., BRUYB B.W. eds. *Handbook of Clinical Neurology*, Part II, vol. 17. American Elsevier Publishing Co., Inc., New York, 1974.

FINE B.S., YANOFF M. *Ocular Histology: a Text and Atlas.* Harper and Row, Hagerstown 1979.

GASS J. D. M. *Differential Diagnosis of Intraocular Tumors.* C. V. Mosby, St. Louis, 1974.

HOGAN M. J., ZIMMERMAN L. E. *Ophthalmic Pathology. An Atlas and Textbook.* Saunders, Philadelphia 1962.

HOPPING W., MEYER-SCHWICKERATH G. *Ocular and Adnexal Tumors.* Boniuk M. Ed., C.V. Mosby, St. Louis, 1964.

JENSEN R. D., MILLER R. W. *Retinoblastoma: epidemiologic characteristics.* JAMA 285, 307, 1971.

OFFRET G., DHERMY P., BRINI A., BEC P. *Anatomie Pathologique de l'oeil et des ses annexes.* Masson, Paris 1974.

REESE A. B. *Atlas of Tumor Pathology.* Washington D.C., Armed Forces Institute of Pathology, 1956.

REESE A. B. *Tumours of the Eye.* Harper and Row, New York 1963.

ROSSI A. *Clinica dei tumori dell'occhio e dell'orbita.* Relaz. 61° Congr. Soc. Oftal. Ital., SATE, Ferrara, 1981.

RUSSELL D. S., RUBINSTEIN L. J. *Pathology of Tumours of the Nervous System.* Edward Arnold, London 1959.

YANOFF M., FINE B. S. *Ocular Pathology. A Text and Atlas.* Harper and Row, Hagerstown 1975.

Chapter 11

OCULAR TRAUMA

BOUDET C. *Plaies et Contusion du segment anterieur de l'oeil.* Soc. Fr. Ophtal., Masson, Paris, 1979.

COX M. S., SCHEPENS C. L., FREEMAN H. M. *Retinal detachment due to ocular contusion.* Arch. Ophthalmol. 76, 678, 1966.

EWALD R. A., RITCHEY C. L. *Sun gazing as the cause of foveomacular retinitis.* Am. J. Ophthalmol. 70, 491, 1970.

HAVENER W. H., GLOECKNER S. *Atlas of diagnostic techniques and treatment of intraocular foreign bodies.* C.V. Mosby, St. Louis 1971.

PATON D., SOLDBERG M. F. *Management of Ocular Injuries.* W. B. Saunders, Philadelphia, 1976.

RUNYAN T. E. *Concussive and Penetrating Injuries of the globe and Optic Nerve.* C. V. Mosby, St. Louis, 1975.

SIPPERLEY J. O., QUIGLEY H. A., GAN J. O. M. *Traumatic retinopathy in primates. The explanation of commotio retinae.* Arch. Ophthalmol. 96, 2267, 1978.

Index

Numbers in **bold** print indicate illustrations

A

Adenoma, Fuchs 267 **454, 455**
Adhesions, paravascular 179
Albinism, cirsoid 152, **239, 240**
Angioid streaks 253, **435-438**
— maculopathy 166, **262**
Angioma, cavernous 151, **221, 222**
— retinal 151, **214-219**
Angiomatosis 150-152, **54, 214-240**
— miliary of Leber 51, **223-232**
— retinal of von Hippel 151, **214-219**
Arch, aortic, syndrome 14, **194**
Arteriosclerosis 121, 126, 138, **145, 148, 166, 183-193**
Arteriovenous, crossing 41, 124, 136, 138, **40-43, 152, 166, 177-179, 184**
Arteritis, temporal 146, **206**
Artery, central retinal, occlusion 121, **133 (d), 141-143, 145**
Astigmatism 94, **111**
Atrofy, areolar, senile 165, **258, 259**
— gyrate, choroid 254, **441**
— optic nerve 112, 113, 121, **129, 132-135, 206, 414, 415, 418, 511**

B

Behçet, disease 240, 241, **342, 410-419**
Berlin, retinal edema 285, **486-489**
Best, disease 164, **247-249**
Bird shot, chorioretinopathy 252, **434**
Blood dyscrasias 142, 143, **51, 74, 195-202**
Bonnet P., sign of 41, **42 (d), 43 (c, d)**
Bourneville, syndrome 149, **211**

C

Candida albicans, retinitis 236, **402-404**
Chalcosis 295
Chloroquine, retinopathy 146, **207**

Chorioretinitis 219, 220, **88, 371, 373-375, 378-392**
— Hutchinson 286, **496, 497**
— Jensen 219, 224, **382, 391, 392**
— traumatic 286, **86 (b), 490-493**
Chorioretinopathy, bird shot 252, **434**
Choroid
— atrophy, gyrate 254, **441**
— coloboma 82, 84, **92, 98**
— detachment 258, **442-444**
— elastosis 253, **435-438**
— hemangioma 271, **474**
— hemorrhage 70, **77, 493**
— melanoma 270, 271, **463-470, 485**
— nevus 270, **87, 270, 456-460**
— rupture 293, **506, 507**
— tumors 270-272, **456-475**
Choroideremia 254, **440**
Choroiditis 219, **220, 372, 376, 377-384**
— geographic or serpiginous 249, 250, **432, 433**
Cilioretinal artery 16, 121, **17 (a), 22, 143, 144**
Coats' disease 152, **67 (b), 233-238**
Collagen diseases 121, 146, **203-207**
Coloboma, choroid 82, 84, 98, **92, 98**
— optic nerve head 84, **96-98**
Color, fundus 5, **5, 6**
Commotio retinae 285, **486-489**
Connective tissue diseases 146, **203-207**
Contusion, retinal 285, 286, **486-497**
Cysticercosis 234, **398, 399**
Cytomegalovirus retinitis 238, **407**

D

Degeneration, macular 163-166, 174, **241-267**
— — cystoid **344, 377, 384**
— — disciform 165, 190, 253, 438, **190, 253-257**
— — hereditary 163, 164, **241-252**
— — myopic 93, 166, **115-120, 263-266**
— — senile 164-166, **84 (d), 253-261**
— retinal, colloid 164, **250-252, 257, 258**
— — cystoid senile 165, **260, 261**

— — paving stone 178, **277**
— — lattice 178, **283-288**
— — peripheral 177-179, **277-297**
— — — nonrhegmatogenous 178, 179, **277-281**
— — — rhegmatogenous 178, 179, **282-297**
— — pigmentary 178, **279-281**
— — senile atrophic 165, **258, 259**
— — snail tracks 178, **289-291**
— — vitelliform 164, **247-249**
— tapetoretinal 173, 174, **268-276**
Detachment, choroid 258, **442-444**
— pigment epithelium 165, 211, **99, 253-256, 263, 264**
— retina 194-196, **322-333, 427**
— — exudative 195, 196, **326, 427**
— — idiopathic (rhegmatogenous) 195, 196, **322-325, 330-333**
— — solid 195, 196, **328**
— — traction 195, 196, **327, 335, 337**
Diabetes 123, 126-128, **46, 153-175**
Dialysis, retinal 185, **316**
Disc edema 103-105, 136, **67 (c), 124-131**
Disinsertion, retina 185
Dysproteinemia 142, **47, 55, 147, 201**
Dystrophy, reticular, pigment epithelium 164
Drusen 76, 164, **84, 250-252, 257, 258**
— optic nerve head 86, **101-106**

E

Eales' disease 104, **345-349**
Edema, macular 86, **81, 99, 344**
— — cystoid **81, 344**
— optic nerve head 103-105, **67 (c), 124-131**
— retina 71, 121, 136, **78-82, 141, 142, 146, 164, 167, 179, 180, 186, 227, 486-489**
— — Berlin 285, **486-489**
Elastosis, choroid 271, **474**
Endocarditis, subacute 121
Epitheliopathy, acute posterior multifocal placoid 208, **350-353**
— retinal diffuse 211, **363-367**
Exudate, retinal 71, 72, 142, 143, **80, 82, 83, 198, 199**
— — hard 71, 72, 127, 128, 138, **80 (a)-83, 152-157, 162, 163, 166, 168, 181, 182, 216, 219, 220, 223, 227, 228, 232-237**
— — soft (cotton-wool patches) 71, 127, 128, 136, 146, **82 (b, c, d), 83 (a), 158, 179-182, 203, 204, 498**

F

Fold, retina 199, **334-338**
— — falciform **91, 109 (a, b)**
Foreign body, intraocular 294, 295, **508-510**
Foster-Kennedy syndrome 107, **132**
Fuchs, adenoma 267, **454, 455**
— spot 95, **119-121 (d), 266**
Fundus, albipunctatus 174, **275**
— flavimaculatus 163, 174, **243, 244, 276**

G

German measles 238, **405, 406**
Gunn, sign 41, **41 (c), 42 (b)**

H

Hemangioma, choroidal 271, **474**
— retinal 151, **214-219**
Hemorrhages 64-70, 124, 127, 128, 142, 143, **71-77, 147-158, 161-163, 174, 195-202, 490-493, 512**
— choroidal 70, **77, 493**
— intraretinal 67, **73, 74, 490**
— preretinal 66, **72, 491**
— retinal, traumatic 285, **490-493**
— subretinal 69, **75, 76**
Histoplasmosis, ocular, presumed 235, **400, 401**
Hole, macular 86, 138, 166, 185, 505, **189, 261, 303-306, 415, 497**
— retinal 185, **298-306**
Hutchinson, chorioretinitis 286, **496, 497**
Hypermetropia 93, **110**
Hyperplasia, pseudoadenomatous 267, **454, 455**
Hypertension, arterial 121, 123, 126, 136, **166-168, 176-182, 203, 204**
Hypotension, arterial 141, **194**

J

Jensen, chorioretinitis 219, 224, **382, 391, 392**

L

Leber, miliary aneurysm 151, **223-232**
— Coats' disease 152, **233-238**
Leukemia 123, 142, 271, **51, 74, 196-200, 475**
Lupus, erythematosus 146, **203, 204, 207, 341**
Lysosomal diseases 147, 148, **208, 209**

M

Macula 15, **15 (a-c)**
— cherry red spot 121, 148, 487, **142, 208**
— degeneration 163-166, 174, **241-267**
— — cystoid **344, 374, 384**
— — disciform 165, 253, **190, 253-257, 438**
— — myopic 95, 166, **115-120, 263-266**
— — senile 164-166, **84 (d), 253-261**
— — vitelliform 164, **247-249**
— edema 86, **81, 99, 344**
— hole 86, 138, 166, 185, **189, 261, 303-306, 415, 497, 505**
Macular star 138, **168, 181, 182, 188**
Maculopathy, angioid streaks 166, **262**
— degenerative 163-166, 174, **241-267**
Melanocytoma 279, **477-482**
Melanoma, choroid 270, 271, **463-470, 485**
Membrane, epipapillary 90, **107**
Metabolic errors, inborn 147, 148, **208, 209**
Microaneurysms 57, 58, 127, **65-68, 70, 79, 153-161, 167**

Myopia 94-96, **112-121, 263-266**
— maculopathy 95, 166, **115-120, 263-266**

N

Neovascularization 50, 51, 128, **56-64, 164, 170, 172, 174, 175, 345, 346, 348**
— subretinal 165, **257, 265**
Nevus, choroidal 270, **87, 270, 456-460**

O

Occlusion, arterial, branch 121, **82 (a), 146**
— — central retinal 121, **133 (d), 141-143, 145**
— — cilioretinal **144**
— — posterior ciliary 259, **444, 446**
— venous, branch 124, 128, **67 (a), 152, 346**
— — central retinal 86, 123, 124, 128, **147-151**
Optic, nerve, trauma 296, **511, 512**
— — tumors 279-280, **477-485**
— nerve head 10, **2, 8-14, 122, 123**
— — atrophy 112, 113, **129, 132-135, 206**
— — coloboma 84, **96-98**
— — drusen 86, **101-106**
— — edema 103-105, **67 (c), 124-131**
— — excavation 112, 113, **135, 136, 140**
— — hypoplasia 84, **95**
— — membrane, epipapillary 90, **107**
— — pit 84, 86, **99, 100**
— neuropathy, ischemic 105, **124 (c)**

P

Panarteritis nodosa 146, **205**
Papillitis 103-105, **124 (b), 131, 409, 420, 422, 426**
Pars planitis 201, **343, 344**
Periphlebitis, retinal 45, 201, **52, 339-344**
Phakomatoses 149-152, **211-213**
Photocoagulation 90, 163, 164, 198, 220 (b), 231, 232, **237, 238, 287, 288, 291, 296, 305, 314, 331**
Pigmentation 5, 77, **5, 6, 85-90**
— paravascular 45, **52, 339, 347**
Purtscher, retinopathy 290, **498**

R

Reflex, retinal 9, 7
— vascular 37, 136, 138, **34, 35, 39, 177, 178, 183**
Retina, periphery 30, 96, **1, 30-33**
— — degeneration 177-179, **277-297**
Retinitis 219, 220, **368-370, 402-404**
— circinate 128, 138, **187**
— mycotic 236, **402-404**
— pigmentosa 173, 174, **133 (c), 209, 268-274**
— viral 238, **405-407**
Retinoblastoma 265, 266, **449-453**
Retinochoroiditis 219, 220, **391-394**
— toxoplasmic 229, 230, **86 (a), 386-394**

Retinopathy, arteriosclerotic 121-126, 138, **145, 148 148, 183-193**
— central serous 211, **354-362**
— chloroquine 146, **207**
— diabetic 126-128, **46, 153-175**
— foveal 291, **502**
— hypertensive 136, **166-168, 176-182, 203, 204**
— nephritic 126, 136, **167, 168**
— prematurity 148, **210**
— proliferative 126, 128, **57, 58, 63, 168-175, 349**
— Puttscher 290, **498**
— solar 291, **499-502**
— toxic 146, **203-204**
— toxemia of pregnancy 136
Retinoschisis 192, **317, 318**
— juvenile 163, **241**
Roth, septic retinitis 220
— spot 67, **74, 200**
Rupture, choroidal 293, **506, 507**
— retinal 185, 291, **309-316, 503-505**

S

Salus sign 41, **41 (d), 42 (c)**
Sarcoidosis 240, **408, 409**
Sclerosis choroidal 254, **191, 439**
— tuberous 149, **211**
— vascular 136, 138, **183, 185, 186**
Siderosis 295
Sjögren disease 164
Staphyloma, peripapillary 94, 95, 138, **113, 114, 116, 192**
Stargardt disease 163, **242-246**
Sunset glow fundus **430, 431**
Sympathetic ophthalmia 245, **420, 424**
Synchisis scintillans 263, **447**
Syndrome, triangular 259, **445, 446**
Syphilis 226, **384, 385**

T

Telangiectasia 151, **223-232**
Thrombosis, venous 123, 124, 128, 138, **147-152, 165, 193**
— — branch 124, 128, **67 (a), 152, 346**
Toxocariasis 232, **395-397**
Toxoplasmosis 229, 230, **86 (a), 386-394**
Trauma, choroid 293
— optic nerve 206, **511, 512**
— retina 285-292
Tuberculois 224, **380-383**
Tumor, choroid, primary 270, 291, **456-475**
— — metastatic 271, **476**
— optic nerve 279-280, **477-485**
— retina 265-267, **449-455**

V

Vasculitis, retinal 45, 201, **50, 205, 339-344, 411-419**
Vein, central retinal, occlusion 86, 123, 124, 128, **147-151**
Vessels, retinal 16-29, **16-24**

Vitreous, primary, persistence   90, **108**
— retinal interphase, retraction   166, **267**
Vogt-Koyanagi-Harada disease   246, 247, **425-431**
Von Hippel retinal angiomatosis   151, **214-219**
Von Recklinghausen neurofibromatosis   149, **212, 213**

W

Waldenstrom, macroglobulinemia   142, **47, 55, 147, 201**
White with or without pressure   178, **292, 293**

Fotolito: PROGRAF

Fotocomposizione: COMPOSSELE

Finito di stampare
nel mese di ottobre 1987
dalla GEL Srl - Massalengo (MI) - Italy